Weight Loss

An Alternative Medicine Definitive Guide

by BURTON GOLDBERG
and THE EDITORS *of* ALTERNATIVE MEDICINE

ALTERNATIVEMEDICINE.COM BOOKS
TIBURON, CALIFORNIA

AlternativeMedicine.com, Inc.
1640 Tiburon Blvd., Suite 2
Tiburon, CA 94920
www.alternativemedicine.com

Editor: John W. Anderson
Associate Editor: Shila Alcantara
Research Editor: Laura Taxel
Writers: John W. Anderson with Shila Alcantara and Laura Taxel
Art Director: Janine White
Production Manager: Gail Gongoll
Production Assistance: Victoria Swart

Cover Photo © 1997, Telegraph Colour Library/FPG International LLC

Printed in Canada.

10 9 8 7 6 5 4 3 2

Library of Congress Cataloging-in-Publication Data
Goldberg, Burton, 1926-
    Weight loss: an alternative medicine definitive guide / by Burton Goldberg
        and the Editors of Alternative medicine.
    p.cm.
    Includes bibliographical references and index.
        ISBN 1-887299-19-X (pbk.)
        1. Weight loss. 2. Alternative medicine. 3. Nutrition. 4. Health. I. Title

RM222.2.G5936 2000
613.7--dc21   99-058674

                          CIP

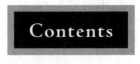

Contents

Part I

Customize Your Weight-Loss Program

Part II

Change Your Lifestyle

Part III

Correct Imbalances

Part IV

Detoxify the Body

Important Information

Burton Goldberg and the editors of *Alternative Medicine* are proud of the public and professional praise accorded AlternativeMedicine.com's (formerly Future Medicine Publishing) series of books. This latest book in the series continues the groundbreaking tradition of its predecessors.

Your health and that of your loved ones is important. Treat this book as an educational tool which will enable you to better understand, assess, and choose the best course of treatment when a health problem arises, and how to prevent health problems such as obesity from developing in the first place. It could save your life.

Remember that this book on weight management is different. It is not a diet book. Unlike the countless fad diets, alternative medicine recognizes that one size does not fit all. Fad diets don't work because they do not address the unique biochemistry of each individual nor do they take into account the underlying imbalances that may have caused you to gain weight in the first place. Rather than simply emphasizing weight loss, this book will instead show you how to correct imbalances and reduce toxicity so that you will gradually return to a healthy weight. This book is about alternative approaches to health—approaches generally not understood and, at this time, not endorsed by the medical establishment. We urge you to discuss the treatments described in this book with your doctor. If your doctor is open-minded, you may actually educate him or her. We have been gratified to learn that many of our readers have found their physicians open to the new ideas presented to them.

Use this book wisely. As many of the treatments described in this book are, by definition, alternative, they have not been investigated, approved, or endorsed by any government or regulatory agency. National, state, and local laws may vary regarding the use and application of many of the treatments discussed. Accordingly, this book should not be substituted for the advice and care of a physician or other licensed health-care professional. Pregnant women, in particular, are urged to consult a physician before commencing any therapy. Ultimately, you must take responsibility for your health and how you use the information in this book.

All of the factual information in this book has been drawn from the scientific literature. To protect privacy, all patient names have been changed. Branded products and services discussed in the book are evaluated solely on the independent and direct experience of the health-care practitioners quoted. Reference to them does not imply an endorsement nor a superiority over other branded products and services, which may provide similar or superior results.

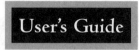

One of the features of this book is that it is interactive, thanks to the following icons:

This means you can turn to the listed pages elsewhere in this book for more information.

Many times the text mentions a medical term that requires explanation. We don't want to interrupt the text, so instead we put the explanation in the margins under this icon.

This tells you where to contact a physician, group, or publication mentioned in the text. This is an editorial service to our readers. All items are based on recommendations from the clinical practice of physicians in this book. The publisher has no financial interest in any clinic, physician, or product discussed in this book.

This sign tells you there may be some risks, uncertainties, side effects, or special contraindications regarding a procedure or substance.

Here we refer you to our best-selling book, *Alternative Medicine: The Definitive Guide*, for more information on a particular topic.

This icon will alert you to an article published in our bimonthly magazine, *Alternative Medicine*, that is relevant to the topic under discussion.

Here we refer you to our book *Alternative Medicine Definitive Guide to Cancer* for more information on a particular topic.

Here we refer you to our book *The Enzyme Cure* for more information on enzymes and how they can be used to relieve health problems.

Here we refer you to our book *The Supplement Shopper* for more information on nutritional supplements for various health conditions.

You Don't Have to
Struggle with Weight

Chances are you have experienced the frustrations of dieting at least once in your life, if you have problems with your weight. Eighty million Americans go on a diet in any given year and up to 95% of them regain any weight they lose within five years. Worse, a third will gain back more weight than they lost, in danger of "yo-yoing" from one popular diet to another. The conventional approach to weight problems, focusing on fad diets or weight-loss drugs, may leave you with just as much weight and the additional burden of ill-health.

Today, an estimated 33% of all adults are obese, up from 25% in 1980—that's about eight extra pounds per person. And our children are following in our heavy footsteps: 21% of children between the ages of 12 and 19 are overweight. Our culture obsesses about staying thin even as we grow fatter, but this isn't about appearances. People who are overweight increase their chances for cancer, heart disease, diabetes, osteoarthritis, and gallbladder disease, and obesity may contribute to as many as 300,000 deaths every year. In addition, the public health costs for obesity are staggering. According to researchers at Harvard University, obesity is a factor in 19% of all cases of heart disease with annual health costs estimated at $30 billion; it's also a factor in 57% of diabetes cases, with health costs of $9 billion per year.

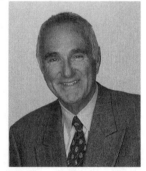

Diet books perennially appear on the best-seller lists, promising a quick-fix for weight problems. Sadly, dieters around the world have discovered the awful truth: diets don't work. Safe, healthy, and permanent weight reduction is what's truly lost among the thousands of popular diet schemes. The problem of being overweight is bad for health but excellent for business. Dieting has become a uniquely American "sport," for which we pay more than $1.5 billion annually to commercial weight-loss centers. The multi-billion dollar diet industry thrives on our inability to find a healthy alternative—until now.

The alternative medicine approach does not focus exclusively on diet, but rather recognizes that obesity is caused by multiple factors that overload your body systems. Unlike conventional medicine, alternative medicine physicians know that it will be impossible to lose weight safely and permanently without first correcting any underlying imbalances. They set about to identify these factors—from colon and liver toxicity to an underactive thyroid or hormone imbalances—through precise, nontoxic tests. Once the underlying factors have been pinpointed, a treatment plan can be designed to address each one. Instead of another fad diet, alternative medicine goes to the root causes and so can provide a real and lasting solution to weight problems.

Instead of a "one size fits all" diet, alternative medicine understands that everyone requires a unique plan to shed weight and regain their health. Use the information in this book and make the commitment to positive change—your health, not just your waistline, depends on it.

In this book, you will learn how over 25 alternative medicine physicians reverse weight problems using an individualized, holistic approach. You will read success stories of people who finally found the answers to their weight problems after years of frustration with dieting and the conventional approach to obesity. Instead of a "one size fits all" diet, alternative medicine understands that everyone requires a unique plan to shed weight and regain their health. Use the information in this book and make the commitment to positive change—your health, not just your waistline, depends on it. God bless.

—Burton Goldberg

Visit our website at
www.alternativemedicine.com

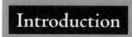

Introduction

Not Just Another Diet Book

By now, you may have been riding the fad diet merry-go-round for quite some time and are ready to jump off. You've followed one regimented diet after another (the Zone, Beverly Hills, or the Atkins diet), eaten the prepackaged or powdered foods, counted calories, given up flavor in favor of low fat, gone to the support groups. And you may have even lost some weight—only to see the pounds reappear after you went off the program. Every year, 80 million Americans go on a diet and up to 95% of them gain back any weight they lose within five years; one-third gain back more weight.[1]

"Fad diets can be a very temporary way to get started, but recognize it's not long-term," says Gary Ewing, M.D., of the University of South Carolina School of Medicine's Department of Family and Preventive Medicine. "Anything you can do in a few days, you can undo in a few days."[2]

The main problem with fad diets, like Barry Sears' Zone diet (30% fat, 30% protein, 40% carbohydrates) or the Cabbage Soup diet (lots and lots of cabbage soup), is that people grow weary of the restrictions and eventually return to their old eating habits. The dietary rules and regulations are too much trouble to maintain in the long run. Many health experts also question the long-term safety of high-protein diets and many of the other popular diets.

Don't continue bouncing from one fad diet to the next. To achieve significant and permanent weight loss, you need to come up with a plan, incorporating healthier eating, exercise, stress reduction, and healing any underlying imbalances, that will last a lifetime. This book is less about dieting and more about regaining a state of health—good health is the key to weight loss. Use this book as a guide to finding a personal plan that you can live with.

We're Getting Fatter

The unmistakable fact is that Americans are getting fatter. According to statistics from the National Institutes of Health,

33% of American adults are considered obese. This number is up from 25% of adults in 1980, a significant increase in such a short period of time,[3] which works out to an average weight gain of eight pounds per person.[4] The overweight problem continues with our children as well. The U.S. Centers for Disease Control (CDC) estimates that 21% of children between the ages of 12 and 19 are overweight, up from 15% in the late 1970s.[5] Children who have overweight parents tend to be overweight themselves, and overweight children tend to have weight problems as adults.[6]

We are growing more and more overweight even as we obsess about our appearance and particularly about staying thin. But this isn't just a matter of appearances: obesity (weight that is 20% above normal for your height) is thought to contribute to a wide range of health problems, including diabetes, heart disease, and cancer.

The unmistakable fact is that Americans are getting fatter. According to the National Institutes of Health, 33% of American adults are considered obese.

■ Diabetes—The incidence of Type II (adult-onset) diabetes has tripled in the last 40 years—about 15 million Americans have the disease—and continues to rise.[7] A vast majority (80%) of those with adult-onset diabetes are overweight. Studies have found that losing weight helps diabetics control their disease with less reliance on medications. Losing weight also reduces the risk of developing diabetes.[8]

■ Heart Disease—Obesity increases your chances of getting high blood pressure and other forms of heart disease, independent of other risk factors. One study concluded that obesity tripled the chances of developing hypertension in people between the ages of 20 and 75.[9] Another study of over 100,000 women found a direct link between weight gain and the likelihood of stroke, particularly strokes caused by blood clots; as more weight was gained, the risk of stroke increased.[10] Obesity also contributes to high total cholesterol and lower levels of high-density lipoproteins or HDLs, the so-called good cholesterol.[11]

■ Cancer—Obesity is an independent risk factor in the development of cancer. Studies have found that overweight men have a higher incidence of colon and prostate cancers, while obese women have higher rates of liver, cervical, and ovarian cancers.[12]

■ Other Conditions—Obesity may be a contributing factor in a number of other health problems, including osteoarthritis, gallbladder disease, gout, and cataracts.

For more on **diabetes and obesity**, see Chapter 8: Strengthen Your Sugar Controls, pp. 184-201.

The health costs associated with obesity are staggering, according to researchers at Harvard University. Obesity is a factor in 19% of the cases of heart disease, with annual health costs estimated at almost $30 billion; 57% of adult-onset diabetes cases ($9 billion); 10% of cases of musculoskeletal disease ($3.75 billion); 30% of gallbladder disease ($3.2 billion); and 23% of cancer cases ($0.67 billion).[13] Obesity may be a contributing factor in as many as 300,000 deaths each year.[14]

What Causes Weight Gain?

What causes weight gain is pretty straightforward: you consume more calories from food than the body uses or burns off in its daily tasks. But whether or not a person becomes obese depends on a number of factors, including genetics, societal influences, amount of physical activity, and psychological makeup.[15]

■ Researchers have found that obesity tends to run in families. This may be partially due to genetics, but could also be influenced by dietary and lifestyle habits learned as a child, including the kinds of food you tend to eat (for example, high-fat or processed foods) and how often you eat.

■ We're exercising too little: the amount of exercise you get on a regular basis will strongly affect your weight. Our lives in general are less physically active than for previous generations and most people aren't getting enough exercise to make up for it. Children in America now spend an estimated two-and-a-half hours per day watching television.[16] A quarter of the population is completely sedentary while 55% are "inadequately active," according to the CDC.[17]

■ Perhaps, living in the "consumer culture" of the United States, it is our just reward to be consuming ourselves to death. Not only are we eating more, but the kinds of foods we consume—fast foods, processed, and high-fat—offer the least nutrition and the most potential for adding fat to our hips. And we're eating too much, period: average calorie intake is over 2,000 calories per day compared to 1,800 calories in the 1970s.[18] The food industry is doing its part to keep us "living large"—it spends $36 billion every year on advertising and a typical child sees up to 10,000 food commercials every year.[19]

■ Psychology may play a significant role in weight gain: many people who overeat do so in response to stress, anger, sadness, boredom, or other emotional factors unrelated to hunger or nutritional needs.[20] Foods affect moods by triggering the release of endorphins, the body's natural pain-killers, and the brain chemical serotonin, a mood regulator. Unfortunately, these foods (chocolate, carbohydrates, sweets) not only elevate your mood but also trigger cravings for more.[21] This kind of "emotional eating" can contribute significantly to weight gain if you lead a stressful life or have unresolved emotional issues.

For more on **exercise programs for weight loss**, see Chapter 6: Start Exercising, pp. 138-155. For the role of **emotions in weight problems**, see Chapter 7: Heal Your Emotional Appetite, pp. 156-182. For **food allergies and weight gain**, see Chapter 11: Break Food Allergies and Addictions, pp. 244-270. For more on **hormones**, see Chapter 10: Restore Hormonal Balance, pp. 220-243.

- Everybody is different. You probably know individuals who can eat anything they want and never seem to gain an ounce, while you have to watch everything you eat. That's because each of us has a different metabolism, the way our bodies extract and use energy from food. And our metabolism changes as we age: hormonal changes and reduced activity levels lead to a slower metabolism, potentially causing weight gain.[22] In other words, the way you put on the pounds and the ease or difficulty with which you lose them is unique to you.

- In addition, alternative medicine practitioners look for underlying imbalances that may contribute to weight gain, including an underactive thyroid, hormone imbalances, food allergies, yeast infections, and parasites.

The Diet Craze

No doubt you've fallen for one or more of the diet-of-the-week schemes over the years, promising quick and painless weight loss. Over the last 30 years, we've seen quite a few of these diets come and go: the Grapefruit diet, Atkins diet, Pritikin Plan, Fit for Life, Beverly Hills diet, the Rotation diet, Scarsdale diet, Ornish plan, Cabbage Soup diet, the Zone—the list goes on and on. Every time you look, there's another diet book on top of the best-seller lists or the latest diet "guru" promising miracles on the talk shows.

First, you're told to count calories. Then, it's not about calories but about eating low-fat foods. Others told you that the magic formula for weight loss was eating lots of protein and cutting back on carbohydrates. Still others advocated high-carbohydrate diets. What you end up with is a glut of confusing and conflicting messages about weight loss.

A recent survey by the Calorie Control Council found that 27% of adult Americans are on a diet, while another 39% are trying to control their weight but do not consider themselves to be dieting. "Dieting is now perceived as a quick-fix, short-term, on-again, off-again solution to a weight problem," concludes John Foreyt, Ph.D., director of the

Bingeing and the Low-Calorie Diet

The average individual will begin to lose weight when they eat fewer than 1,500 calories per day. However, low-calorie diets, such as the Cambridge, Liquid Protein, Optifast, and Protein-Sparing Modified Fast, often go much lower than this amount, some to as low as 300 calories per day. Many who try to bring their calorie intake down to this level frequently develop overeating or "bingeing" behaviors. Bingeing is when a dieter uncontrollably eats a large quantity of food in a short period of time. Studies have shown that 46% of individuals who participate in weight-loss programs regularly binge.[23]

Bingeing is not a sign of weakness or lack of willpower, but rather a response to the biochemical disruptions caused by a low-calorie diet. Among the disruptions is reduced thyroid gland activity. When food intake is

For the **role of the thyroid in weight gain,** see Chapter 9: Overcome a Sluggish Thyroid, pp. 202-219.

reduced, the thyroid responds by secreting fewer hormones, thus lowering metabolism and conserving the body's energy resources. This slowing of metabolism works against the dieter's goal, as less body fat will be burned when metabolism slows. In time, the body will attempt to correct the imbalance and restore thyroid function. Often these attempts take the form of binge behavior. "Because the thyroid gland is the single most important controller of metabolic rate, the body may initiate overeating as a way to increase thyroid hormone to stimulate the metabolic rate," explains Carol Simontacchi, C.C.N., M.S., a clinical nutritionist in Vancouver, Washington, and author of *Your Fat Is Not Your Fault*. "In other words, binge eating may be a compensatory mechanism for a reduced thyroid function."[24]

Nutrition Research Clinic at Baylor College of Medicine in Waco, Texas. However, those trying to control their weight "see weight control as something to be permanently incorporated into their lifestyle, recognizing that to be successful at maintaining a healthy weight, they'll have to develop lifelong habits incorporating diet and exercise."

In this same survey, people were asked why they had failed to stay at their desired weight. The number one answer was that they weren't getting enough exercise (56%). The fad diets, by concentrating on food restrictions of one sort or another, ignore the importance of incorporating physical activity into one's life. Other reasons given for failure: bingeing on favorite foods (41%) and watching only fat intake and not calories (34%). "Counting fat at the exclusion of calories and bingeing are two symptoms of a diet gone awry," says Dr. Foreyt. "The fact that dieters are more prone to these behaviors is further evidence that diets usually fail."[25]

According to a study done by researchers at *Consumer Reports* magazine, commercial diet programs don't work either. *Consumer Reports* evaluated programs offered by Diet Center, Jenny Craig, Nutri/System, Physicians Weight Loss Centers, Health Management Resources, Medifast, Optifast, and Weight Watchers. Most of these programs prescribe a low-calorie diet of about 1,000-1,500 calories a day, exercise, and counseling. The *Consumer Reports* study found that, "most individuals who go through a commercial diet program typically regain half their lost weight in a year and much of the rest in another year." In general, the researchers concluded, "there is no evidence that commercial weight-loss programs help most people achieve significant, permanent weight loss."[26]

"Diets make you think that if you just had more willpower, you'd be able to lose weight," says Dr. Foreyt. "If you stick to a restrictive diet for a few weeks, you lose weight and think the diet 'works.' Then you start to feel uncontrollable cravings and you relapse. But that's because of the calorie re-strictions, not because you lost your willpower. It's not your fault."[27] (See "Bingeing and the Low-Calorie Diet," p. 18.)

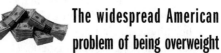

The widespread American problem of being overweight is bad for health but excellent for business, explains Michael Fumento, author of *The Fat of the Land*. Fumento is resident fellow at the American Enterprise Institute in Washington, D.C., and he thinks "Americans are the fattest people in the industrial world." Whether or not this is statistically true, many are cashing in on the financial bonanza presented by the near epidemic of overweight people in the U.S. According to Fumento, each year Americans spend more than any other country on weight-loss programs, most of which don't work.

In 1995, Americans handed over $1.78 billion to commercial weight-loss centers, whose liquid diets and powdered formulas guaranteed "permanent" weight loss. But despite the appealing hyperbole about pounds to be shed, the results of most of these programs have been poor at best, says Fumento. Thirteen centers making "long-term weight loss" or weight-loss "cure" claims were recently forced to back down from these promises because of a suit filed by the Federal Trade

Commission. Nevertheless, many weight-loss centers rely on marketing scams that continue to lure clients. Fumento describes how one center, Medifast, Inc., used a kickback scheme that paid doctors up to $1,000 for each client referral. "We're losing the [overweight] war as the industry is booming," says Dr. Foreyt.

The pharmaceutical industry has reaped considerable dividends at the expense of consumer health, Fumento contends. Redux and fenfluramine (half of the drug combination, known as fen-phen), two popular diet pills, netted distributor Wyeth-Ayerst Laboratories, Inc., billions of dollars before the products were taken off the market in September 1997, due to high blood pressure risks and heart damage to users.[28]

Success Story: The Individual Approach to Weight Loss

Claire, 41, was a retired executive who had fought with her weight her entire life. She was 5'7" and weighed 340 pounds. Her body mass index or BMI was 53 (body mass index is a ratio of your weight to your height; a BMI of 27 or higher is considered overweight). After she turned 40, Claire began to have more problems with her weight and her physician told her that she had high blood pressure, high cholesterol, and that she was diabetic. Her physician recommended medications for each of these problems, but Claire wanted another option.

She came to see Frances Gough, M.D., and Teresa Girolami, M.D., of Sound Weight Solutions in Bellevue, Washington. Claire was put on a comprehensive program of dietary changes, exercise, and counseling. "Our philosophy is that life is a series of decisions and choices and being enabled to make good, confident decisions about diet and exercise leads to success," says Dr. Gough. "Positive changes need to be a priority and worked at every day."

Claire's diet consisted of large amounts of meat, cheese, and butter. She disliked vegetables of any type and incorporated few of them into her diet. Dr. Gough instructed her to keep a food diary, writing down everything she consumed for a week. "The diet diary helps people understand what they're actually eating," says Dr. Gough. "They're quite surprised when they write it down—they forgot about that cookie they grabbed on their way out the door and little things like that."

Claire then met with a holistic nutrition specialist for a full assessment of her food intake. The nutritionist used a special computer program to design dietary guidelines specifically for Claire. She was advised to convert to a whole foods diet, primarily vegetarian with five servings of fruits and vegetables every day, and cut back on meat consumption to once or twice weekly. She discovered that, while she disliked cooked vegetables, she actually enjoyed eating raw ones. Claire was quite enthusiastic about the vegetarian approach and even bought a rice cooker to start eating more rice and vegetables. One session with the nutritionist involved a trip to the grocery store to help Claire make healthier choices when shopping for foods as well.

Claire participated in weekly group therapy sessions to help with the emotional issues surrounding weight problems and trying to lose excess weight. The therapy program also focuses on lifestyle changes (in behavior, attitude, and self-esteem) that are helpful in maintaining weight loss. Items that might be discussed in a typical therapy session include: issues of loneliness, depression, and isolation and how they relate to food bingeing; sabotage from others—family members who bring home high-calorie foods, chocolates, cookies, and other snacks; and how to stay on a healthful eating plan while maintaining a hectic schedule or eating on the run. Peer support greatly improves the chances of maintaining weight loss, according to Dr. Gough. "Some type of therapy, particularly in a group, is highly beneficial and helps solidify their motivation and their feelings about what they're going through," she says.

Claire also began an exercise program with a personal trainer, working out for one hour three times per week. Her program began with a body composition assessment using bioelectric impedence, in which a small electric current is passed through the body to measure Claire's levels of body fat and lean body mass. This measurement is more specific than simply stepping on a scale, allowing the person to see how much fat they may be losing and muscle they're gaining from an exercise regimen. Based on this analysis, the trainer then designed an exercise program for Claire, including both cardiovascular exercises and weight training.

In nine months on this program, Claire lost 60 pounds. That amounted to a 5% reduction in body fat and a 5% increase in lean body mass. Her BMI dropped from 53 to 42. Her blood pressure dropped from 160/110 to 130/80 and her cholesterol, triglycerides, and blood sugar levels were all within normal ranges. More importantly, Claire learned to incorporate these healthy changes into her life and continues to lose weight.

Frances Gough, M.D., and Teresa Girolami, M.D.: Sound Weight Solutions, 14730 N.E. 8th Street, Suite 110, Bellevue, WA 98007; tel: 425-747-6000; website: www. soundweight.com.

"You could say that the supplement we use is an educational supplement," explains Dr. Gough. "Education to

For information on **dietary recommendations**, see Chapter 2: Healthy Eating, pp. 50-75. For more on the **emotional/psychological aspects of weight problems**, see Chapter 7: Heal Your Emotional Appetite, pp. 156-182. For more on **exercise**, see Chapter 6: Start Exercising, pp. 138-155.

help people make the choices they need to make to get out of the situation they're in. We help them make good choices nutritionally, good choices behaviorally, and good choices in terms of exercise."

Why This Book is Different

This book is not a diet book. Alternative medicine offers you an approach that helps you lose weight and keep it off while improving your overall health and fitness. It is essential to understand the factors that went into creating a weight problem in each person, because obesity is never caused by one thing alone and no two people have exactly the same causal factors. Alternative medicine employs a battery of diagnostic tools—physical examination, dietary assessment, tests for immune, digestive, and detoxification function, and emotional evaluation—to build an individualized picture of a person's condition. Skilled alternative practitioners take the time needed to find the root causes of obesity and the patient also becomes actively involved in their treatment. Alternative medicine not only respects differences between individuals, but concentrates its diagnosis and treatment plan around this "customized" approach. Rather than giving you one more fad diet, we provide you with the tools you need to individualize your diet, make better food choices, use supplements wisely, start an exercise program that works for you, deal with any emotional issues, and correct any underlying imbalances or toxicity that may be contributing to your weight gain.

Part 1: Customize Your Weight-Loss Program

■ The conflict among the diet experts regarding the right combination of protein, carbohydrate, and fat has left those trying to lose weight at a loss over what to eat. Fad diets don't take into account individual physiology. One diet does not fit all people: different body types (determined by genetics, physiology, metabolism, and other factors) require unique dietary and nutrient recommendations. Alternative medicine honors individuality, recognizing that each individual has a different biochemistry and different nutritional requirements. The key is to match the diet to individual physiological needs. In Chapter 1: Individualize Your Diet, we show you how to match your body type to a diet that will help you lose weight and stay healthy.

■ Healthy eating is the best way to reach and maintain a healthy body weight. A whole foods diet—containing a variety of vegetables, fruits, and grains; raw seeds and nuts; beans; fermented milk products; and fish, poultry, and tofu—is the best prescription for reaching your ideal body weight. Chapter 2: Healthy Eating provides you with helpful tips for choosing the right foods and avoiding the detrimental ones.

■ A good weight-loss plan must be based on a well-rounded diet, as a deficiency in one or more nutrients may be interfering with your weight-loss goals. In Chapter 3: Supplements for Weight Loss, we show you how to identify which nutrients may be missing from your diet and what you can do to restore the levels of these substances in your body.

■ Proper digestion is essential for maintaining a healthy, well-nourished body. When this process is impaired, body weight will almost surely increase. As we explain in Chapter 4: Enzymes and Weight Loss, enzyme supplementation and dietary alterations can repair a weakened digestive system, restoring the body to health and helping you shed unwanted pounds.

■ The body, when healthy, burns rather than stores excess calories in a process called thermogenesis. Focusing on dieting and exercise to control weight can fail if your calorie-burning process isn't working. Chapter 5: Optimize Your Calorie Burning shows you how a careful combination of herbs, nutrients, and exercise can get your calorie-burning fires on the job again.

Part 2: Change Your Lifestyle

■ Exercise helps to burn off excess calories and starting a regular exercise program is critical for long-term weight reduction. But physical activity does not have to be excessive or overly strenuous to be effective, as you will discover in Chapter 6: Start Exercising. Less vigorous activities, such as focused breathing, yoga, and *tai chi*, not only burn calories, but have a balancing and harmonizing influence on every body system.

■ Although weight gain is often the outcome of an underlying physiological problem (toxic liver, blood sugar imbalance, food allergy), each of these physical causes also has a distinct emotional dimension. However, emotions are not simply the effects of the physical illness, they can also be the cause. Mind/body treatments, outlined in Chapter 7: Heal Your Emotional Appetite, enable you to examine what may be unconsciously driving you to gain weight and help raise your awareness regarding what you choose to eat and why. They can also help relieve stress, alleviate depression, and, in turn, help you to lose weight permanently.

Part 3: Correct Imbalances

Alternative medicine does not look at obesity as an isolated problem, as a matter of just losing a few pounds. Being overweight may be due to underlying imbalances in the body. Correcting these imbalances will not only help shed the pounds, but will help improve your overall health.

■ Insulin is the hormone responsible for managing how our bodies use the sugars and starches we eat. When the body's insulin balance is disrupted, starches and sugars are turned into fat rather than being burned as a fuel. If left unchecked, the condition can result in serious illnesses, including diabetes and heart disease. In Chapter 8: Strengthen Your Sugar Controls, you will learn how proper diet, nutritional supplements, and alternative therapies can help to restore insulin health which, in turn, will keep your blood sugar levels in check and control your appetite.

■ The thyroid gland plays a key role in weight control through its regulation of metabolism, as discussed in Chapter 9: Overcome a Sluggish Thyroid. However, diseases of the thyroid are often overlooked by medical doctors in relation to obesity. Alternative healthcare practitioners employ diagnostic tools that can quickly and accurately assess thyroid function, and restore the gland to health using natural treatments.

■ When hormone levels in the body become imbalanced, one of the primary results for both men and women is a steady rise in body weight. Aging, stress, and an increasingly toxic environment are some of the main factors causing hormonal disruption. In Chapter 10: Restore Hormonal Balance, learn how you can balance hormonal levels with natural therapies, which can contribute to a weight-loss program.

■ Do you find certain foods irresistible? Are you often a victim of uncontrollable bingeing? If so, you may be suffering from a food allergy. Although largely ignored by mainstream medical practitioners, food allergies affect millions of Americans, causing a variety of symptoms, including weight gain. Pinpointing hidden food allergies may be the key to finally realizing permanent weight loss and a healthier life. In Chapter 11: Break Food Allergies and Addictions, we describe ways to detect and eliminate allergies, so that you can return to good health.

Part 4: Detoxify the Body

Other contributing factors to weight problems include yeast infections, parasites, and the accumulation of toxins in the body. These factors block the body's normal detoxification processes, often leading to an increase in body fat. Alternative medicine can help you determine if you have a buildup of toxins and help you detoxify your body systems.

■ A healthy colon teems with beneficial microorganisms that contribute to the healthy digestion and absorption of food. However, years of poor diet, medications, stress, and other factors can throw our intestinal ecology severely out of balance, causing a number of illnesses that contribute to weight gain. In Chapter 12: Detoxify the Colon, discover natural, gentle, and effective methods provided by alternative medicine that can restore the intestinal environment and facilitate weight loss.

■ *Candida albicans* is a yeast-like fungus that's normally present in the body. When there's an unhealthy overgrowth of these microbes, it can have a body-wide impact, resulting in a variety of conditions and symptoms including increased appetite, out-of-control food cravings, and weight gain. Yeast overgrowth and yeast-related disorders often go undetected for years. As you will see in Chapter 13: Eliminate Yeast Infections, for many individuals, correctly diagnosing and treating the problem is the key to health and a healthy weight.

■ Few people are aware of the health risk that parasites can present. Contrary to popular belief, parasites are more common than you may think. Travelers drinking water of questionable quality are at risk, but so is anyone who eats seafood, poultry, or meat that is not carefully cleaned and cooked. Parasites cause our bodies to lose their biological balance by secreting toxins and damaging vital organs. This invasion of parasites and subsequent imbalance throughout the body may lead to significant weight gain. Chapter 14: Eradicate Parasites will show you what symptoms to look for that result from a parasitic infestation and how to safely and naturally eliminate them.

■ The liver serves as a filter for the toxins that the body absorbs from food, air, and water. Unhealthy lifestyles, poor diet, and exposure to industrial chemicals and pesticides can overload the liver with poisons, creating toxic conditions in the body that cause a buildup of fat. As described in Chapter 15: Cleanse the Liver, once you have cleared toxins from the liver, you can finally shed the weight you have been struggling to lose and begin enjoying a more healthy life.

■ The lymph system is part of the body's internal plumbing, helping it to dispose of wastes and other debris generated by muscles and other body tissues. Like the blood in the circulatory system, lymph fluid circulates in the body in an elaborate network of channels and vessels. As you will see in Chapter 16: Get the Lymph Flowing, a variety of factors can cause lymph fluid to become heavy and thick, which restricts its flow and causes it to clog and back-up in the body. Such blockages can cause excess body weight and a number of other serious diseases. Alternative medicine practitioners frequently focus on the lymph as part of a comprehensive approach to weight loss, helping to unblock and restore the ability of the lymph to drain wastes from the body.

No matter what health-care practitioners you consult, chances are they will tell you that the only way to achieve a healthy weight is to look closely at your life and change the things that are not serving your best interests. Depending as much on your personality as on your condition, this could be as simple as eating better, starting an exercise program, finding a creative outlet, learning how to express your emotions, or getting a dog to walk every night. Your life is a series of choices, some of them healthy, others unhealthy—only you know what makes you feel good. To achieve lasting weight loss, you must make a commitment to change. Your health, not just your waistline, depends on it.

Are You Overweight?

You probably know if you're overweight—your clothes seem a little tight or your body just feels uncomfortable or bulky to you. A quick look in the mirror may confirm the extra pounds. However, an ideal weight for you should be based on how healthy you feel, not on how you or others think you should look. One of the easiest ways to get a general picture of where you are on the weight scale is to use the guidelines issued by the U.S. Department of Health and Human Services. These general guidelines give normal weight ranges based on height and age.

When you've found your correct weight range, keep in mind your frame size (small, medium, or large) and gender when considering where you fall in a given range. Specifically, those with smaller frames should be on the lower end of a given range, while those with larger frames will be on the higher end. Men will generally fall on the higher end of each weight range (because they tend to have higher muscle and bone mass) and women will be on the lower end of the range. Again, these are meant as general guidelines, not as absolute numbers—you need to always bear in mind your unique physiology.

Height	Weight (in pounds)	
	Ages 19-34	Ages 35 and up
5' 0"	97-128	108-138
5' 1"	101-132	111-143
5' 2"	104-137	115-148
5' 3"	107-141	119-152
5' 4"	111-146	122-157
5' 5"	114-150	126-162
5' 6"	118-155	130-167
5' 7"	121-160	134-172
5' 8"	125-164	138-178
5' 9"	129-169	142-183
5' 10"	132-174	146-188
5' 11"	136-179	152-194
6' 0"	140-184	155-199
6' 1"	144-189	159-205
6' 2"	148-195	164-210
6' 3"	152-200	168-216
6' 4"	156-205	173-222
6' 5"	160-211	177-228
6' 6"	164-216	182-234

Weight Ranges for Older Adults

Some physicians like Reubin Andres, M.D., of Johns Hopkins University in Baltimore, Maryland, and clinical director of the National Institute on Aging, believe that some weight gain is normal as we get older. "It's acceptable, possibly even beneficial, for normal, healthy adults to gain gradually about a pound a year beginning around age 40," states Dr. Andres. Using data from over four million subjects, Dr. Andres has estimated what he considers medically sound weight ranges specifically for older adults. (see p. 28)

The middle of the weight range for each age and height is considered the ideal weight, according to Dr. Andres.[29]

Body Mass Index (BMI)

Calculating your body mass index is another way to determine if you are overweight, with a little more precision than the height-weight charts. The BMI is the ratio of your weight to your height. The BMI

Height	Weight (in pounds) Ages 50-59	Weight (in pounds) Ages 60 and up
5' 0"	114-142	123-152
5' 1"	118-148	127-157
5' 2"	122-153	131-163
5' 3"	126-158	135-168
5' 4"	130-163	140-173
5' 5"	134-168	144-179
5' 6"	138-174	148-184
5' 7"	143-179	153-190
5' 8"	147-184	158-196
5' 9"	151-190	162-201
5' 10"	156-195	167-207
5' 11"	160-201	172-213
6' 0"	165-207	177-219
6' 1"	169-213	182-225
6' 2"	174-219	187-232
6' 3"	179-225	192-238
6' 4"	184-231	197-244

is based on the metric system, so pounds and inches will need to be converted to kilograms and meters.

1. Multiply your weight in pounds by 704. For example, if a person weighs 160 pounds, multiply 160 by 704, which equals 112,640.

2. Convert your height to inches (5'10" equals 70 inches), then multiply it by itself. In this example, 70 inches multiplied by 70 inches equals 4,900.

3. Divide the answer from step 1 by the answer in step 2: 112,640 divided by 4,900 equals 22.99, which should be rounded to the nearest whole number. This is your BMI. So, our 5'10" person who weighs 160 pounds has a BMI of 23.

The higher your BMI, the greater your health risk. Physicians generally consider a BMI between 20 and 25 to be acceptable; those with a BMI from 27 up to 30 are considered overweight and at a higher risk for weight-related diseases; those with a BMI of 30 and higher are considered obese.[30]

BMI should not be used as a weight guide by pregnant women, body builders or other competitive athletes, children, or the elderly (particularly those who are sedentary or frail).

Body Mass Index (BMI) Chart

Weight (pounds)	Height							
	5'0"	5'2"	5'4"	5'6"	5'8"	5'10"	6'0"	
	6'4"							
125	24	23	22	20	19	18	17	16	15
130	25	24	22	21	20	19	18	17	16
135	26	25	23	22	21	19	18	17	16
140	27	26	24	23	21	20	19	18	17
145	28	27	25	23	22	21	20	19	18
150	29	28	26	24	23	22	20	19	18
155	30	28	27	25	24	22	21	20	19
160	31	29	28	26	24	23	22	21	20
165	32	30	28	27	25	24	22	21	20
170	33	31	29	28	26	24	23	22	21
175	34	32	30	28	27	25	24	23	21
180	35	33	31	29	27	26	24	23	22
185	36	34	32	30	28	27	25	24	23
190	37	35	33	31	29	27	26	24	23
195	38	36	34	32	30	28	27	25	24
200	39	37	34	32	30	29	27	26	24
205	40	38	35	33	31	29	28	26	25
210	41	39	36	34	32	30	29	27	26
215	42	39	37	35	33	31	29	28	26
220	43	40	38	36	34	32	30	28	27
225	44	41	39	36	34	32	31	29	27
230	45	42	40	37	35	33	31	30	28
235	46	43	40	38	36	34	32	30	29
240	47	44	41	39	37	35	33	31	29
245	48	45	42	40	37	35	33	32	30

Are You an Apple or a Pear?

In addition to your BMI, it is important to determine where you carry your fat. People generally fall into either of two basic body shapes, apples or pears. Apple-shaped people tend to gain weight above the waist and in the abdominal area. "Apples" are more prevalent among men and they need to be most concerned with developing health problems related to obesity. Pear-shaped people carry extra fat on their hips, thighs, and buttocks. More women follow this pattern of weight gain and "pears" have a lower risk of developing heart disease, diabetes, and other weight-related diseases.[31]

To more precisely determine which body shape you have, measure your waist-to-hip ratio. First, measure your waist at its narrowest point (just above the navel). Then measure your hips at their widest point around your buttocks. Divide your waist measurement into your hip measurement. For example, a woman with a waist size of 35" and a hip size of 38" would have a waist-to-hip ratio of 0.92. If this number is higher than 1.0 for men or 0.8 for women, then your weight gain is of the "apple" variety and you are potentially at risk for weight-related health problems. Men with a waist circumference of more than 40" and women with waists larger than 36" are also at greater risk.[32]

Body Fat or Body Lean?

All of these charts, measurements, and calculations are intended to help you determine if you have a weight problem. They are relatively easy ways of estimating your body fat based on standards for your height and age. Overall weight is used as an indicator of excess body fat. However, there are ways to more directly measure your body fat (as opposed to lean body tissue such as muscle and bone).

"Experts are beginning to realize that the best measure of overall health is not weight-to-height-to-sex-to-age ratios, but the ratio of body fat to body lean tissue," states Daniel B. Mowrey, Ph.D., director of the American Phytotherapy Research Laboratory, in Lehi, Utah. Dr. Mowrey believes that putting aside the old concept of weight management in favor of fat management is more useful.[33]

There are a number of ways of measuring body fat, all of which are generally performed in a physician's office, health club, or weight-loss clinic. One method uses calipers to measure skinfold thickness at various points on the body. Another method is called hydrostatic weighing, whereby a person is weighed repeatedly both in and out of water; since fat is lighter than water, the proportion of fat to other tissues can be calculated. A third way of determining body fat is through bioelectric impedance, in which a small electric current is passed through the body; because fat tissue is a poor conductor compared to lean body mass, the percentage of fat in the body can be estimated. Cost and convenience may be factors in whether or not you choose to use one of these methods.

How Do You Feel?

The last determinant of whether or not you have a weight problem is how you feel. Your level of health and vitality is the final measure of your ideal weight. So, answer a few questions about your overall state of health:

- Do you have plenty of energy or would you like to have more?
- What health problems do you have?
- Does your weight hamper your movements or activities?
- Do you feel comfortable with your size?
- Are you victimized by eating behaviors, like compulsive overeating, that leave you debilitated physically and emotionally?
- Would you like to feel better than you do?

Take an honest look at how excess weight may factor into your general state of health. Keep in mind that being overweight or obese can contribute to a variety of health problems, including heart disease, adult-onset diabetes, and cancer, among others.

If you have tried to lose weight before, consider what you did in the past that did not work for you and start from a different place. Establish realistic, healthy goals for yourself and, as best as you can, be clear about the reasons why you are undertaking this process again and what you are willing to do to achieve success. You know yourself well, and what does and does not work for you. Give yourself the tools, knowledge, and support to reach your goal. Ultimately, you are the one who must decide if losing weight and making other lifestyle changes will improve your health.

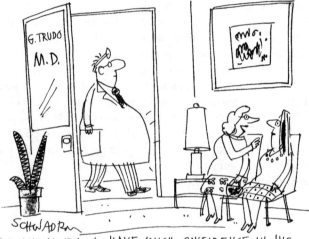

"FRANKLY, I DON'T HAVE MUCH CONFIDENCE IN HIS DIET BOOK EITHER."

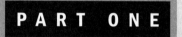

PART ONE

Customize Your Weight-Loss Program

1 Individualize Your Diet

THE CONFLICT among the diet experts and the resulting confusion of dietary recommendations has left many people trying to lose weight at a loss over what to eat. Alternative medicine honors individuality, recognizing that each person has a different biochemistry and different nutritional requirements. The key is to honor individual physiological needs. Once you determine your body type, you can match it to a diet that will help you lose weight and stay healthy too.

The Diet Debate

In this era of diet fads, you may be overwhelmed by the number of dietary regimens out there. Much of the debate among weight-loss experts focuses on what proportion of protein, carbohydrate, and fat should be included in a diet. Some claim a high-carbohydrate, low-fat diet is best, while others argue that carbohydrates need to be balanced by some protein and fat. Dean Ornish, M.D., author of *Eat More, Weigh Less*, advocates a high-carbohydrate, very low-fat (mostly vegetarian) diet for weight loss. His diet instructs people to eat to satiety but strictly limiting animal proteins and fats, based on the idea that, eating fat makes you fat.

Barry Sears, Ph.D., recommends the "Zone" diet—30% fat, 30% protein, and 40% carbohydrates. Dr. Sears faults the high-carbohydrate diets for misleading people into overconsuming carbohydrates, which can lead to an insulin imbalance. Once that happens, fewer carbohydrates are burned off as fuel and more calories are stored as body fat. By eating more protein, Dr. Sears believes, the metabolism is stimulated and burns stored body fat rather than recently consumed carbohydrates. However, researchers estimate that approximately 25% of the population can eat a high-carbohydrate diet without causing an imbalance in their insulin levels—a fact that Dr. Sears acknowledges.[1] For the remaining 75%, however, a diet that emphasizes carbohydrates at the expense of protein or fats may be the wrong approach.

Robert C. Atkins, M.D., author of *Dr. Atkin's Diet Revolution*, says that a diet high in protein and low in carbohydrates is the way to go for similar reasons, that by consuming a lot of protein, the body is able to shed fat more efficiently as it is burning off excess body fat and not just dietary calories. High carbohydrate or low carbohydrate? High protein or no protein? Which of these experts is right? Who should you believe?

This conflict and controversy exists only among mainstream experts. Alternative medicine practitioners recognize that individuals have different nutritional requirements. As Ralph Golan, M.D., author of *Optimal Wellness*, explains, "A successful weight-loss regimen requires a diet tailored to individual needs. A majority of Americans may lose weight and thrive on a high-protein, low-carbohydrate diet, whereas others get results on a high-complex-carbohydrate, low-protein diet."[2] The key is to match the diet to individual physiology. It is also important to understand that your individual needs are not static, but change according to the conditions of your life. Illness, stress, or exposure to environmental toxins increase requirements for different nutrients. All of these factors must be taken into account in making the right dietary decisions. So how to go about tailoring a diet to fit your individual needs? The first step is to look more closely at your body type.

Different Body Types, Different Diets

Many of you have probably already learned the hard lesson that one diet does not fit all. What none of the hundreds of diets on the market can tell you is what diet is the correct one for your individual biochemistry or body type. Just like fingerprints, each of us has a unique metabolism, that is, how we convert food into energy for running all of the body's processes. In fact, many chronic illnesses may be simply symptoms of an underlying disturbance in metabolism. Your body

"We are all biologically different and our nutritional needs vary for each person," says nutrition researcher Harold J. Kristal, D.D.S.

type could be the key to your health. The way to discover this biochemical "fingerprint" is metabolic typing.

Body types are used by many alternative medicine practitioners as a guide to help patients tailor their own diet plans. One of the most detailed body-typing systems is called metabolic typing, which is based on research done by George Watson, Ph.D., William Donald Kelley, D.D.S., Francis Pottenger, M.D., and others. They all believed that each individual has a particular metabolic type that determines how quickly—or slowly—your body burns off the calories you consume, and how and even where you are likely to store fat. Your type is determined from a series of diagnostic tests that reveal which physiological systems tend to drive your body.

What is Metabolic Typing?

"We are all biologically different and our nutritional needs vary for each person," says nutrition researcher Harold J. Kristal, D.D.S., of Corte Madera, California, who has been studying metabolic typing for many years. "Once a person's metabolic type is determined, specific foods and supplements can be recommended that address a person's unique biochemistry."

The first step in looking at one's biochemistry is determining the acid/alkaline state, or pH, of the individual's blood. Ideal blood pH is slightly alkaline at 7.46. A blood pH above this is considered alkaline and below 7.46 is acid. "Blood pH reflects the biochemical balance and metabolic efficiency for an individual," states Dr. Kristal. Blood pH indicates your state of health and your body type will predispose you to being more acidic or more alkaline. When you are too acid or too alkaline, your body doesn't absorb or use nutrients as well, which can lead to an array of problems, including weight gain, fatigue, allergies, high blood pressure, and many other chronic illnesses.

Each body type requires specific foods and dietary supplements to help rebalance the pH. "Foods themselves are not acidifying or alkalinizing to the body," says Dr. Kristal. "Rather they will produce an acid or alkaline effect depending on the body's metabolic type." In other words, any food or nutrient can have opposite effects on a person depending on their metabolic type. Is it any wonder that the one-size-fits-all diets don't work?

To further understand this typing system, it is important to understand its two primary criteria: the autonomic nervous system and oxidation rate.

■ Autonomic Nervous System—Each of our bodies has a unique way of functioning, determined by genetics and controlled by the autonomic nervous system (ANS). The ANS can be likened to your body's automatic pilot. It keeps you alive through breathing, heart rate, and digestion, without your being aware of it or participating in its activities. The ANS has two divisions: the sympathetic and the parasympathetic. The sympathetic nervous system expends energy and is associated with action, arousal, and stress. It prepares us physically, or energizes us, by increasing our heart rate, blood pressure, and muscle tension as it prepares the body for action; the thyroid, pituitary, and adrenal glands are sympathetic-influenced. The parasympathetic nervous system conserves body energy, slows heart rate, and increases intestinal, liver, and pancreas activity as it reduces the energy the body expends. People tend to be dominant in either sympathetic function or parasympathetic function. Sympathetic dominance makes the body more acid, while parasympathetic dominance tends toward alkalinity.

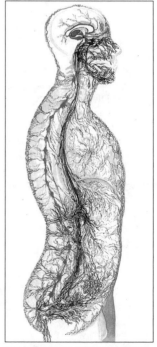

■ Oxidation Rate—Oxidation refers to the process of converting food into energy. All foods—proteins, fats, and carbohydrates—are converted into energy (measured in calories) which are then burned off by the body. Ideally, your calorie intake matches the amount of calories you use as energy. But if your oxidation rate is too fast, it tends to acidify the blood, and if your oxidation is too slow, it alkalinizes your blood pH. An imbalance will also tend to convert food into fat instead of using it as energy.

Both of these systems will affect your metabolism and how efficiently you are burning off calories you consume—or how you are storing excess calories as body fat. One of these systems will be dominant and influence all of your body's processes. "Dominance" means that while ANS influence and oxidation rate complement one another, one of these systems tends to be in

THE AUTONOMIC NERVOUS SYSTEM.

A Brief Survey of Body Typing

The idea that each of us has a specific body type is not a new one. Ayurvedic medicine, the 5,000-year-old traditional medicine of India, describes three metabolic, constitutional, and body types (*doshas*), in association with the basic elements of nature—*vata* (air and ether, rooted in the intestines), *pitta* (fire and water/stomach), and *kapha* (water and earth/lungs). Ayurvedic physicians use these categories (which also have psychological aspects) as the basis for prescribing individualized programs of herbs, diet, massage, breathing, meditation, exercise, and detoxification techniques.

Traditional Chinese medicine (TCM) originated in China over 5,000 years ago and is a comprehensive system of medical practice that heals the body according to the principles of nature and balance. A Chinese medicine physician considers the flow of vital energy (*qi*) in a patient through close examination of the patient's pulse, tongue, body odor, voice tone and strength, and general demeanor, among other elements. Underlying imbalances and disharmony in the body are described in terminology analogous to the natural world (heat, cold, dryness, or dampness). TCM employs a body-typing paradigm called the Five Element Theory, which holds that each individual expresses the energy of the elements of fire, wood, air, water, and metal in different measures and that an interplay of *yin* (passive, watery, stationary, dark, calming) and *yang* (active, fiery, moving, bright, energizing) energies influences one's health.

Modern science is now catching up with these concepts. One recent body-typing system is glandular types, developed in the early 1980s by Eliot D. Abravanel, M.D., of Los Angeles, California, author of *Dr. Abravanel's Body Type Diet*. This approach is based upon the idea that each one of us has a "dominant" endocrine gland that controls the workings of our internal chemistry, namely how our bodies process and use proteins, carbohydrates, and fats. It also determines our general body shape, fat distribution, food preferences, and energy level, and is associated with a distinctive set of personality traits and behavior patterns, according to Dr. Abravanel. The main types are adrenal, pituitary, thyroid, and gonadal.

Another body-typing system was developed by James D'Adamo, N.D., founder of the Institute for the Advancement of Natural Therapy in Toronto, Canada, who pioneered the idea that blood type is a determinant of individual nutritional requirements. His observations of more than 3,000 patients led him to conclude that the four basic blood groups—O, A, B, and AB (plus six additional subtypes)—have different physiological and nutritional needs. Dr. D'Adamo's work on blood type and diet has been continued by his son, Peter D'Adamo, N.D., author of *Eat Right for Your Type*. Although wide-ranging in their origins and principles, all these systems share a belief that everyone has a distinct physiological "fingerprint" that cannot be ignored.

control. This concept of dominance in metabolic typing was first observed by William L. Wolcott, a metabolic typing researcher and founder of Healthexcel, Inc., in Winthrop, Washington, an organization that performs metabolic typing evaluations. Knowing whether you are predominantly oxidative or autonomic will provide a lot of information that can help identify your metabolic type and also guide you in selecting the foods that will enable you to maintain a healthy weight, without rigid dieting or excessive physical activity.

Success Story: Body Typing Promotes Weight Loss

Greg, 49, was overweight at 211 pounds. He had been faithfully avoiding "fattening" foods such as fatty meats, butter and oils, and dairy, but still remained overweight. He came to see Dr. Kristal because of his frustration at being unable to lose the extra pounds. The metabolic typing tests revealed that Greg was a Fast Burner, a type that tends to be acid. Greg's diet consisted of large amounts of carbohydrates—he was eating pasta just about every night. Wheat, in particular, is unhealthy for this type as it tends to further acidify their system. "Fast Burners have to stay away from wheat," says Dr. Kristal. "It's the only grain that's acidifying—it's just putting pounds on them. Fast Burners need more proteins and more fats."

Dr. Kristal immediately recommended dietary changes. The Fast Burner can eat more proteins (40% of diet) and fats, but needs to cut back on carbohydrates. Greg could eat proteins—beef, chicken, fish (tuna, mussels, mackerel, abalone, salmon), and dairy—at every meal. Nuts and seeds (almonds, flaxseeds, pecans, sesame, walnuts) and oils (canola, olive, sesame, and sunflower) were also recommended. These are the very foods that Greg had been avoiding.

Greg needed to reduce the amount of carbohydrates he ate, but he could include some vegetables (asparagus, carrots, cauliflower, peas, spinach, squash, beans, and lentils) and fruits (bananas, apples, and pears). All food choices should be whole, natural foods, not canned or processed foods. Snacks should be proteins, not carbohydrates, as this type needs to limit carbohydrate consumption.

Dr. Kristal recommended that Greg take a supplement of digestive enzymes. He also put him on a fiber supplement to be taken before lunch and dinner to help curb his appetite and prevent overeating. In just two months, Greg lost 17 pounds and his pH (acid/alkaline level) is more balanced now. "He's a happy camper," says Dr. Kristal. "He's had a tremendous response. That's what happens when you eat the right things—what your body really wants."

Determining Your Type

Metabolic body typing uses a number of tests to identify an individual's biochemistry before creating a program of appropriate diet and exercise. These tests provide information that, taken together and analyzed by an experienced health practitioner, can more accurately identify your type.

■ Blood pH—Testing will reveal if you are acid, below the norm of 7.46, or alkaline, above that same level. Knowing whether you are acid or alkaline will determine the foods that will work with your metabolism, and it will also influence the type of vitamins that are best for you.

■ Blood Typing—Blood is classified into four blood types or groups according to the presence of type A and type B antigens on

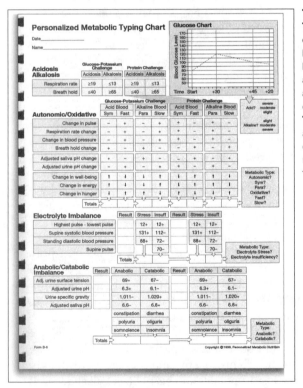

The Metabolic Typing Chart tracks changes in pH, blood glucose levels, respiration, and other indicators after a glucose challenge test. These measures are useful for determining metabolic type.

the surface of red blood cells. These antigens are also called agglutinogens and pertain to the blood cells' ability to agglutinate, or clump together. Type O blood (containing neither type) is found in 47% of the Caucasian population; type A, 41%; type B, 9%; type AB, 3%. Blood type is considered relevant to metabolic typing because agglutination also occurs in the body in response to a type of protein called lectin. Lectins are found in 30% of the foods we eat; they have characteristics similar to blood antigens and can thus sometimes become "an enemy" when they enter the body. Nutritionist Ann Louise Gittleman, M.S., C.N.S., author of *Your Body Knows Best*, notes that there are 65 different lectins known to have an agglutination reaction in the body.[3]

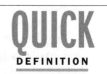

QUICK DEFINITION

Glucose, a type of sugar, is the main fuel used by the brain. After a meal is eaten, the pancreas produces insulin to enable sugars to be metabolized. If you are eating a lot of carbohydrates, your body will become accustomed to producing a lot of insulin and over time, you may experience insulin resistance. The result is your body may store the carbohydrates as fat rather than be made available as "fuel" that can be burned off by your body as energy.

■ Glucose Metabolism—During a glucose (SEE QUICK DEFINITION) tolerance test, a drink rich in sugars is given and saliva and urine samples are taken and measured to determine how quickly or slowly the body is "burning off" or oxidizing the sugars. The person's sense of well-being, hunger, and energy are noted prior to taking the drink and at intervals over the next two hours. The readings form a pattern to further establish if a person is one of five metabolic types.

■ Oxidative or Autonomic—Your blood pressure, heart rate, pulse, and respiratory rate will be recorded at the beginning of testing to see what they are in a fasting state and again measured after the glucose test is administered. Changes in the readings will reflect if you are oxidative or autonomic.

■ Body Temperature—Known as the basal temperature, this provides a clue as to whether your metabolism, essentially the internal "furnace" that burns the calories you are consuming, is operating efficiently. You can measure your own basal temperature at home—for three consecutive days, take a thermometer and place it in your mouth first thing in the morning for about ten minutes (digital thermometers will take less time) to record your body temperature. The normal range is 97.8°-98.2° F. If your temperature falls below this level, your thyroid and, in turn, your metabolism may be underactive. Women who are menstruating are likely to have an elevated temperature and should begin recording their temperature after the third day of their cycle.

- Food Diary—The diary provides a detailed list of all the foods consumed over a 3-day period. This includes all the snacks and foods eaten on the run that you may have forgotten you consumed.
- Hair Analysis—Your hair is analyzed to reveal what minerals you may be lacking. Much like the rings on a tree, hair provides a nutrient history. This information reveals what supplementation may be needed to restore your health.
- *Candida*—The presence of the yeast-like fungus *Candida albicans* will provide more information regarding any food allergies and the resulting symptoms of fatigue or incomplete digestion and absorption of foods.
- Photos of Your Body—Photos are used to record what parts of your body tend to store fat. This is based in part on Abravanel's body typing system (see "A Brief Survey of Body Typing," p. 38), which states that distinct physiological types predispose you to gain and carry excess weight in certain areas of your body.
- General Health—An extensive survey with questions regarding what you eat, what snacks you crave, sleeping habits, and general outlook on life is also given. This inventory reveals general tendencies and any obvious imbalances, such as intense cravings for salty snacks or interrupted sleep. For the same reason, an electro-acupuncture test is administered to determine if any of your organs, such as liver, thyroid, or spleen, are underactive or overstimulated.

Taken together, these tests give an overview of your general health and if any of your body systems are creating imbalances that will affect your metabolism.

The Five Metabolic Types

With all of this information, an experienced practitioner can determine the person's metabolic type as one of the following:

Fast Burners—Fast Burners (fast oxidizers) have a tendency to burn off their carbohydrates too quickly for their energy needs. At the same time, they are poor at converting fats to fuel that can be used by the body. They have acid blood and do best on a whole foods diet including whole grains, extensive animal protein, and full-fat dairy foods. Wheat is to be avoided as it is too acid-forming.

Slow Burners—Slow Burners (slow oxidizers) are alkaline and do well eating a diet limiting high-fat, high-purine animal proteins. Low-fat dairy foods and whole grains are allowable, but wheat should be favored as it is acid-forming.

Energizers—Energizers (sympathetic dominant) tend to have acid blood and their bodies are dominated by the thyroid, pituitary, and adrenal glands. They do well on a low-protein, relatively low-fat diet.

Conservers—Conservers (parasympathetic dominant) do well on a diet including full-fat dairy foods, with more animal protein. This type is characterized by increased activity in the liver, intestines, and, pancreas.

Balanced—A small number of people are blessed with balanced, well-functioning endocrine systems. They maintain a healthy weight and eat intuitively, selecting foods that provide them with a steady supply of energy that discourages overeating.

What Your Type Means for Your Health

Fast Burners, who tend to be acid, need to be given alkaline-forming foods to help balance their system, while Slow Burners (alkaline) should be given acid-forming foods and nutrients. But the Energizers and Conservers are just the opposite: although Energizers tend to be acid, they require acid-forming foods in order to alkalinize their systems, while Conservers, being alkaline, need alkaline-forming foods in order to acidify their systems. Without knowing your specific body type, your eating habits and supplements could be making your health worse. For example, eating an orange may calm down one metabolic type and result in an alkaline shift, whereas in a different metabolic type, the same orange can be found to cause a hyper response and result in an acidic shift.[4]

Once an individual's metabolic body type is identified, imbalances can be corrected, allowing the body to return to a healthy weight without rigid dieting. A good example of an imbalanced Fast Burner is Suzanne, 35, who was 100 pounds overweight. "She was eating everything low-fat and trying to stay away from meats, especially fats," says Dr. Kristal. "People like this need a lot of the right kind of fats. Actually, fats make them thinner." Dr. Kristal placed Suzanne on a diet consisting of relatively high protein (40%) and relatively low carbohydrates, which, along with supplementation, resulted in immediate weight loss. Within a month, she lost ten pounds and reported she felt "wonderful" and had more energy. "What happens is they lose fat," says Dr. Kristal of Fast Burners like Suzanne. "She was approximately 60% body fat and we really want to

William L. Wolcott: Healthexcel, Inc.; tel: 650-325-1840; website: www. metabolictyping.com. **Harold J. Kristal, D.D.S.:** Personalized Metabolic Nutrition, 520 Tamalpais Drive, Suite 205, Corte Madera, CA 94925; tel: 415-924-2571; fax: 415-927-4664; website: www. bloodph.com.

Are You a Candidate for Metabolic Typing?

Consulting a dietitian or other health practitioner regarding your diet is always a good idea, but there are basic warning signals that your diet may be working against you (and your metabolic type), causing you to go further out of balance and gain weight:

■ Appetite—Are you always hungry no matter how frequently or how much you eat?

■ Digestion—After you eat, do you experience any bloating, gas, or indigestion? Do you find it difficult to digest certain foods, such as dairy, meats, or wheat products?

■ Energy Levels—Are you excessively tired a few hours after eating? Or do you have sustained energy and are able to perform tasks that require concentration and alertness?

■ Cravings—Do you crave certain foods such as salty snacks or sweets, caffeine or fat?

■ Regularity—Do you have a daily bowel movement? Do you experience any constipation or difficulty in completely detoxing on a daily basis?

■ Sleep—Are you able to fall asleep fairly easily and do you feel rested in the morning? Are you sleeping too much and feel lethargic or sleeping too little and edgy from fatigue?

■ Sense of Well-Being—Do you feel well? Or do you experience mood swings or any depression?

If you responded negatively to more than two of the above questions, you may want to consider metabolic typing to help you choose the right foods for your particular biochemistry and to restore a healthy balance in your life.

get her down to under 28%." During the course of the program, Dr. Kristal continued to monitor her progress and notes that she will probably lose about 5-6 pounds a month.

In another case, Peter, a 17-year-old boy who weighed 220 pounds and had a body fat of 50%, was brought in to see Dr. Kristal by his parents. He was unable to participate in sports at his school because of his excess weight. After using the metabolic typing protocol to test him, Dr. Kristal determined him to be an imbalanced Fast Burner, a type that tends to metabolize their carbohydrates too rapidly. This can lead to overeating as this type may feel hungry all the time. Also, they are not efficient in releasing their fat stores to be used as fuel, which can contribute to further weight gain, explains Dr. Kristal. He started Peter on high-protein foods. His diet included high-purine meats, such as beef, chicken (dark meat), fish with dark meat (tuna, abalone, mackerel), and lamb, which take longer to digest, thereby providing a feeling of satiety and energy for a longer period of time. Dr. Kristal also had him start to supplement with essential fatty acids to improve his metabolism and digestive aids to ensure he was absorbing the nutrients from his food. As a result of these changes to his diet, Peter's weight dropped to 201 pounds, a loss that resulted in a body fat reduction from 50% to 42%. And his energy level was greatly improved, enabling him to play sports again comfortably.

Sizing Up the Popular Diets

Walk into any bookstore and you will find hundreds of books on dieting. While the most popular diets have enthusiastic fans who have shed pounds following their programs, others have not been as successful at keeping weight off. The problem, again, is that these programs try to assign everyone to only one diet.

Dean Ornish, M.D., author of *Eat More, Weigh Less*, is among the leading advocates of a high-carbohydrate, low-fat diet for weight loss. According to his diet plan, your fat intake should not exceed 10% of your caloric intake. He also believes that the majority of calories (70%) should come from carbohydrates and only 20% from proteins. Dr. Ornish therefore recommends that dieters follow a mostly vegetarian diet, as meat contains high levels of fat and cholesterol.[5] Disdaining dietary fat and proclaiming essentially that eating fat makes you fat, the Ornish diet emphasizes grazing throughout the day and avoiding fat of any kind, whether from meats, fish, nuts, seeds, or oils.

Unfortunately, eating too many carbohydrates can lead to insulin imbalance and turn your body into a fat-storing machine. "Overconsumption of carbohydrates can create excess insulin," explains Ann Louise Gittleman, M.S. "Excess insulin production blocks the fat-burning glucagon [SEE QUICK DEFINITION] from doing its job, which results in more fat being stored."[6] Aside from the possibility of upsetting your body's insulin and glucagon balance, the extremely low-fat diet may not be suitable for women. "Anyone following this diet long-term should increase the fat amount, especially women, because inadequate fat consumption can affect a woman's hormone levels," states Monika Klein, C.C.N., who runs a nutritional counseling practice in Malibu, California.[7]

Barry Sears, Ph.D., author of *The Zone*, advocates a diet higher in fat and protein—specifically, 30% fat, 30% protein, and 40% carbohydrate. Dr. Sears argues that high-carbohydrate diets cause the body to manufacture large quantities of insulin, a hormone secreted by the pancreas that allows the

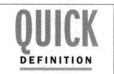

DEFINITION

Glucagon is secreted by your pancreas and helps to "unlock" the body's fat stores to be burned as fuel. If too much insulin is present in the bloodstream, such as following a steady diet of carbohydrates, glucagon is blocked. Fat is not freed up to be used and the dieter often craves more carbohydrates as he or she may feel lethargic, unable to gain access to the energy locked in the body's fat stores.

body's cells to burn carbohydrate as fuel. Excessive insulin causes an imbalance that breaks down the body's ability to use carbohydrates, causing more of them to be converted into fat rather than burned as a fuel. According to Dr. Sears, a diet higher in protein and fat helps to keep insulin levels in check, and thus reduces the conversion of carbohydrates into fat.

The same can be said for the high-protein, low-carbohydrate diet advocated by Robert C. Atkins, M.D., in *Dr. Atkin's Diet Revolution*. Eating a high-protein, low-carbohydrate diet will put the body in a state of ketosis, forcing it to burn stored fat for fuel, instead of using carbohydrates from daily consumption. By increasing the metabolism and balancing blood sugar levels, this diet has had some success, Klein says, and many people can benefit from eating fewer carbohydrates. However, much of the weight loss on this diet comes from water weight and this can put added stress on the liver and kidneys. Ketosis can also cause some unpleasant side effects, such as headaches and mental fatigue. More significantly, weight loss may come from lean body mass instead of fat as the body converts muscles into glucose.[8] Ultimately, however, Klein agrees with Dr. Atkin's recommendation that people are best supervised on this diet by a physician.

As for the Zone diet designed by Dr. Sears, its 40% carbohydrates, 30% protein, and 30% fats formula is designed to alter levels of the hormones insulin and glucagon to burn off stored carbohydrates rather than turn them into fat. However, the notion that a 40/30/30 diet can significantly alter these hormone levels is not supported by the scientific literature. As with most fad diets, the food restrictions of the Zone diet limits its long-term effectiveness because people have difficulty staying on the diet. "Even though people lose weight on this diet, its calorie restrictions leave people hungry, especially those who are physically active," notes Klein.[9]

Lastly, there is the blood type diet designed by James D'Adamo, N.D., in *The D'Adamo Diet*, which assigns each blood type a specific diet. As with many diets, there are varied opinions. Klein believes D'Adamo's diet has some merit and application to certain types of people. "I have seen success with this diet in my practice: people have lost weight, cleared sinus conditions, improved bowel function, and balanced blood sugar. It is better suited to people interested in clearing up existing health conditions, such as arthritis or allergies, and maintaining their health."[10] Others, however, question if there is sufficient scientific research to back up the claims of this dietary regimen.

Selecting a diet that works in harmony with your specific metabolism will enable you to stop the dieting merry-go-round, eat freely within your specific food group, and gradually return to a healthy weight—permanently.

Nutrition for Your Body Type

By eating in a way that works best with your particular metabolism, you may notice improved energy levels and not experience as many cravings between meals. Eat a wide variety of foods within your food plan and try to avoid eating the same foods every day. Always eat protein with every meal and even with snacks; do not eat carbohydrates alone. Eat at least three meals a day, following a regular meal schedule and, whenever possible, eating at the same times each day. Eat only whole, natural foods, avoiding processed, canned, preserved, packaged, synthetic, artificially colored foods or foods processed with hormones. Begin each day with three cups of water, but avoid drinking liquids with meals and never have cold drinks; to do so dilutes the digestive juices in your stomach, making it more difficult for your body to assimilate the foods you have consumed. Whenever possible drink only distilled or water purified by some other means, such as reverse osmosis (SEE QUICK DEFINITION). Once you have learned how to eat according to your biochemistry, it will become second nature. Rather than adhering to a rigid diet, you will be able to eat comfortably within your food group and see your weight gradually drop to a healthier level.

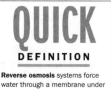

QUICK

DEFINITION

Reverse osmosis systems force water through a membrane under pressure. They are most effective against inorganic pollutants like nitrates and metals like lead. (Deonization resins are also used to accomplish this purpose.)

Group 1 Foods and Nutrients

Group 1 is primarily a vegetarian diet, with low fat intake, to acidify Slow Burners and to alkalinize Energizers. This is a diet consisting of 55% carbohydrates, 25% protein, and 20% fats.

■ Emphasize all types of whole grains, favoring wheat as this grain is very acid-forming, as well as vegetables and fruits, but limit dairy foods. Avoid caffeine, salt, high-fat foods, avocado, artichoke, beans, peas, lentils, cauliflower, spinach, asparagus, high-purine meats, organ meats, butter, alcoholic beverages, soft drinks, sugar, and artificial sweeteners. Minimize salt intake and avoid commercial salt.

■ Eat limited animal and seafood proteins and cook by boiling, broiling, or baking. Do not eat microwaved or fried food. Include chicken and turkey breast meat, lean pork, ham; catfish, cod, crab, crayfish, flounder, haddock, lobster, perch, scrod, shrimp, sole, and white tuna. Select dairy from non- or low-fat milk (cheese, cottage cheese, milk, yogurt); eggs. Limit milk-based foods due to calcium content.

■ Nuts, seeds, and oils should be used sparingly. Do not eat roasted nuts or hydrogenated nut butters. Avoid margarine, hydrogenated oils, fat substitutes, and butter. Use only fresh, raw nuts and seeds, but in small quantities.

■ Eat only whole grains. Baked goods should be made from whole-grain flours. Select from all varieties, especially wheat, and including amaranth, barley, buckwheat, millet, oat, quinoa, rice, rye, and triticale.

■ Eat only fresh, frozen, or dried vegetables and use organic whenever possible. Consume them raw, boiled, or lightly steamed. Emphasize leafy vegetables over root vegetables, but avoid carrots; choose from beets, broccoli, Brussels sprouts, cabbage, cucumber, eggplant, leafy greens, onions, peppers, potatoes, scallions, all types of squash, turnip, and yams.

■ Consume only fresh or frozen fruits, but no juices. All fruits are allowed, including apple, apricot, berries, cherry, citrus, grape, melon, peach, pear, pineapple, plum, and tomato.

■ Drink only purified water. Do not drink tap water.

Group 2 Foods and Nutrients

Group 2 emphasizes proteins and fats, and limits carbohydrate consumption, to alkalinize Fast Burners and to acidify Conservers. This diet consists of about 30% carbohydrates, 40% protein, and 30% fats.

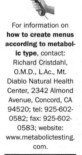

For information on **how to create menus according to metabolic type**, contact: Richard Cristdahl, O.M.D., L.Ac., Mt. Diablo Natural Health Center, 2342 Almond Avenue, Concord, CA 94520; tel: 925-602-0582; fax: 925-602-0583; website: www.metabolictesting. com.

■ Favor high-fat meats, poultry, and fish. Protein should be eaten with every meal. Cook by baking, boiling, or broiling. Do not overcook or eat blackened, charred meat. Eat a variety of meats, selecting from beef, duck, goose, fowl, kidney, lamb, liver, pork rib, chicken (dark meat), red meats, sweet bread, tongue, tripe, veal, venison; abalone, caviar, clams, crab, crayfish, herring, lobster, mackerel, mussels, oysters, octopus, salmon, sardines, scallops, shrimp, and dark tuna.

- Avoid candy, pastry, fruit, citrus jam, jelly, ice cream, potatoes, zucchini, ketchup, white rice, pastas, refined flour breads, crackers, refined or processed cereals, soft drinks, coffee, black tea, and beer, wine, or any alcoholic beverages.
  - Eat limited amounts of dairy from whole milk (cheese, cottage cheese, milk, yogurt); eggs.
  - Use oils sparingly in your diet. Avoid margarine, hydrogenated oils, or fat substitutes. Use only natural, cold-pressed oils, including almond, canola, flax, peanut, olive, sesame, sunflower, and walnut. Butter and ghee are also allowed.
  - Avoid commercial salts. Also avoid artificial sweeteners and generally limit sugar.
    - All nuts and seeds are allowed. Avoid roasted nuts and hydrogenated nut butters. Eat only fresh, raw nuts and seeds, including almonds, Brazil, filberts, macadamia, peanuts, pecans, walnuts, flax, sesame, pumpkin, and sunflower.
    - Eat only whole grains and in moderate amounts. Avoid refined carbohydrates and baked goods should be made from whole grain flours; however, avoid wheat breads or white rice.
    - Use only fresh, frozen, or dried vegetables and use organic whenever possible; consume raw, boiled, or lightly steamed. Select from artichoke, asparagus, carrots, cauliflower, celery, mushrooms, peas, spinach, squash; lentils, tofu, and other fresh or dried beans.
- Limit fruit intake and use only fresh or frozen. Avoid citrus, dried or very ripe fruit, and juices. Select from avocado, bananas, apples, and pears, preferably unripe or green. Watch for hypoglycemic reactions (SEE QUICK DEFINITION) to carrots, starches (grains), and fruits.

Note: Balanced types can eat freely from both food groups and are striving for a diet that is 45% carbohydrates, 30% protein, and 25% fats. Again, despite this dietary freedom, any excessive eating of any one particular food group may create an imbalance that requires correction.

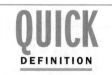

DEFINITION

Hypoglycemia, or low-blood sugar, is a condition often associated with diabetes. Symptoms include anxiety, weakness, sweating, rapid heart rate, dizziness, headache, irritability, and poor or double vision, among others. These symptoms commonly occur in mid-afternoon, when most people experience a slight drop in blood sugar (glucose) levels.

2 Healthy Eating

LOW-CALORIE diets and exercise have been the typical solution to losing weight. With thousands of diets and a multi-million dollar industry dedicated to weight control, shedding a few pounds should be easy. Unfortunately, the weight lost by dieters is almost always regained. As a result, many dieters fall into the "yo-yo trap," a repetitive cycle of weight loss and gain.

Susan Kano, a national speaker and author on dieting and eating disorders, tells a story about a friend who had not only been trying to lose weight for years, but was also in the dieting business. Initially she struggled to get from 165 pounds down to 120 pounds. After a while, her weight returned to the 165-pound mark. Over the years, as she tried one diet after another, her weight yo-yoed up and down. Today, she continues to diet and weighs over 200 pounds.

There are several reasons why this happens and why food restriction for the purposes of weight loss should be avoided. "We have gotten fatter as a culture over the last few years," says Kano, "partly because of dieting." Whenever the body is deprived of food, whether from famine or dieting, it ensures survival by decreasing the metabolic rate in order to compensate for fewer calories. Energy is stored so efficiently in fat tissues that someone of normal weight can survive for weeks without eating. The desire to binge after food restriction, although disheartening to dieters, is another built-in survival mechanism intended to click on after a famine.[1] "Our innocent cellular metabolism has no way to tell the difference between self-imposed starvation and life-threatening famine," says Nancy Dunne, N.D., of Missoula, Montana.

Proper diet and exercise are the most effective ways to lose weight. However, it is not a matter of how much a person eats, but what they eat that is important. "Although it is commonly assumed that obesity is due to overeating, there is, in fact, a complex interaction between one's culture, environment, exercise habits, and eating styles, as well as one's genetic makeup and biochemical individuality," according to Timothy Birdsall, N.D., of Sandpoint, Idaho.

Rather than restrictive dieting, simply learning how to eat in a healthy and balanced way can have a major impact on weight. Whether or not you decide to follow the dietary recommendations based on your metabolic type (covered in the previous chapter), incorporating healthier eating habits into your lifestyle can improve your overall health and help you achieve a healthy body weight for the rest of your life.

The Healthy Eating Plan

Both alternative and conventional medicine agree that Americans should consume less fat, animal protein, and processed foods, and eat more complex carbohydrates, especially whole grains rich in fiber, and at least five servings daily of fruits and vegetables. Buck Levin, Ph.D., R.D., Assistant Professor of Nutrition at Bastyr University in Seattle, Washington, offers a simple prescription for a healthy diet—one of natural, whole foods. "By whole foods we mean consuming a diet that is high in foods as whole as possible, with the least amount of processed, adulterated, fried, or sweetened additives," says Dr. Levin.

A whole foods, whole grain, high–complex carbohydrate, low-fat, high-fiber diet is recommended by Dr. Birdsall. He suggests a maximum of 25% of the daily food intake be in the form of fat. In general, this amounts to 45-50 grams per day, which represents about 450 calories. He believes lowering dietary fat and increasing exercise are the two key factors to weight loss. A whole foods diet is generously filled with a wide variety of different colored vegetables, fruits, and grains; raw seeds and nuts and their butters; beans; fermented milk products such as yogurt and kefir; and fish, poultry, and bean products like tofu. It should also be lower in animal meats, fats, and cheeses. Eating well-balanced meals at regular times during the day (four to five hours apart) will stabilize your blood sugar and help you control your appetite.

For information on **carbohydrate addictions and weight gain**, see Chapter 11: Break Food Allergies and Addictions, pp. 244-270.

Carbohydrates—Carbohydrates consist of simple sugars, complex carbohydrates, and fiber. They are the preferred source of energy for all bodily functions. The typical American diet includes more refined and processed foods than the diet of any other nation. It is estimated that refined sugars comprise one-fifth of all calories consumed daily by Americans.[2] When food is refined and processed, not only is fiber removed but simple sugars often replace complex carbohydrates. A diet low in fiber and high in simple sugar can be a major contributing factor to excess weight gain as well as diabetes, heart disease, and cancer. Foods rich in complex carbohydrates include vegetables, whole grains, rice, potatoes, legumes, milk, and dairy products (be sure to use foods raised or processed under organic conditions).

Dietary fiber can have a major impact on weight gain as evidenced by the almost complete lack of obesity in cultures that consume a diet high in fiber.[3] Fiber has been shown to not only reduce serum cholesterol, but to also pull dietary fat from the body into the feces. Other benefits of roughage include increasing chewing time, thus slowing down the eating process and inducing satiety, preventing constipation, and stabilizing blood glucose levels.[4] Whole grains (wheat, oats, rice, rye, barley, millet) have the highest level of fiber, followed by legumes, nuts and seeds, root vegetables (potatoes, turnips, beets, carrots), fruits, and leafy, green vegetables.

Proteins—Protein is one of the most plentiful substances in our body (second only to water). It is a major component in muscles, skin, hair and nails, the heart and brain, many hormones including insulin, red blood cells, antibodies, and enzymes. Proteins are present in nearly every cell and fluid in the body. Structurally, protein is made up of linked amino acids (SEE QUICK DEFINITION). Proteins are necessary for growth and repair of body tissues and the regulation of bodily activities.

Healthy sources of protein are foods that contain all the essential amino acids, the building blocks of proteins. These "complete" proteins are milk, eggs, cheese, meat, fish, and poultry. Green, leafy vegetables, grains, and beans (legumes) are a source of some important amino acids, but not all, and are therefore referred to as "incomplete" proteins. These proteins can be combined with complementary foods, such as brown rice, corn, nuts, seeds, or whole-grain wheat, to form complete proteins. Vegetarians, in particular, need to be aware of food combining in order to obtain adequate amounts of protein in their diet. Nutritionist Maile Pouls, Ph.D., of Santa Cruz, California, generally recommends obtaining proteins from vegetable sources. Of the animal proteins, she says that poultry and fish are healthier sources than red meat and dairy (which are higher in saturated fats), which should be eaten less frequently and in small portions. Again, be sure to choose organic sources for all dietary proteins.

Fats—Elson Haas, M.D., of San Rafael, California, author of *Staying Healthy With Nutrition*, points out that certain people will do better on different types of diets, with the one consistent factor being that the diets are low in fat. "For instance, some people will do better on a low-carbohydrate diet, instead of one that is high in carbohydrates," he says. "As long as the fat content of the diet remains low, the overweight person can have success." A Cornell University study showed that when women were allowed to eat as much as they wanted, with the only restriction being that they had to consume low-fat foods (only 20%-25% of calories from fat), they lost weight.[5] This is because fat contains more than twice as many calories per gram as protein or carbohydrates. A Swiss study also revealed that, unlike carbohydrates, approximately 90% of extra fat consumed during a meal is converted to body fat.[6] Very fatty foods may also encourage overeating because more needs to be consumed in order to maintain the body's natural storage of glucose.[7] Weight loss should therefore be directed toward a change in eating habits rather than dieting.

Contrary to popular belief, some fats are good for you, but not all fats are created equal. Of the three kinds of fats (saturated, polyunsaturated, and monounsaturated), polyunsaturated are the healthiest because they are a dietary source of essential fatty acids, unsaturated fats required in the diet. Additional information on incorporating healthy fats into your diet and avoiding the unhealthy ones is provided later in this chapter.

Alcohol should also be avoided or minimized, since it has been found to act like a fat in the body and promote weight gain. J.P. Flatt, Ph.D., from the University of Massachusetts Medical School, estimates that one ounce of alcohol represents one-half ounce of fat in the diet.[8] Cigarettes, which are used by many people to manage their weight, also appear to steer extra fat to the abdomen. In addition, both of these sub-

QUICK

DEFINITION

Amino acids are the building blocks of the 40,000 different proteins in the body, including enzymes, hormones, and the brain chemical messengers called neurotransmitters. Eight amino acids cannot be made by the body and must be obtained through the diet; others are produced in the body but not always in sufficient amounts. The body's main "amino acid pool" consists of: alanine, arginine, aspargine, aspartic acid, carnitine, citrulline, cysteine, cystine, GABA, glutamic acid, glutamine, glycine, histidine, isoleucine, leucine, lysine, methionine, ornithine, phenylalanine, proline, serine, taurine, threonine, tryptophan, tyrosine, and valine.

The Maligned Egg

Avoiding eggs because you're worried about their cholesterol content is a mistake. Dietary sources of cholesterol account for very little of the cholesterol in your blood. In fact, the liver manufactures about 3,000 mg of cholesterol in any 24-hour period, a quantity equivalent to the amount contained in ten eggs. This occurs regardless of how much cholesterol is ingested through food. Doctors at Princeton Associates for Total Health (PATH), a clinic in Princeton, New Jersey, call the egg a "much maligned" food and insist that the presence of other nutrients (such as lecithin) moderate its cholesterol-raising properties. They also consider eggs to be one of the best sources of complete protein. "To consider cholesterol content only is misleading," writes PATH physician Eric Braverman, M.D., "because the ratio of cholesterol to other nutrients is what is important."

Nevertheless, how an egg is cooked can make all the difference as to whether or not you should eat it. Excessively high temperatures cause the fats and cholesterol in eggs to become oxidized; eating oxidized fat may damage artery walls. To minimize oxidation, soft-boiling (the best choice), scrambling, or baking eggs is recommended instead of hard-boiling or frying them.[9]

stances should be avoided especially by those who are prone to glucose intolerance. A sense of balance is important in approaching one's diet. If the majority of meals are comprised of whole, fresh foods, then a little junk food, an occasional alcoholic drink, or a piece of candy won't hurt. But when too few whole foods are consumed, as compared to "stressor" foods (those lacking in nutritional value), the body's physiology is damaged.

Eating Lower on the Food Chain

While it is preferable that a whole foods diet be as plant-based as possible, it is not necessary to become a complete vegetarian, eliminating meats and other animal foods from the diet totally. Today, many kinds of dairy products and animal foods have reduced levels of fat. In addition, whole milk, eggs, and meats provide amino acids and other important nutrients necessary for health. Even so, meats and other animal products should be eaten in moderation and always choose the leanest meats possible, raised without the use of antibiotics and other drugs, as this will cut down effectively on calories, weight gain, and toxic exposure.

There are many reasons to stick to a more plant-based diet. First, important antioxidant nutrients, including vitamin C, beta carotene, vitamin E, and many cancer-fighting substances known as phytochemicals, are found in fruits, vegetables, and grains. These antioxidant nutrients are considered the best protection against age- and environmental-related diseases, from dandruff, bad breath, and wrinkling to cataracts, cancer, diabetes, and heart attacks. In many studies, they have been associated with increased immune response.[10] Also, the high-fiber content of plant foods helps keep the digestive tract clean by absorbing and eliminating many potentially dangerous toxins. Plant foods also tend to have a lower toxicity than animal foods to begin with, because they are lower on the food chain and as such have had less exposure to accumulating toxins.

Medical and scientific evidence also points to the benefits of moving toward a vegetable-based diet. Dean Ornish, M.D., of the University of California at San Francisco, demonstrates that a diet low in animal protein, along with exercise and stress-reduction measures, can actually reverse heart disease.[11] James Anderson, M.D., has brought Type II diabetics off of insulin with a vegetarian diet. In 1988, the American Dietetic Association published research showing that a vegetarian lifestyle reduces the risk of heart disease, diabetes, colon cancer, hypertension, obesity, osteoporosis, and diverticular disease.[12]

Repetition vs. Variety in the Diet

Nutritionist Lindsey Berkson, M.A., D.C., of Santa Fe, New Mexico, sees today's typical American diet as containing too few foods. "Unfortunately, most Americans tend to avoid variety and commit the dietary sin of monotony," she says, "eating the same foods meal after meal, only disguised by different names." They also consume food not according to what is best for them but according to what tastes best to them.

According to Dr. Berkson, the American menu is actually made of various combinations of the same foods, usually wheat, beef, eggs, potatoes, and milk products. For example, she points out, a breakfast of eggs, sausage, white toast, and hash browns is the same as a lunch of a hamburger, white bun, and fries, which is the same as a dinner of steak and potatoes or white pasta. All of these meals, besides the fact that they are high-fat, high-calorie, low-fiber, and filled with toxins, are strikingly devoid of fruits and vegetables. They are also low in many of the essential nutrients. Such repetition can build deficiencies into the body.

Daily consumption of the same foods also tends to produce allergies and hypersensitivities to those foods, according to experts in envi-

Avoid These Foods	Use These Foods Instead
Refined sugars: white sugar (sucrose), fructose, corn syrup, sorbitol, mannitol. Synthetic sugars: NutraSweet™ and saccharin.	Natural sweeteners: fruit juice, raw honey, organic maple syrup, molasses, barley malt, sucanat (organic sugar cane). Avoid if diabetic or sugar intolerant.
Refined flours: white, unbleached, bleached, enriched flour and products containing these flours.	Organic whole grains: best are heirloom (genetically unaltered) grains such as kamut, quinoa, amaranth, and spelt. Grain-intolerant people may do well on heirlooms.
Synthetic fats: margarine, hydrogenated or partially hydrogenated oils, vegetable shortening, Mocha Mix™, Olestra™.	Unsaturated oils (olive, flaxseed, safflower); butter, preferably raw and organic.
High levels of saturated fats (from meats, butter, palm and coconut oils).	Use unsaturated oils such as cold-pressed grapeseed, olive, corn, canola, and safflower oils. Oils must be fresh and cold-pressed; rancid oils can be harmful.
Homogenized, pasteurized, nonfat, or *acidophilus* milk, and processed cheese.	Raw, whole milk (contains vitamin A), cultured milk products (kefir, yogurt, buttermilk), and goat's milk; unprocessed cheese. Use in moderation if you are lactose intolerant.
Nuts and seeds: commercial, oiled, sugared, and salted. Beware of aflatoxin mold on peanuts.	Preferably organic nuts and seeds. Must be soaked (6 hrs), blanched, or roasted to destroy enzyme inhibitors.
All commercial red meat and poultry.	Lamb or organic beef, organic free-range poultry. Fish is fine if it is not from polluted waters.

Avoid These Foods		Use These Foods Instead
Commercial eggs or egg substitutes.		Organic eggs (no chemicals, drugs, or hormones) from free-range chickens or ducks.
Canned, pre-cooked, microwaved, or processed fast foods, and junk foods.		Buy fresh, organic foods first, fresh nonorganic second, frozen third, and canned if that is the only food available.
Drinks: commercial, sugared fruit juices, juice drinks, and soft drinks (both diet and regular).		Raw juices: juice your own or buy 100% juice, preferably raw and organic. Natural spritzers containing only fruit and carbonated water.
Canned coffee and commercial decaffeinated coffee.		Grind your own beans, preferably organic. Use only Swiss water-processed decaffeinated beans. Don't exceed three cups daily. Try organic black or herbal teas.

ronmental medicine. Instead of nourishing the body, these foods may start to act against it. Eating a varied diet minimizes these problems. The optimal diet should consist of more vegetables, fruits, and whole grains than any other foods.

Benefits of a Whole Foods Diet

According to Dr. Levin, a whole foods diet promotes health by decreasing fat and sugar intake and increasing fiber and nutrient intake. Ideally, it means more satisfaction and less overeating.

More Fiber: Most animal products, like meat, cheese, milk, eggs, and butter, contain no fiber, compared to brown rice, broccoli, oatmeal, or almonds, which have 6-15 grams per serving. Low fiber intake has been associated with weight gain, due to fiber's effect on insulin levels and its ability to promote satiety.[13] Fiber is also the transport system of the digestive tract, moving food wastes out of the body before they have a chance to form potentially cancer-causing and mutagenic chemicals. These toxic chemicals can cause colon cancer or pass through the gastrointestinal membrane into the bloodstream and damage other cells.

Less Fat: On a percentage-of-calories basis, most vegetables contain less than 10% fat, and most grains contain from 16%-20% fat. By comparison, whole milk and cheese contain 74% fat. A rib roast is 75% fat and eggs are 64% fat. Low-fat milk or a skinned, baked chicken breast still has 38% fat. Not only do animal foods have more fat, but most of these fats are saturated. In addition, a lower fat, whole foods diet means fewer calories, since an ounce of fat contains twice as many calories as an ounce of complex carbohydrates. Studies have shown that a diet containing fewer calories can increase health and extend life.[14]

Decreased Sugar Consumption: Eating a diet high in natural complex carbohydrates tends to be more filling and decreases the desire to consume processed sugars. Lower sugar consumption also decreases overall food intake. As with fat, sugar is a hidden and unwelcome ingredient in many processed foods. "When you eat sugar, your body uses up whatever vitamins and minerals it has to burn these foods off," says Linda Lizotte, R.D., C.D.N., a registered dietitian and weight-loss consultant from Trumbull, Connecticut. "Body stores of these nutrients decline and metabolism is more likely to become sluggish. One has difficulty losing weight, because the body lacks the nutrients to burn off fat."[15]

More Nutrients: Plant foods are richer sources of nutrients than their animal counterparts. Compare wheat germ to round steak: ounce for ounce, wheat germ contains twice the vitamin B2, vitamin K, potassium, iron, and copper; three times the vitamin B6, molybdenum, and selenium; 15 times as much magnesium; and over 20 times the vitamin B1, folate, and inositol. The steak only has three nutrients in greater amounts—vitamin B12, chromium, and zinc.

Increased Variation: A greater variety of vegetables also exposes the consumer to, literally, more colorful foods—red beets, chard, yellow squash, red peppers, cabbage. "This is more important than you may have imagined," says Dr. Berkson. "Variations in color are due to various minerals, vitamins, and other nutrients that perform important health-promoting functions in the human body." The color variations in vegetables are due to carotenes, naturally occurring pigments that are converted into vitamin A in the body. Carotenes act as antioxidants and may be helpful for cancer prevention.

Fore more on **dietary sugars and their effect on insulin**, see Chapter 8: Strengthen Your Sugar Controls, pp. 184-201.

More Food Satisfaction and Less Over-Eating: Foods such as vegetables, whole grains, and beans that are dense in nutrients and fiber, require more eating (chewing) time, and result in consumption of fewer calories. Eating whole foods makes a person satisfied more quickly, which means he or she eats less.[16]

Making the Transition to Whole Foods

Eating better means living better. The types of dietary changes that you make should not be threatening, limiting, or difficult to live with. Most Americans were raised eating meat and the transition to a more vegetable-oriented, whole foods diet may seem daunting. However, this change may be easier and more pleasurable than imagined and, considering the enormous health benefits, is worth it. Here are some tips:

- Eat more high-fiber plant foods like grains, legumes, nuts, and seeds.
- When dining out, try more exotic vegetarian dishes. Most ethnic restaurants—Indian, Chinese, Thai, Japanese, Mexican, Latin American, African, Middle Eastern—offer wonderful dishes with vegetables and grains. You can also prepare many of these at home. Experiment with spices and seasonings and invest in vegetarian or ethnic cookbooks for the secrets to the exotic flavors found in vegetarian cooking.
- Choose range-fed, hormone-free, additive-free meats.
- Cook protein foods by one of the following methods: bake, broil, poach, stir-fry, saute, or steam. Avoid frying as much as possible, as it adds calories and may add to the toxic load in the body. Do not overcook meats, which diminishes their nutritional value.[17]
- Don't be rigid about your diet. Move toward a whole foods diet gradually.
- Achieve rhythm in your diet. Eating regularly provides your body with a consistent intake of nutrients and avoids the stress associated with skipping meals and overeating.

At the Market

Choosing the ingredients for an ideal diet in today's marketplace requires a healthy dose of skepticism, diligence, and a certain amount of fortitude to resist slipping into old convenience patterns. But the improvements you make in your food choices will pay off in better health. Here are some shopping guidelines:

- Read labels—The package label is the last place one is apt to find the truth about a product. Bold statements such as "100% Natural" or "98% Fat-Free" might be legal, but could be deceiving. Go directly to the ingredient list and nutritional analysis. New labeling regulations now mean better and more accurate information for consumers.
- Think complex carbohydrates—The "main dish" approach centering on protein and a high-fat sauce is out. Replace those large portions of meat loaf and baby back pork ribs with whole grains,

Low-Fat Fallacies

Low-fat and nonfat food products are marketed to individuals who are health and weight conscious. Ironically, manufacturers often add a variety of unhealthy and artificial ingredients to these foods. For example, various viscous substances are added to low-fat salad dressings to mimic the thickness and smooth texture of oil. "These fat-mimickers do not occur naturally and they cannot be metabolized by our bodies," explains Paul McTaggert, of Los Angeles, California, an expert in the biochemistry of food. "They stay in our systems, thick, gooey, and paste-like. [Salad dressing] is a good example of how a not-so-great product was made into a worse one, and marketed as a better choice for health and weight."

Low-fat foods often lack flavor. To make them more palatable, some manufacturers load them up with extra sugar, which boosts the product's calorie content while still maintaining a reduced fat content. Others use artificial sweeteners such as aspartame (Nutrasweet™) or saccharin. These sugar substitutes, while lower in calories, are no guarantee to weight loss and may actually cause weight gain. Researchers at Harvard's School of Public Health, found that "sugar substitutes have not proved helpful in curbing weight." Studies have shown that saccharin use actually leads to weight gain rather than weight loss.[18]

beans, and fresh vegetables, balanced with moderate amounts of lean animal proteins.

■ Buy organic foods—Organic farming doesn't use artificial fertilizers, pesticides, herbicides, growth regulators, and livestock feed additives. Crop rotations, animal and "green" manures, organic wastes, mineral-bearing rock, and biological pest controls are used by organic farmers to raise whole, natural foods.

■ Buy seasonal foods—By definition, foods grown out of season must be treated or manipulated to grow using artificial means. Often, the foods are imported from countries where pesticides banned in the U.S. continue to be used. Seasonal foods are healthier, more abundant, and less expensive.

■ Eat colorfully—Instead of being concerned with getting all the right vitamins and minerals in perfect ratios, focus on eating a colorful diet. By making an effort to get at least three different colored vegetables or fruits at both lunch and dinner, you will ensure the best exposure to appropriate nutrients.

Dietary Fats— The Real Story

Low-fat dieting has become a national obsession and has given rise to whole new lines of low-fat or nonfat products. But sometimes adding fats to your diet will help you lose weight—if they're the right fats. Certain fats, particularly the essential fatty acids, are vital for the healthy functioning of our bodies (including the maintenance of proper body weight), while hydrogenated fats like margarine may actually contribute to your difficulties with losing weight.

The relationship of dietary fat to body fat is grossly misunderstood, according to Lizotte. "Fat makes fat—it sounds right, it makes a good headline, and it's easy to understand, but it's simplistic and incomplete," she says. Similarly, nutritionist Gittleman explains that Americans actually lack certain fats. "Many overweight Americans are fat-deficient," she says. "While there's no doubt that eliminating unhealthy fats from the diet is important, eating the right kinds can help with weight management."

Why We Need Fats

What the low-fat fanatics fail to tell us is that some fats are needed to support the functioning of the brain, nervous system, and immune system. They comprise the building blocks of hormones, assist in the absorption and transport of certain vitamins in the body, and are vital to maintaining a healthy metabolism (SEE QUICK DEFINITION), which controls how quickly the body burns calories. "Fats are like vitamins and minerals," explains nutritional biochemist and author Jeffrey Bland, Ph.D., of Gig Harbor, Washington. "When we don't get what we need, either from the food we eat or from supplements, metabolic activity diminishes."

Metabolism is an important determinant of body weight. In order to avoid accumulating pounds, the amount of calories we eat must be balanced by the amount we burn via metabolism. When we burn fewer calories than we eat, the excess calories get stored as body fat; conversely, if we burn more calories than we eat, we lose weight. Low-fat diets attempt to tip the body's calorie balance in favor of weight loss by cutting out calorie-rich fats. However, because metabolism slows when fat intake is reduced, dieters can still end up burning fewer calories than you ingest, particularly since many low-fat foods are still notoriously high in calories from added sugars (see "Low-Fat Fallacies," p. 60), which can affect your insulin levels.

Another problem with fat-free diet programs is that they tend to be high in carbohydrates (starches and sugars), which often serve as the primary energy

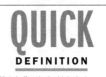

QUICK DEFINITION

Metabolism is the biological process by which energy (measured in calories) is extracted from the foods consumed, producing carbon dioxide and water as by-products for elimination. Biochemically, metabolism involves hundreds of different chemical reactions, necessitating the involvement of hundreds of different enzymes. There are two kinds of metabolism constantly underway in the cells: catabolic and anabolic. The catabolic function controls digestion, disassembling food into forms the body can use for energy, while the anabolic function produces substances for cell growth and repair.

For more about **sugars and insulin**, see Chapter 8: Strengthen Your Sugar Controls, pp. 184-201. For more about **metabolism and body weight**, see Chapter 5: Optimize Your Calorie Burning, pp. 122-135.

source in such diets. However, too many carbohydrates will actually cause you to accumulate fat rather than lose it. The reason has to do with the fact that all carbohydrates are converted to sugar in the body. If there is more sugar in the blood than the body can use, the excess gets converted directly into body fat. High-carbohydrate meals tend to send blood sugar levels skyrocketing, causing the body to store the sugar as fat. Dietary fats, on the other hand, tend to moderate blood sugar levels, which helps to control weight gain.

Fats also help manage weight by controlling appetite. "Fats delay hunger because they take longer to digest, and thus slow the emptying time for the stomach," says Gittleman. "They leave you satisfied longer." Gittleman, once a staunch anti-fat advocate, has since recognized the importance of fat in the diet. While serving as the director of nutrition at the Pritikin Longevity Centers (SEE QUICK DEFINITION), she observed the health and weight problems brought on by a non-fat diet. "There were complaints about weight gain and feeling hungry all the time no matter how much food was eaten," she explains.[19]

Essential Fatty Acids: The Good Fat

Fatty acids are the chemical molecules that make up all fats. The body needs a regular supply of certain fatty acids, appropriately called essential fatty acids (EFAs—see "A Quick Guide to Fats," pp. 64-65), in order to stay healthy. The body cannot synthesize these from other nutrients, but must obtain them directly from food. Individuals deficient in essential fatty acids may experience a number of health problems, including weight gain. Unfortunately, many individuals today do not obtain the EFAs that they need. Dr. Bland says that an increasing number of Americans suffer from essential fatty acid deficiency. He attributes the trend to the popularity of low-fat diets. "There's no question," he says, "that the current overemphasis on low-fat eating, coupled with a lack of understanding about fats and the role they play in health, has led to a dramatic rise in essential fatty acid deficiency."

Even though Americans now consume about 40% more fats per day than our forebears did around 1900, the "mass commercial refinement of fats, oil products, and the foods containing them has effectively eliminated the essential fatty acids from our food chain," observes naturopathic physician and educator Michael T. Murray, N.D. Because of this, he estimates that Americans may be consuming only 10% of the EFAs required for good health. Nutritionist Gittleman believes that the trend in essential fatty acid deficiency is causing increases in obesity. "Believe it or not," she says, "almost 80 million Americans are too fat and yet fat-deficient." Gittleman claims that a diet that includes EFAs is a key step for achieving a healthy and permanent weight loss.[20]

Essential fatty acid deficiencies contribute to weight gain by increasing appetite and reducing energy levels, thereby making exercise more difficult. EFAs also boost the metabolic rate, increase energy production, and help move cholesterol out of arteries and tissues. "I can't say that if you take essential fatty acid supplements, you will lose weight for sure," says Tammy Geurkink-Born, N.D., a naturopath from Grand Rapids, Michigan, "but what I can say with certainty is that when the body is supplied with essential fatty acids, in the proper amount and proportion, it functions better. You will be less fatigued, less hungry, and have fewer sweet cravings. This will allow you to exercise and eat normally."

> "When the body is supplied with essential fatty acids, in the proper amount and proportion, it functions better," says Tammy Geurkink-Born, N.D. "You will be less fatigued, less hungry, and have fewer sweet cravings. This will allow you to exercise and eat normally."

EFAs—Use With Caution

Lita Lee, Ph.D., a nutrition specialist from Lowell, Oregon, cautions people against an excess intake of unsaturated oils. "Most people are aware of the detrimental health effects of hydrogenated oils, such as margarine, but few know about the toxic effects of a diet high in unsaturated oils (excluding extra virgin olive oil)," says Dr. Lee. She summarizes some of the potentially detrimental effects of excess unsaturated fats:

■ Unsaturated oils can inhibit enzymes essential to digestive and metabolic processes required for health and immune protection.[21]

■ Unsaturated oils affect important enzyme processes, including the digestion of protein and the healthy function of the thyroid gland.[22]

■ Circulating unsaturated oils can lead to insulin resistance and a diet high in safflower oil may cause diabetes.[23]

A Quick Guide to Fats

Fat or oil (*lipid* is the biochemical term) is one of the six basic food groups. Fats and oils are made of building blocks called fatty acids. Structurally, a fatty acid is a chain of carbon atoms with a certain quantity of hydrogen atoms attached; the more hydrogen atoms attached, the more "saturated" the fat. Fats come in three natural forms (saturated, monounsaturated, and polyunsaturated) and one synthetic form (called hydrogenated or trans fats).

Saturated Fats—Saturated fats are solid at room temperature and are primarily found in animal foods and tropical oils, such as coconut and palm oils. A fatty acid that has its full quota of hydrogen atoms is a saturated fatty acid. The body produces saturated fats from sugar, which is one reason why low-fat foods do not decrease body fat—their high sugar content is converted into stored fat in the body. Although high fat intake from animal sources has been associated with heart disease, some amount of saturated fat in the diet is necessary to help the body's cells remain healthy and resistant to disease.

Unsaturated Fats—Unsaturated fatty acids (both monounsaturated and polyunsaturated) are liquid at room temperature. Most vegetable oils are unsaturated. Unsaturated means some of the carbon molecules are not filled with hydrogen.

■ Monounsaturated Fats: When a fatty acid lacks only two hydrogen atoms, it is a monounsaturated fatty acid. Monounsaturated fats are considered healthier than polyunsaturated fats because of their ability to lower blood levels of "bad" cholesterol and maintain or raise levels of "good" cholesterol. Canola oil and olive oil are naturally high in monounsaturated fats. Olive oil is the best oil for cooking, because it does not break down easily into singlet oxygen molecules (free radicals) like most oils do when they are heated. Olive oil is probably the most widely used oil, both for cooking and raw on salads, on a worldwide basis.

■ Polyunsaturated Fats: Oils high in polyunsaturated fats include flaxseed and canola oils, as well as pumpkin seeds, purslane, hemp oil, walnuts, and soybeans, which contain omega-3 and omega-6 essential fatty acids. A fatty acid lacking four or more hydrogen atoms is a polyunsaturated fatty acid. They can be found in both healthy and unhealthy fats and oils.

Hydrogenated and Trans Fats—These terms refer to a synthetic process in which natural oils are broken down into a semi-solid fat by adding a hydrogen atom to an unsaturated fat molecule. This process is widely used to prolong the shelf life of commercial baked goods, packaged foods, most salad oils and dressings, margarine, and cooking oils. The molecules that make up these fats, called trans-fatty acids, are known to interfere with the healthy functioning of our bodies due to their unusual molecular shape.

Essential Fatty Acids (EFAs)—Unsaturated fats required in the diet are called essential fatty acids. Omega-3 and omega-6 oils are the two principle types of EFAs and a balance of these oils in the diet is necessary for good health. The primary omega-3 oil is alpha-linolenic acid (ALA), found in flaxseed and canola oils, as well as pumpkin seeds, walnuts, and soybeans. Fish oils, such as salmon, cod, and mackerel, contain the other important omega-3 oils, DHA (docosahexaenoic acid) and EPA (eicosapentaenoic acid). Linoleic acid is the main omega-6 oil and is found in most vegetable oils, including safflower, corn, peanut, and sesame. The most therapeutic form of omega-6 oil is gamma-linolenic acid (GLA), found in evening primrose, black currant, and borage oils. Once in the body, omega-3 and omega-6 are converted to prostaglandins, hormone-like complex fatty acids that affect smooth muscle function, inflammatory processes, and constriction and dilation of blood vessels.

Dr. Lee recommends the use of extra virgin olive oil, organic butter, and coconut oil. Coconut oil, in particular, appears to have weight-loss benefits.

EDITOR'S NOTE
The position on unsaturated fats presented here is a controversial one. Many physicians advocate the dietary use and supplementation of essential fatty acids in the form of fish, primrose, borage, and flaxseed oils, among others, in the unsaturated category. There is research to support both positions.

Diagnosing an Essential Fatty Acid Deficiency

The first step in seeing if your weight problem is linked to your intake of fats is to identify any essential fatty acid deficiencies. Then proper dietary changes and nutritional supplementation can be recommended. In addition to getting a symptom history and assessing dietary habits, alternative medicine practitioners use a number of laboratory tests for nutrient status, which can provide detailed and practical information on EFA status.

For more about **coconut oil**, see this chapter, p. 74-75.

■ Pantox Antioxidant Profile™—A lipid panel measures the level of blood fats, including cholesterol. The Pantox test includes a comprehensive lipid panel as well as an analysis of serum levels of antioxidant micronutrients. Using a small blood sample, this test measures the status of more than 20 nutritional factors, specifically, lipoproteins (cholesterol and triglycerides), antioxidants, and iron balance. The test must be ordered by a health-care professional.

■ Body Bio Blood Chemistry/Red Cell Membrane Fatty Acid Test—Two other blood tests for determining EFA deficiencies are the Body Bio Blood Chemistry, which provides information on 44 different blood biochemical levels, and the Red Cell Membrane Fatty Acid Test, which reveals the status of 67 fatty acids in the blood by examining their presence in the membrane of a single red blood cell. Together, these tests provide a picture of the whole biochemistry specific to the patient. The red cell fatty acid analysis charts 12-16 weeks of an individual's lipid metabolism, useful for accurately determining the fats, vitamins, and minerals the patient requires.

■ Individualized Optimal Nutrition (ION)—Using a blood and urine sample, the ION Panel measures 150 biochemical components. It is useful for physicians needing detailed biochemical assessments of patients with immune disorders, heart disease, multiple chemical sensitivities, or obesity. The ION test checks for nutritional status of fatty acids, lipid peroxides, vitamins, minerals, amino acids, general blood chemistries (cholesterol, thyroid hormone, glucose), and antioxidants.

■ FIA™ (Functional Intracellular Analysis)—This is a group of tests (Comprehensive Profile 3000, B-Complex Profile 1100, Primary Profile 1500, Cardiovascular Profile 1600, Antioxidants Profile 1400) that measure the function of key vitamins, minerals, fatty acids, antioxidants, amino acids, and metabolites (choline, inositol) at the cellular level. They also assess carbohydrate metabolism in terms of insulin function and fructose intolerance.

Avoiding the Bad Fats

Most of the negative reports about fat have to do with saturated fat and cholesterol. Diets high in these two substances are considered to be a leading cause of obesity and heart disease. However, the medical establishment's focus on saturated fats and cholesterol is not altogether warranted—it represents only a portion of the larger causal mechanism pushing up the rates of obesity and heart disease. "Few of us realize that heart attacks hardly occurred in this country at the beginning of this century. The total fat consumption [at that time] was nearly the same as in 1961, when death from heart attack was at an all-time high," states Ralph Golan, M.D.[24] More evidence confounding claims that fat causes heart disease comes from other cultures whose diets are traditionally high in saturated fats and cholesterol. For example, the Atiu-Mitario peoples of Polynesia and the Eskimos of Greenland both have diets high in saturated fats, yet are virtually free of heart disease, says Dr. Golan.

So why the relatively recent increase in heart attacks and heart disease in the United States? The rise in cigarette smoking is one sure reason. However, many experts believe certain food processes, such as hydrogenation (used to increase the shelf life of fats), are also to blame. Such processes are known to damage fats by destroying the EFAs they contain, while creating new types of harmful substances.

"You can't get the kinds of fats your body needs from denatured, heated, and hydrogenated oils," says Lizotte. "The fats we should be eating are those that have not been tampered with or have been minimally processed without heat, as these are the only ones that still contain essential fatty acids." Nutritionist Gittleman insists that consumers need to know that processing, refining, and even certain cooking methods make fats, including unsaturated ones, unhealthy to eat. "Avoiding damaged fats will assist you in optimizing weight loss and immune function, as well as protect you from degenerative diseases," says Gittleman.[25]

Hydrogenated Fat

"In the interest of staying slim, people reject butter and cream in favor of margarine and other hydrogenated (semi-solid) fats. Saturated hydrogenated fats (also called trans-fatty acids) create havoc in a person's biochemistry, negatively affecting every system of the body," says Patricia Kane, Ph.D., a nutritional biochemist based in Millville, New Jersey. At the same time, using only or mostly hydrogenated fats leads to nutrient depletion because the body is not given the kind of fat it needs

The French Paradox

The French are known to enjoy a diet filled with rich patés, cheeses, cream, and butter. All of these foods are high in saturated fat—the kinds of foods thought to be sure killers by the U.S. medical establishment as well as significant contributors to weight gain. But only 8% of the French population is considered obese, compared to a 19% rate in Germany and 33% in the United States.[26] The French also have less than half the rate of heart disease as the United States. Some researchers attribute low heart disease rates among the French to their affinity for red wine, which contains substances (phenols) that protect the heart and arteries from damage, while others claim that the low level of hydrogenated fat (like margarine) in the French diet is responsible.[27] Still others have adopted a sugar theory, claiming it is the low sugar consumption of the French that is responsible (they eat 70% less sugar per year than Americans).

Nutritionist Ann Louise Gittleman, M.S., is an advocate of the sugar theory. "Too much sugar can be stored as saturated fat in the tissues," says Gittleman. But whatever the cause, she notes that the French experience is proof that fat is not the universal evil it has been made out to be by doctors and the media. "If we take a lesson from the French," she says, "fat may not be the bad guy after all."[28]

Not All Cholesterol is Harmful

Cholesterol is a steroid found in meat, egg yolks, and dairy products. In addition to obtaining cholesterol from these dietary sources, we manufacture cholesterol in the liver (about 3,000 mg per day). Despite all the bad press it has received, cholesterol is needed by the body to maintain and repair cells. When cholesterol levels get too low, depression, lung disease, and even cancer can result. There are two types of cholesterol. Low-density lipoproteins (LDLs) circulate in the blood and act as the primary carriers of cholesterol to the cells of the body. An elevated level of LDLs, often called "bad" cholesterol, contributes to atherosclerosis, a buildup of plaque deposits on the inner walls of the arteries. A diet high in saturated fats can increase levels of LDLs in the blood. High-density lipoproteins (HDLs) readily absorb cholesterol and related compounds in the blood and transport them to the liver for elimination. HDLs, or "good" cholesterol, may also be able to take cholesterol from plaque deposits on the artery walls, thus helping to reverse the process of atherosclerosis. A higher amount of HDL compared to LDL cholesterol in the blood is associated with a reduced risk of cardiovascular disease.

(essential fatty acids) for proper body function. When your diet no longer supplies the necessary raw materials—some of them derived from fats—for running the body efficiently, many things go wrong and the body starts to shut down. In the contrast between trans-fatty acids and essential fatty acids, you have the cause of many of these problems.

"The production of trans-fatty acids for human consumption is the most devastating nutritional mistake ever made," says Dr. Kane. "In the effort to make foods last longer in the supermarket, all traces of essential fatty acids are obliterated from processed foods, and trans-fats or partially hydrogenated oils take their place." A trans-fatty acid sits like a heavy blob inside you, shutting down fatty acid metabolism and replacing the good, necessary fats (omega-3s and omega-6s) with something harmful to health. "You can't do anything with a trans-fatty acid except burn it for calories, and its activity poisons your system and generates an abnormal, undesirable biochemistry," says Dr. Kane. Similarly, Dr. Lee says trans-fatty acids inhibit the action of liver enzymes that convert cholesterol into harmless salts; this contributes to high blood levels of cholesterol and leads to weight gain.

Homogenization

Another process that damages fat is homogenization, a technique used to make milk uniform in texture. Homogenization breaks up fat globules found in the cream fraction of milk into very small particles, which

Common Foods That Contain "Bad" Fats

Trans-fatty acids are widely available in the American diet and impair the functioning of many of the body's vital systems. John R. Lee, M.D., of Sebastopol, California, laments that few individuals are aware of the dangers of these substances. "Unknowingly," he says, "we are poisoning ourselves." Margarine is one common type of hydrogenated fat, but it is not the only source. "If steering clear of margarine were all you had to do, your job would be easy," says Dr. Golan, "but food companies use partially hydrogenated oil in more foods than you can imagine."[29] Indeed, a great many processed food products contain hydrogenated oils. The average American consumes 8-28 grams of these altered fats a day, or about 20% of their total daily fat intake.[30] Read the labels of packaged food before you buy to determine if they contain hydrogenated fats. In the list of ingredients, you will see them described as either "hydrogenated" or "partially hydrogenated" oils. The "Nutrition Facts" label will also provide you with amounts of saturated and unsaturated fats. Some of the more common foods that contain hydrogenated fats are:

- Diet foods
- Mayonnaise
- Crackers and chips
- Cookies, cakes and cake mixes, pastries, and doughnuts
- Candy
- Pudding
- Packaged breads
- Canned, creamed soups
- Breakfast cereals and frozen waffles
- Microwave popcorn
- Frozen entrees, French fries, fish sticks, and chicken nuggets

remain suspended in the milk rather than floating on top of it. William Campbell Douglass, M.D., author of *The Milk Book: How Science is Destroying Nature's Nearly Perfect Food*, explains that, because of homogenization, natural whole milk is virtually unknown in the United States today. "Most Americans under the age of forty have never seen milk in its natural state with a cream layer," he says.

Patricia Kane, Ph.D.,:
Body Bio Corporation,
Five Osprey Drive,
Suite 9, Millville,
NJ 08332;
tel: 888-320-8338 or
609-825-9554;
fax: 609-825-2143.

While we have become accustomed to drinking milk without a cream layer, what we don't know is that we increase our fat buildup and risk of heart disease with each glass. The problem is that the tiny globules of fat, which result from homogenization, allow a deadly enzyme called xanthine oxidase to get into the body. In the bloodstream, xanthine oxidase damages artery walls, causing lesions to occur on the lining. These lesions attract cholesterol deposits, which eventually clog the artery. Dr. Haas explains that "cholesterol goes wherever there's an irritation or inflammation in the body. It acts as a tissue healer and pro-

If you have high levels of cholesterol or other fats in your blood, it does not simply mean you're eating too much fat. It actually can be an indication that your body is not processing foods properly, a condition which may stem from liver toxicity or from too much insulin in your blood. For more about **liver toxicity and weight problems**, see Chapter 15: Cleanse the Liver, pp. 330-346. For more about how **insulin affects fat levels**, see Chapter 8: Strengthen Your Sugar Controls, pp. 184-201.

tector." When there is no damage, cholesterol is less likely to adhere to artery walls.

All milk fat, excluding that from humans, contains xanthine oxidase. However, as Dr. Douglass explains, the normal-sized fat globules from cream are too big to easily pass through the lining of the intestines and enter the bloodstream. Since xanthine oxidase is chemically bound to these fat molecules, the enzymes go wherever the fat globules go. When the fat is a normal size, xanthine oxidase is expelled out of the body along with the fat.[31] Homogenization, however, makes the globules small enough to squeeze through the intestinal lining and into the blood.

Oxidation

In addition to hydrogenation and homogenization, fats can also be damaged by oxygen. Fats combine with oxygen in a process called oxidation. During oxidation, fats become rancid and form new substances called oxysterols and peroxides, which are two types of free radicals (unstable, toxic molecules that cause considerable damage to the body's cells). Oxidized oils are loaded with free radicals, which may cause a variety of chronic, degenerative diseases.[32]

Oxidation occurs very rapidly when an oil is heated during cooking. The most common source of oxidized fats is food fried in deep-fat fryers, such as those used at many fast food restaurants. The oils used in these fryers are subjected to very high heat for prolonged periods and, consequently, they are almost always rancid and contaminate the foods cooked in them with oxidized oil. Simply exposing them to the air will cause fats and oils to oxidize. This means that as soon as an oil is pressed from a nut or seed it becomes vulnerable to oxygen damage. In their natural state, many unsaturated fats contain antioxidants that protect them from oxidation, but these are often removed or destroyed when oils are refined. They then become more vulnerable to oxidation from prolonged exposure to air.

Choosing the Right Fats

Average Americans get approximately 40% of the calories they eat from fat. A major source of this fat is animal fat, specifically beef, dairy products, fish, and chicken. The fat contained in these foods is not only very difficult for our bodies to digest, but it also contains arachidonic acid, which can cause higher levels of "bad" (pro-inflammatory) prostaglandins. The current recommendation from groups such as the American Heart Association and the American Cancer Society is to reduce daily fat consumption to 30% of total caloric intake, with an emphasis on substituting unsaturated fats like olive oil for saturated ones such as butter. While this is a step in the right direction, many health-care experts believe that for long-term health and weight control, fats should constitute between 15%-20% of your daily calories. They should also be selected carefully, making sure to exclude all harmful fats.

In general, you should choose vegetable and seed oils that are cold-pressed. This means that the oils were extracted from their sources with a minimum of heat, a process that protects the oils from damage. You should always check the expiration date of any oil you buy; many high-quality oils have a short shelf life (3-4 months). In addition, look for dairy products that have not been homogenized. Most butters available on your supermarket shelf are made from homogenized milk, but in response to increased consumer demand, many stores are also beginning to carry raw butter, made from non-homogenized milk.

As you start to replace the unhealthy fats in your diet with healthy ones, you may experience an immediate drop in weight. Weight-loss consultant Lizotte explains how many of her patients experienced a weight-loss breakthrough upon correcting their fat intake. "They'd lose about half the weight they needed to and then hit a brick wall," she says. "They'd be very upset, feeling as though it was their fault somehow. I would get them eating some healthy fats and give them

Understanding Fat Content Information

Most food package labels contain information regarding fat content, but this information can often be misleading. For example, "daily value" is one statistic that often appears on most food packages: it is an estimate of the amount of fat the food is expected to contribute to an individual's daily diet, based on the assumption that an individual consumes between 2,500 to 3,000 calories per day with 30% of those calories coming from fat. If the daily value, for example, is listed at 20%, it does not mean the product contains 20% fat; instead, it means that the food provides 20% of the total amount of fat calories you are expected to consume in one day. If you want to know how much fat is in a product, ignore the daily value column. Instead, divide the amount of calories from fat by the total number of calories. If there are 70 calories from fat and a total of 100 calories in a product, then 70% of what's inside the package is fat.

an essential fatty acid supplement. They immediately began losing again, and felt better too."

Here are some general dietary recommendations from Dr. Kane for supplying the body with nourishing, healthy fats:

■ Use liberal amounts of unprocessed sesame oil blended with coconut oil; also recommended are avocado, almond, or grapeseed oils (cold-pressed).

■ Reduce carbohydrate intake and avoid all refined sugars, processed foods, margarine, hydrogenated oils, and gluten-containing foods such as wheat, oats, and barley.

■ For better mineral density, increase the consumption of ground raw nuts and seeds (especially sesame), seaweeds, fish, tempeh (fermented soybeans), poultry, avocado, and legumes.

■ Incorporate spices and herbs into the diet such as fresh ground black or red cayenne pepper, thyme oil, and ginger; these foods contain substances that will help stabilize fats in the cell membranes.

■ Avoid all fats and oils containing very long-chain fatty acids, such as mustard, peanut butter, and peanut oil.

Adding Essential Fatty Acids to Your Diet

Essential fatty acids can be obtained from foods and edible oils, as well as supplements. Here is a guide to the two major groups:

Omega-3 Fatty Acids—The primary omega-3 fatty acid is alpha-linolenic acid, which comes from plant oils such as safflower, peanut, sunflower seed, walnut, sesame, and olive. DHA (docosahexaenoic acid) and EPA (eicosapentaenoic acid) are other omega-3 fatty acids that come from fish oils, such as salmon, cod, and mackerel. Beans, especially great northern, kidney, navy, and soy, also supply omega-3 fatty acids.

Flaxseed oil is a particularly good source of omega-3 fatty acid (58% alpha-linolenic acid). It is also a flavorful oil and can be used with lemon juice on salads or drizzled on vegetables and grains after cooking. The recommended dosage of flaxseed oil is 1-2 tablespoons daily (capsules are also available). Absorption of the oil is enhanced if it's taken with a tablespoon of cottage cheese. In addition to the oil, the flaxseeds themselves can also be sprinkled on foods, from oatmeal to casseroles (the seeds should be freshly ground to help release the oil). Flaxseed oil is especially prone to oxidation and can easily turn rancid in the presence of light or air, even in its capsule form. Refrigerate it in tightly-sealed, dark glass bottles. Olive oil is another good source of omega-3 fatty acids and contains high quantities of monounsaturated fats. Studies have demonstrated that this type of fat is excellent for lowering blood cholesterol levels. You can use olive oil liberally on salads. As with flaxseed oil, olive oil should always be kept in a tightly sealed container.

High temperature cooking, such as frying, destroys the EFA content of certain oils. Flaxseed and walnut oils should only be used for baking or added to soups or salads. When frying foods, use more heat-stable oils, such as canola, grapeseed, avocado, peanut, and olive.

Omega-6 Fatty Acids—There are two forms of omega-6 fatty acids: linoleic acid and gamma-linolenic acid (GLA). Linoleic acid is found in flaxseed, pumpkin seeds, walnuts, and wheat germ. GLA is difficult to obtain from food sources and is best taken as a supplement. GLA is useful for increasing the body's resting metabolism; that is, the rate at which it burns calories while not exercising. Resting metabolism is what maintains the body's internal temperature, with heat generated primarily in areas of dense brown fat. Brown fat is one of the types of stored body fat and is different from common body fat (known as yellow fat). We do not gain brown fat in the same way as yellow fat; rather, we are born with a given amount of brown fat and slowly lose it as we age. GLA raises the rate of heat-generating activity within brown fat, a process known as thermogenesis. A rise in the body's thermogenesis level causes more calories to be burned off as heat energy and fewer of them to be stored as fat.[33]

Normally, the body can convert linoleic acid into GLA. However, stress, alcohol, aging, hypothyroidism, illness, and a diet high in saturated fats or damaged oils can block this conversion, resulting in a GLA deficiency. Evening primrose oil is a good source of GLA, containing both omega-3 and omega-6 oils (suggested dosage is 500 mg daily).

Too much linoleic acid can be harmful, leading to an overproduction of arachidonic acid and "bad" prostaglandins. Arachidonic acid is a fatty acid found primarily in animal foods and to a lesser extent in fish and vegetables. When the diet is abundant with arachidonic acids, these are stored in cell membranes. While arachidonic acid is important particularly for the brain, if other EFAs are deficient, these stored acids are transformed into prostaglandins that instigate inflammation. Consequently, some physicians recommend avoiding daily use of safflower, sunflower, and corn oils, which are rich in linoleic acid. Instead, use unrefined sesame, rice bran, and flaxseed oils, which contain lesser quantities of linoleic acid.

Medium-Chain Triglycerides (MCTs)

Similar to GLA, medium-chain triglycerides, or MCTs, have also been shown to promote weight loss. MCTs are a form of natural fat found in certain seeds. Like GLA, they tend to accelerate metabolism while lowering blood levels of cholesterol. They also improve absorption of vitamin E, calcium, and magnesium, protect against hypoglycemia (low blood sugar), and benefit those with digestive disorders. A good source of MCTs is grapeseed oil, available at most health food stores; use it

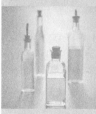

Vegetable Oils: The Good and the Bad Fats

All vegetable oils contain levels of unsaturated and saturated fats. Generally, oils with a higher percentage of unsaturated fats are more healthful.[37]

Oil	Monounsaturated	Polyunsaturated	Saturated
Olive	72%	9%	14%
Flax	72%	19%	9%
Pumpkin seed	57%	34%	9%
Hempseed	80%	12%	8%
Safflower	12%	75%	9%
Canola	62%	32%	6%
Peanut	46%	32%	17%
Corn	24%	59%	13%
Soybean	23%	59%	14%
Sunflower	20%	66%	10%
Sesame seed	40%	40%	18%
Butter	29%	4%	62%
Coconut	6%	2%	87%

CAUTION

Diabetics and those with liver disorders should approach the use of MCTs with caution, as the fat tends to be burned very rapidly in the liver. Individuals with these conditions should avoid MCTs entirely or use them only under a doctor's supervision.

uncooked on salads. Because MCT oils don't spoil easily and have a high burn-point, they are also good for cooking.

Coconut oil has long been considered to be harmful due to its high saturated fat content. Nevertheless, some health experts insist coconut oil, which is 65% MCTs, is a good source of dietary fat. People who consume large amounts of coconut oil as part of their normal diet have not shown increases in health problems. For example, the Polynesian population of Trobriand island (off the coast of Australia) eat a diet of steamed vegetables, fresh fish, and yams, and their primary source of fat is coconuts. Yet, in addition to being relatively free of heart disease, these islanders have an extremely low incidence of obesity. "Coconut oil is less likely than other oils to cause obesity," says nutritionist Gittleman, "because the body easily converts it into energy rather than depositing calories as body fat. You won't get a spare tire around your midsection just from eating foods containing coconut oil."[34]

Coconut oil is more stable than other oils and does not become rancid as easily. Dr. Lee says that coconut oil, unlike many other oils, does not readily oxidize, either inside or outside the body. Because of undeserved media criticism of saturated fats, says Dr. Lee, people are no longer enjoying the health benefits of incorporating coconut oil into their diet, including the following:

For information on **MCT oil**, contact: Sound Nutrition, P.O. Box 555, Dover, ID 83825; tel: 800-844-6645 or 208-263-6183. For **grapeseed, walnut, flax, and pumpkin seed oils**, contact: Spectrum Naturals, 133 Copeland Street, Petaluma, CA 94952; tel: 707-778-8900.

■ Coconut oil lowers cholesterol, a direct result of its thyroid-stimulating properties. In the presence of adequate thyroid hormone, cholesterol is converted by enzymes to the anti-aging steroids pregnenolone, progesterone, and DHEA. These substances are required to help prevent heart disease, senility, obesity, cancer, and other chronic degenerative diseases.[35]

For more about **thermogenesis**, see Chapter 5: Optimize Your Calorie Burning, pp. 122-135.

■ Coconut oil has properties that promote weight loss—another result of its thyroid-stimulating attributes and ability to raise metabolism. Farmers discovered this when they used coconut oil to fatten their animals but found instead that it made them lean, active, and hungrier. That's why they switched to soybeans and corn, which are high in unsaturated oils.[36]

CHAPTER

3

Supplements for Weight Loss

STRANGE AS IT SOUNDS, if you have trouble losing weight, you may not be eating enough food. A good weight-loss plan must be based on a well-rounded diet, as a deficiency in one or more essential nutrients may be interfering with your weight-loss goals. These nutrients are often referred to as micronutrients because they are required in much smaller quantities than proteins, carbohydrates, or fats. A deficiency in any one of them can cause an imbalance that increases appetite and slows metabolism, both of which lead to fat storage. For example, a deficiency in the nutrient choline (a vitamin B complex co-factor) is known to cause an insatiable appetite. "A person who always has a ravenous appetite that doesn't correspond to their activity level may have a deficiency of choline," explains Jeremy Kaslow, M.D., of Garden Grove, California. "It's that deficiency and not their appetite that must be addressed in order to achieve lasting weight loss."

The diet is the best way to obtain the nutrients needed for weight loss, but it is also important to pursue a supplement program tailored to your specific nutritional deficiencies. Although a program of nutritional supplementation should be individualized, this chapter discusses the

In This Chapter

- Overconsumptive Undernutrition
- Detecting a Nutritional Deficiency
- Success Story: Addressing Nutrient Deficiencies Leads to Weight Loss
- Getting the Nutrients You Need for Weight Loss
- Essential and Accessory Micronutrients
- Vitamins
- Minerals
- Amino Acids
- Other Nutrients for Weight Loss

most common nutrient deficiencies associated with weight gain, along with recommendations for preventative dosages. You will also learn how to obtain these nutrients both through food and as supplements.

Overconsumptive Undernutrition

Many leading health professionals approach the problem of weight loss by assessing micronutrient deficiencies. They understand that the growing problem of obesity in the United States is due to a nutrient-poor diet. "The truth is, with the crippled condition of our national diet, we are compelled to overfeed ourselves to get a little nourishment," said the late Hazel Parcells, N.D., D.C., Ph.D., former director of the Parcells Center in Santa Fe, New Mexico. "We may look well-fed, but I believe we are basically undernourished."[1]

Statistics from the U.S. Department of Agriculture (USDA) confirm this contention. According to the USDA, most Americans receive less than 70% of the U.S. Recommended Daily Allowance (RDA) for vitamin A, vitamin C, B-complex vitamins, and the essential minerals calcium, magnesium, and iron.[2] While these figures are alarming, it is important to note that most nutritional experts consider the RDA standards to be below what is needed for optimum health. Consequently, the extent to which we have been starving our bodies of vital nutrients is even worse than what the USDA figures suggest.

To understand why we have become so malnourished, it is necessary to look more closely at how our diet has changed. In comparison to the early part of this century, Americans now eat 50% fewer nutrient-rich foods, such as whole grains, unrefined cereals, fruits, and vegetables; 150% more refined sugars; and 500% more sweetened beverages, such as soda.[3] The startling increase in sugar consumption has been matched by a corresponding rise in harmful fat consumption, such as trans-fatty acids (SEE QUICK DEFINITION). Today, two-thirds of the average American diet consists entirely of high-calorie sugars and fats. The result is that, while we are eating more, we are getting less of what we need to stay healthy and trim. Jeffrey Bland, Ph.D., a biochemist and nutrition expert based in Gig Harbor, Washington, calls it a problem of "overconsumptive undernutrition."

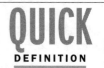

QUICK DEFINITION

A **trans-fatty acid (TFA)** is a chemically and structurally altered hydrogenated vegetable oil (such as margarine), which is combined with hydrogen to lengthen shelf life. Trans-fatty acid (TFA) composition of commercially prepared hydrogenated fats varies from 8% to 70% and comprise about 60% of the fat found in processed foods. It is estimated that Americans consume over 600 million pounds annually of TFAs in the form of frying fats. TFAs can increase the risk of heart disease when consumed as at least 12% of the total fat intake. TFAs also reduce production of prostaglandins (hormones that act locally to control all cell to cell interactions) and interfere with fatty acid metabolism.

For more on the **role of fat in the diet**, see Chapter 2: Healthy Eating, pp. 50-75.

While the decline in the American diet can be attributed, in part, to the popularity of "junk foods," even some so-called healthy food choices fail to deliver adequate quantities of nutrients. For example, canned vegetable soup, considered by most to be a healthy choice, generally contains few nutrients. Although the ingredients used in these foods may be high in vitamins, enzymes, and other nutrients, high-heat processing often destroys their value. Sherry Rogers, M.D., author of *Wellness Against All Odds*, says that any preservation method that uses high-heat processing denatures and destroys essential nutrients.[4] While some manufacturers try to compensate for the destruction of nutrients in their products by artificially adding back some of the nutrients, this method rarely is able to restore the nutritive value available in the raw, unprocessed food.

Food quality has also been affected by changes in agricultural practices. Over the past century, commercial farmers have adopted intensive cropping methods that rely on large quantities of synthetic chemical fertilizers. The fertilizers return only a fraction of the vital minerals from the soil that growing plants remove. Consequently, the mineral content of American soils, along with the nutritive value of plants, has steadily declined. Paul Bergner, clinical director of the Rocky Mountain Center for Botanical Studies in Boulder, Colorado, has charted the mineral content of plants grown in the United States over the past 50 years. His data shows that, since 1948, levels of the essential minerals iron, manganese, and copper have declined significantly in a variety of crops. The iron content of lettuce, for example, has dropped from an average of 52 mg per 100 grams in 1948 to a mere 0.5 mg today. Bergner warns that this serious depletion of nutrients from the country's food supply is "leading our entire nation down the road to malnutrition and disease."[6]

Total Nutrition in a Box?

Some boxed cereal manufacturers claim that you can obtain all the nutrients you need for an entire day by eating one bowl of their product. Researchers at Tufts University took issue with these claims and demonstrated that the nutrients added to boxed cereals (which are sprayed onto the surface of the flakes) are not efficiently absorbed by the body. For example, the researchers showed that only 2% of the supplemental iron added to cereal is effectively absorbed by the body. Zinc is even more difficult for the body to absorb, as it is inhibited by the presence of fiber in the cereal and the calcium in milk. Richard Wood, Ph.D., of the Tufts Human Nutrition Center, says that not one milligram of zinc will be absorbed in the presence of milk.[5]

Detecting a Nutritional Deficiency

So what supplements should you take? The answer is that it depends on your individual biochemical needs. It can take years of personal research and experimentation to put together a good dietary and supplement program. To eliminate a lot of the guesswork and frustration, consult a qualified health professional trained in the intricacies of nutritional biochemistry, who can help you assess your needs and develop an effective, individualized dietary and nutritional supplement program. The following tests can be used to analyze your nutrient status, pinpoint specific deficiencies, and serve as the basis for recommending supplement dosages that best suit your needs.

Many mainstream physicians assess nutritional status using blood tests. These tests measure nutrient concentrations only in the blood serum, the liquid fraction of blood, and not in the blood cells (the globular or non-liquid fraction of blood). The cells are generally separated out and discarded. Unfortunately, a good deal of information about an individual's nutritional status is thrown out along with these cells. "It's important to understand that ordinary tests on blood serum levels don't provide the correct data," says John Dommisse, M.D., a nutritional medicine specialist based in Tucson, Arizona. "What must be measured are whole blood levels." Whole blood analysis, which examines both the serum and the blood cells, is not commonly done since most mainstream physicians are looking at blood primarily to diagnose a disease, and serum testing is generally adequate for that purpose. As most mainstream physicians are oriented towards using drugs to treat symptoms, they have no interest in nutritional status and are thus not inclined to order the proper tests. "Many doctors, unschooled in nutritional medicine, are reluctant to order such tests," says Dr. Dommisse, "especially those practicing within the strictures of an HMO."

In addition to whole-blood analysis, a variety of other test procedures can help assess nutrient status. These include hair analysis, the Individualized Optimum Nutrition Panel, and the Functional Intracellular Analysis.

For **referrals to physicians trained in nutritional and preventative medicine,** contact: American College of Advancement in Medicine (ACAM), P.O. Box 3427, Laguna Hills, CA 92654; tel: 714-583-7666.

■ Hair Analysis—Hair analysis measures the body's levels of various minerals, including calcium, iron, magnesium, potassium, and zinc, among others. As the hair is considered a storage organ, it provides a biochemical record of nutritional status over a period of several months. This is why many health-care practitioners consider hair analysis to pro-

For more about **hair analysis**, contact: Omegatech, 24700 Center Ridge Road, Cleveland, OH 44145; tel: 800-437-1404 or 440-835-2150; fax: 440-835-2177. For the **Functional Intracellular Analysis**, contact: Spectracell Laboratories, 515 Post Oak Blvd., Suite 830, Houston, TX 77027-9409; tel: 800-227-5227. For the **ION Panel**, contact: MetaMetrix Medical Laboratory, 5000 Peachtree Industrial Blvd., Suite 110, Norcross, GA 30071; tel: 770-446-5483 or 800-221-4640; fax: 770-441-2237.

vide a better picture of underlying mineral imbalances than most blood or urine tests. Hair analysis does not assess vitamin deficiency, however, so other testing procedures are needed to supplement the findings of a hair analysis.

■ Individualized Optimal Nutrition (ION) Panel— The Individualized Optimal Nutrition Panel, from MetaMetrix Medical Laboratories in Norcross, Georgia, uses blood and urine samples to measure 150 biochemical components. Specifically, ION checks for nutritional status in categories including vitamins, minerals, amino acids, fatty and organic acids, lipid peroxides, general blood chemistries (cholesterol, thyroid hormone, glucose), and antioxidants. Each patient's nutritional level is then compared with what is considered the healthy norm. In addition, ION can provide supplement recommendations based on the individual's test results.

■ Functional Intracellular Analysis (FIA)—Another accurate and comprehensive technique is the Functional Intracellular Analysis, available through Spectracell Laboratories in Houston, Texas. The FIA measures how micronutrients are naturally functioning within the activities of living white blood cells rather than simply measuring the micronutrient levels in the blood. This nutritional assay must be ordered by a health-care professional, but the lab will refer individuals to nutritionally oriented practitioners in their area.

Success Story: Addressing Nutrient Deficiencies Leads to Weight Loss

Marilyn, 50, weighed 303 pounds and suffered from severe fatigue. "I experienced shortness of breath so extreme I couldn't walk and breathe at the same time. I was so tired that there were days I could not get out of bed at all," she said. Marilyn also had night sweats, disturbed sleep, loss of concentration, colds, fevers, sore throats, and felt constantly hungry. Although she tried to control her eating habits, she frequently would go on an eating binge. "I inhaled food," she said, "I felt as though I couldn't get enough."

Marilyn sought treatment from John Dommisse, M.D., a nutritional medicine specialist in Tucson, Arizona. After taking Marilyn's complete history and having her undergo a comprehensive nutritional analysis, Dr. Dommisse determined that Marilyn was seriously deficient in vitamin B12 and the mineral chromium and had a slight manganese deficiency. These deficiencies had severely impaired Marilyn's metabolism, making it difficult for her to burn fat. Dr. Dommisse immediately began giving Marilyn vitamin B12 shots, along with chromium and manganese. Within three days, she stopped having hunger pangs. She also began feeling full after eating an ordinary meal and felt satisfied between meals.

For more on **Candida**, see Chapter 13: Eliminate Yeast Infections, pp. 294-309.

Dr. Dommisse also had Marilyn eliminate all white flour and sugar from her diet and continue on a regimen of supplements that included vitamins A, C, and E, iron, beta carotene, lysine, and garlic. Since Marilyn had also tested positive for *Candida*, a type of yeast fungus, he also prescribed anti-fungal agents for two months, including dosages of caprylic acid and *acidophilus*. After several weeks, Marilyn began to respond. Her energy returned and her hunger subsided. In six months, she lost 63 pounds.

John V. Dommisse, **M.D.**: 1840 East River Road, Suite 210, Cambric Corporate Center, Tucson, AZ 85718; tel: 520-577-1940; fax: 520-577-1743.

Getting the Nutrients You Need for Weight Loss

The best way to get the nutrients your body needs to lose weight is in your diet. The key is to carefully consider the quality of the food you eat. In other words, forget about calories and start focusing on whether the food you are eating is wholesome and rich in essential nutrients. Judith DeCava, C.N.S., a certified nutritional consultant, wellness counselor, and author of *Overcoming Overweight*, describes the approach this way: "Don't count calories—instead make calories count."[7] The place to start is with a whole foods diet.

"By whole foods, we mean consuming a diet with the least amount of processed, adulterated, fried, or sweetened additives," says Buck Levin, Ph.D., R.D., a registered dietitian and Assistant Professor of Nutrition at Bastyr University in Seattle, Washington. A whole foods diet is filled with a wide variety of vegetables, fruits, and grains; raw seeds and nuts and their butters; beans; fermented milk products such as yogurt and kefir; and fish, poultry, and bean products like tofu.

Yet even a whole foods diet may not succeed in satisfying all of your nutritional requirements. As stated previously, the declining nutrient content of plants makes it difficult to obtain an adequate intake of essential nutrients. In addition, exposure to environmental toxins, such as exhaust fumes, industrial chemicals and wastes, and

For more on the **whole foods diet**, see Chapter 2: Healthy Eating, pp. 50-75.

agricultural pesticides, puts a heavy demand on the body's detoxification systems, which tends to deplete nutrient reserves even further. Moreover, if you diet and restrict your calorie intake to 1,500-2,000 calories per day, you are unlikely to consume even the Recommended Daily Allowance (RDA) of most essential vitamins and minerals.[8] All of these factors make nutritional supplementation essential to maintaining good health and controlling body weight.

Essential and Accessory Micronutrients

"Essential nutrients are those nutrients derived from food that the body is unable to manufacture on its own," says Dr. Bland. These nutrients are absolutely necessary for human life and include at least thirteen vitamins and fifteen minerals. Essential vitamins are broken up into two groups, fat-soluble and water-soluble. The fat-soluble vitamins include vitamins A, D, E, and K. The water-soluble essential vitamins are C (ascorbic acid), B1 (thiamine), B2 (riboflavin), B3 (niacin), B5 (pantothenic acid), B6 (pyridoxine), B12, folic acid, and biotin. The essential minerals include calcium, magnesium, phosphorus, iron, zinc, copper, manganese, iodine, chromium, potassium, sodium, and a number of trace elements. They make up part of the necessary elements of body tissues, fluids, and other organs and play an active role in the body's regulatory functions.

In addition to the essential nutrients are the "accessory nutrients," co-factors that work in harmony with the essential nutrients to aid in the breakdown and conversion of food into cellular energy and help support all of the body's physical and mental functions. According to Dr. Bland, some of the key accessory nutrients include the vitamin B complex co-factors choline and inositol, coenzyme Q10 (a close relative of the B vitamins), and lipoic acid. Other accessory nutrients that have demonstrated preventative functions include B-complex co-factor PABA (para-aminobenzoic acid) and bioflavonoids (substances that enhance the beneficial effects of vitamin C).

Vitamins and minerals that work to control body weight can be separated into two general categories: energy nutrients, which are principally involved in the conversion of food to energy; and protector nutrients, which help defend the cells against damaging toxins derived from drugs, alcohol, radiation, environmental pollutants, or the body's own enzyme processes. Each of these groups is vital to the management of body weight. Without enough energy nutrients, calories cannot be burned in the body's cells and instead are stored as fat. Similarly, when the protector nutrients are scarce, cells are damaged by free radicals and other harmful substances, resulting in impaired metabolism and weight gain.

"Magnesium and the B-complex vitamins are examples of energy nutrients," says Dr. Bland. "They activate specific metabolic facilitators called enzymes, which control digestion and the absorption and use of proteins, fats, and carbohydrates. These nutrients often work synergistically, each enhancing the other's function." Examples of protector nutrients are vitamins C and E, beta carotene, and the minerals zinc, copper, manganese, and selenium, which play a critical role as antioxidants in preventing the effects of damaging free radicals.

For more on **enzymes**, see Chapter 4: Enzymes and Weight Loss, pp. 98-120. For **supplements that increase thermogenesis**, see Chapter 5: Optimize Your Calorie Burning, pp. 122-135.

Below is a brief summary of the key weight-loss micronutrients. Review it to understand how each substance works in your body and to become familiar with standard daily dosages as well as the best dietary sources of each nutrient.

Vitamins

A good quality multivitamin formula is helpful for general dietary support. In addition, a number of vitamins have been shown to be useful specifically for weight loss.

Vitamin A and Beta Carotene—Vitamin A facilitates the efficient absorption of nutrients by strengthening the lining of the digestive tract. Along with vitamins C and E, it strengthens the immune system and thus makes the body more resistant to infection from parasites and yeast overgrowth, two common causes of weight gain. Vitamin A is also necessary for the production of thyroxin, a thyroid hormone, and helps the thyroid (SEE QUICK DEFINITION) to absorb iodine, a key nutrient.[9] The healthy functioning of the thyroid is essential to maintaining metabolism and preventing the accumulation of body fat. The body obtains vitamin A from food sources or manufactures it through the conversion of carotenes (alpha, beta, gamma). Because high levels of vitamin A can be toxic, it is usually safer to boost intake of carotenes, which will be converted by the body into sufficient amounts of vitamin A.

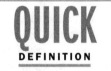

DEFINITION

The **thyroid gland**, one of the body's seven endocrine glands, is located just below the larynx in the throat, with interconnecting lobes on either side of the trachea. The thyroid is the body's metabolic thermostat, controlling body temperature, energy use, and, for children, the body's growth rate. The thyroid controls the rate at which organs function and the speed with which the body uses food; it affects the operation of all body processes and organs. Of the hormones synthesized in and released by the thyroid, T3 (tri-iodothyronine), represents 7%, and T4 (thyroxine), accounts for almost 93% of the thyroid's hormones active in all of the body's processes. Iodine is essential to forming normal amounts of thyroxine.

For more about the **thyroid and weight gain**, see Chapter 9: Overcome a Sluggish Thyroid, pp. 202-219. For more on **yeast overgrowth and parasites**, see Chapter 13: Eliminate Yeast Infections, 294-309 and Chapter 14: Eradicate Parasites, 310-328.

Beta carotene is a precursor to vitamin A and it also has additional antioxidant properties not found in vitamin A.[10] For most people, beta carotene is the preferred source of vitamin A (most vitamin A supplements found in health food stores are actually beta carotene). The only exception is individuals whose thyroid is impaired, because they cannot effectively convert beta carotene to its biologically usable form.

Food sources of vitamin A: fish oil (such as cod liver oil), liver, chili peppers, carrots, dried apricots, sweet potatoes, and leafy greens.[11] Supplements: Those with impaired thyroid function typically should take 10,000 IU to 20,000 IU of vitamin A daily in a form that is already pre-converted from beta carotene. Precautions: Very high levels of vitamin A can cause headaches and irritability and can be toxic; high levels should be avoided during pregnancy.[12] Unless closely supervised by a physician, your intake of pure vitamin A should at no time exceed 25,000 IU per day. Food sources of carotenes: all yellow and green vegetables, including carrots, beet greens, spinach, and broccoli. Supplements: most multivitamins contain beta carotene; typical dose: 100,000-300,000 IU.

Vitamin B Complex—The B vitamins (collectively known as B complex) nutritionally support the brain, eyes, intestines, liver, muscles, and skin. The B vitamins act as a team to help maintain healthy energy metabolism, which is crucial for burning off calories and avoiding weight gain. Stress levels, diet, and lifestyle can deplete the body's store of B vitamins.

■ Vitamin B1 (thiamin) and vitamin B2 (riboflavin) primarily serve in the maintenance of mucous membranes, formation of red blood cells, and metabolism of carbohydrates. Deficiencies of vitamin B1 may lead to blood sugar imbalances. Food sources: brewer's yeast is an excellent source of both of these vitamins. Supplements: B1 and B2 are commonly found in B-complex supplements.

■ Vitamin B3 (niacin) is necessary for oxygen transport in the blood, and fatty acid and nucleic acid formation. It is also vital to the actions of more than 150 enzymes in the body—without these enzymatic reactions, our body's energy production would quickly shut down. Low levels of B3 can cause muscle weakness, fatigue, skin sores, irritability, and depression. Eating a diet high in refined sugar as well as prolonged use of antibiotics will deplete B3 reserves in the body. Food sources: meat, chicken, fish, peanuts, wheat germ, brewer's yeast, and whole grains, particularly rice. Supplements: niacin is the natural form of vitamin B3 available in supplement form. When taken in dosages of over 100 milligrams, niacin can cause a very distinctive flushing, tingling, and redness that begins in the lower part of the body and moves up to the face, hands and head.[13] Niacinamide causes no flushing and is the form found in many supplements.[14] Typical therapeutic dose: 50 mg. Precautions: Liver enzymes may be affected when utilizing high levels of B3 or niacinamide. Use of inositol hexoniacinate has shown no toxicity and may be the best choice for this supplement.

- Vitamin B5 (pantothenic acid) is vital for the synthesis of hormones and support of the adrenal glands. Pantothenic acid deficiency can cause fatigue, insomnia, and depression.[15] Some researchers claim that vitamin B5 also increases the rate at which fat and carbohydrates are metabolized. In one study, 100 overweight individuals between the ages of 15 and 55 took 2.5 g of vitamin B5 four times daily. The average reported weight loss was 2.6 pounds per week.[16] Food sources: liver, meat, chicken, whole grains, and legumes. Eating a variety of foods can ensure adequate levels of vitamin B5. Typical therapeutic dose: 10 mg to 2,000 mg.

- Vitamin B6 (pyridoxine) strongly influences the immune and nervous systems. It aids in fat and protein metabolism and the conversion of the amino acid tryptophan to the brain neurotransmitter serotonin, which helps to control appetite.[17] B6 is also essential in the production of prostaglandins, which influence a variety of biological processes, including strengthening the immune system and controlling inflammation. A prostaglandin imbalance may cause some individuals to develop food sensitivities and allergies, leading to addictive behaviors and other reactions that frequently lead to weight gain. Deficiencies occur as a result of eating a diet high in fats and low in fruits and vegetables. Food sources: brewer's yeast, whole grains, legumes, nuts, and seeds. Supplements: there are two forms of B6, pyridoxine hydrochloride and pyridoxal-5-phosphate (the most active form). For efficient absorption of pyridoxal by the body, sufficient levels of riboflavin and magnesium should be present.[18] Typical recommended dose: 50 mg. Precautions: High levels of pyridoxine can cause toxic side effects.[19]

- Vitamin B12 (cobalamin) is virtually absent in vegetable food sources, which means vegetarians are likely to be deficient in this vitamin. B12 is essential for normal formation of red blood cells and the maintenance of the nervous system and mucous membrane linings. These linings are important for the proper absorption of nutrients and to pre-

For more about **food allergies**, see Chapter 11: Break Food Allergies and Addictions, pp. 244-270.

vent parasites and other pathogens (disease-causing substances) from entering the body. Food sources: meats, most fish (especially trout, mackerel, and herring), egg yolks, and yogurt. Supplements: B12 can be given in injectable form or as an oral supplement. Typical recommended dosage: 10-500 mcg daily.

■ Choline is a B vitamin that helps the body break down fats and transport them in and out of cells. It is particularly important in helping to clear the liver of fats, by keeping cholesterol from solidifying in the gallbladder. Food sources: choline is found in lecithin, used as a thickener in some foods, and is also present in high amounts in egg yolks, meat, milk, whole grains, and soybeans. A good source of lecithin is lecithin granules, which can be sprinkled on salads, cereals, and casseroles. Lecithin is also present in the herb chickweed (*Stellaria media*). Supplements: choline is available in lecithin capsules or as phosphatidyl choline. The average recommended dose of choline is 100-200 mg per day, or one to two tablespoons of lecithin granules per day.[20]

■ Folic acid (folacin, folate; members of the B vitamin family) is important for red blood cell formation, breakdown and utilization of proteins, and proper cell division, which is especially important in the early stages of pregnancy (folic acid prevents spina bifida and neural tube defects). It is also useful for anemia, atherosclerosis, fatigue, immune weakness, infection, and osteoporosis. Food sources: green leafy vegetables such as spinach and kale, asparagus, broccoli, lima beans, green peas, sweet potatoes, bean sprouts, whole wheat, cantaloupe, strawberries, and brewer's yeast. Supplements: the folic acid content in foods can be depleted by cooking, so supplementation may be necessary. Typical recommended dose: 400 mcg daily.

■ Inositol is important for bone marrow, eyes, and intestines. It assists in metabolizing fats in the blood and liver and lowers cholesterol. Inositol helps control arteriosclerosis (hardening of the arteries) and hypertension. Food sources: whole grains, citrus fruits, brewer's yeast, liver, cabbage, and some nuts. Caffeinated beverages can deplete the body of inositol. Supplements: inositol is best taken in combination with other B vitamins.[21] Typical dose: 500 mg daily.

■ Para-aminobenzoic acid (PABA) is important for the skin, hair pigment (color), and blood cell formation. PABA aids in the metabolism and assimilation of amino acids (proteins) and is essential for the growth of "friendly" intestinal bacteria and supports their production of vitamin B12. Food sources: brewer's yeast, wheat germ, whole grains, and eggs. Supplements: PABA should be taken in a time-released form. Typical recommended dosage: 50-100 mg, three times daily.

Vitamin C (Ascorbic Acid)—Vitamin C is an important antioxidant and also helps to keep the adrenal glands (the endocrine glands located above the kidneys) and the thyroid healthy and functioning. Vitamin C is particularly important when the body is under stress, as stress severely impacts the adrenal glands.[22] Damage to the adrenals, in turn, can cause shortages of protective hormones, such as DHEA, leading to diminished energy and overeating or undereating. This may deprive the body of essential nutrients and, in turn, prompt urgent food cravings. A vitamin C deficiency can also cause capillaries in the thyroid to bleed, and normal cells in the gland to multiply abnormally—a condition called hyperplasia.[23]

For more on **stress and the adrenal glands**, see Chapter 7: Heal Your Emotional Appetite, pp. 156-182.

Food sources: most fruits and vegetables, including oranges, grapefruit, kiwis, lemons, avocado, parsley, red chili peppers (have over seven times more vitamin C than oranges), leafy greens, kale, collard, and broccoli. Supplements: Esterified vitamin C, often called ester C, is a combination of several forms of vitamin C. It has all of the same healthful properties and benefits as standard vitamin C, but is more quickly absorbed by the body. Because it is non-acidic, ester C is also less likely to cause gastrointestinal distress.[24] Typical recommended dose: Michael Murray, N.D., author of *Natural Alternatives for Weight Loss*, recommends 500-9,000 mg a day of vitamin C (to bowel tolerance) in divided doses.[25]

Vitamin E (Alpha Tocopherol)—Vitamin E is one of the primary agents used to protect cell membranes against the damage caused by environmental pollutants. Since chemical exposure can lead to a toxic liver, lymph, or colon—three conditions that contribute to weight gain—vitamin E should be an important component of any weight-loss program. Some studies have also suggested that fat tissue may trap alpha-tocopherol, the active ingredient in vitamin E, making the vitamin unavailable for use by the body. Consequently, if you are overweight, it is likely that you are deficient in vitamin E. A study of teenage boys found that those who were overweight (more than 30% over their ideal weight) had half the blood levels of vitamin E than teenage boys of normal weight.[26] A vitamin E deficiency can also reduce thyroid iodine absorption. When the thyroid lacks iodine, it secretes fewer hormones, resulting in hypothyroidism and a sluggish metabolism.

CAUTION Prolonged intake of excessive doses of vitamins A, D, niacin, and possibly B6 may produce toxic effects. In addition, anyone currently under medical care, taking medications, or with a history of specific problems should always consult a health-care professional (preferably one knowledgeable about nutrition) before making any changes in diet or using supplements.

Antioxidant Protection

An antioxidant is a natural biochemical substance that protects living cells from the damaging effects of free radicals. Free radicals cause oxidation, the same chemical process that causes metal to rust and apples to turn brown. In the body, if left uncontrolled, free radicals cause cell membranes to erode and die, leading to a variety of degenerative conditions.

Produced as a by-product of cellular activities, free radicals are typically neutralized and rendered harmless by antioxidants. But when environmental and other toxins (poor diet, pollution, stress, cigarettes) introduce an increased burden of free radicals, the body's reserve of antioxidants is quickly exhausted.

Types of Antioxidants—

Amino Acids: cysteine, glutathione, methionine

Bioflavonoids: anthocyanin bioflavonoids (in fruit, especially grapes, cranberries, and bilberries), citrus bioflavonoids (in grapefruit, lemons, and oranges), oligometric proanthocyanidins (OPCs) in pycnogenol (pine bark or grape seed extract)

Carotene: alpha and beta carotene (in red, yellow, and dark green fruits and vegetables), lycopene (in red fruits and vegetables, such as red grapefruit and tomatoes)

Spices: cayenne pepper, garlic, turmeric

Herbs: astragalus, bilberry, ginkgo, green tea, milk thistle, sage

Minerals: copper, manganese, selenium, zinc

Vitamins: A, B1, C, and E, coenzyme Q10, NADH (nicotinamide adenine dinucleotide)

Enzymes: catalase, glutathione peroxidase, superoxide dismutase

Hormones: melatonin

Miscellaneous: lipoic acid

Food sources: cold-pressed polyunsaturated vegetable oils (such as sunflower and safflower), leafy green vegetables, avocados, nuts, seeds, and whole grains. Supplements: Vitamin E is actually a group of compounds called tocopherols. When purchasing supplements of vitamin E, avoid products that contain vitamin E in the DL-alpha tocopherol acetate form—this means that it is a petroleum-based synthetic form of the vitamin. The natural form of vitamin E will be designated with the letter "D". Typical recommended dose: 30 IU daily; for those suffering from hypothyroidism, 800-1,200 IU per day.

Minerals

A combination mineral formula is generally recommended for dietary support and several minerals have specific actions helpful for weight loss.

Chromium —Chromium is a mineral essential for regulating the production of the hormone insulin, which is responsible for stabilizing blood sugar levels and preventing the conversion of blood sugar into fat. Although the body requires only small amounts of this important mineral, Americans are more likely to be deficient in chromium than any other micronutrient. Chromium is found in the outer bran portion of grains, but much of it is lost in the milling and processing of white flour (the staple ingredient in most refined bread and pasta products).

The chromium that we do draw from food sources can be depleted in our bodies by various means, including a high-carbohydrate diet, infections, repeated pregnancies, air pollution, exposure to radiation, and physical and emotional stress. The urinary excretion of chromium can increase as much as fifty-fold under stress.[27] A high intake of white sugar also tends to deplete the body of chromium, as the mineral is used up in removing these sugars from the blood.[28] Regular chromium supplementation is imperative both for general health and weight management.

Food sources: an excellent source of chromium is brewer's yeast (available in powder form or in tablets), wheat germ, beef and chicken, liver, whole grains, potatoes, eggs, apples, bananas, and spinach. Supplements: According to Dr. Bland, chromium and other minerals are better absorbed in the body when bound in a "transporter" molecule, called a chelate. Chelated minerals are protected from damage in the digestive system. Dr. Bland says that the glucose tolerance factor chelate (GTF chromium) tends to be a more bioavailable form of chromium than chromium salts, such as chromium chloride.[29] Chromium polynicotinate is another chelated variety that is chemically bound to niacin, a B-complex vitamin. According to some researchers, this form of chromium is superior to either chromium chloride or chromium picolinate. Typical recommended dosage: 200-300 mcg.

Iodine—Along with the minerals copper, zinc, and selenium, iodine is part of the structure of thyroid hormones (especially thyroxin), which regulate how fast the body burns calories. As the metabolism of all the body's cells (except for brain cells) is influenced by thyroid hormones, iodine's effects are far-reaching. Iodine deficiency most typically results in hypothyroidism, which may subsequently cause weight gain and fatigue. Stephen Langer, M.D., author of *Solved: The Riddle of Weight Loss*, says that for many hypothyroid sufferers, simply adding more iodine-containing foods to the diet is often enough to restore thyroid function.

Food sources: seaweed, kelp, cod liver oil, and fish (haddock, cod, halibut, and herring). In the United States, table salt is iodized, which provides sufficient levels of iodine. People using sea salt as a replacement for table salt should consider supplementing with kelp, a vegetable rich in elemental iodine (the most therapeutic form of iodine).[30] Certain foods, called goitrogens, prevent iodine absorption. These include soybeans, turnips, cabbage, and pine nuts, especially if eaten raw.[31] Supplements: supplements often contain inorganic iodine such as sodium iodide and potassium iodide, which are not as beneficial as elemental iodine, found in iodine caseinate.[32] Typical recommended daily dosage: 100 mcg for women and 120 mcg for men. Precautions: Dr. Langer advises against taking more than these quantities of iodine. He also warns that using too much table salt, another source of iodine, can alter the body's sodium/potassium balance and contribute to serious disorders, such as heart disease, high blood pressure, and obesity. Too much iodine can also suppress the formation of the thyroid hormone T3.

Iron—Iron is essential to red blood cell synthesis, oxygen transport, and energy production. A diet low in iron causes anemia, which has also been found to cause hypothyroidism.[33] An iron deficiency can also decrease hydrochloric acid in the stomach, impairing digestion and contributing to further nutritional deficiencies. Individuals who follow low-calorie diets are particularly vulnerable to developing iron deficiencies.[34]

Food sources: kelp, organ meats, egg yolk, blackstrap molasses, lecithin, certain nuts and seeds, millet, and parsley. Supplements: the form of iron (heme) found in desiccated liver or liquid liver extract supplements is most easily absorbed and has fewer side effects. Of the non-heme forms of iron, ferrous fumerate and ferrous succinate are recommended. Typical dosage: to ensure the proper functioning of the thyroid, you should take 100 mcg per day. Precautions: Ferrous sulfate, commonly used in conventional supplements, can cause the production of free radicals and should not be used. Elevated levels of iron in the blood are associated with an increased risk for heart attacks and other cardiovascular problems, as well as low immunity.[35] Women who are menopausal and those who experience a heavy menstrual flow should consult their physicians. Overdose in infants can be serious or even fatal, so be sure that your iron supplements are out of the reach of children.

Selenium—Selenium plays an important role in maintaining balance among the thyroid hormones.[36] It is an important constituent of the antioxidant enzyme glutathione peroxidase, which protects the body from free-radical damage.[37] Selenium can also protect against the absorption of heavy metals such as aluminum, mercury, and lead.[38]

Food sources: wheat germ, Brazil nuts, bran, and Swiss chard. Supplements: avoid multimineral supplements that contain sodium selenite, an organic salt that is not well absorbed. Organic selenium from yeast or the chelated mineral (seleno-methionine) are better sources. Typical therapeutic dosage: 200-1,000 mcg per day; individuals suffering from thyroid hormone imbalance should take 200 mcg per day. Precautions: Selenium toxicity is possible but rare. An overdose can cause hair loss, nail malformations, weakness, and slowed mental function.[39]

Zinc—Zinc helps in the conversion of the thyroid hormone T4 to T3, increases the sensitivity of cell membranes to these hormones, and serves as a building block of the hormone thyroxin. Zinc is often lacking in a vegetarian diet, because beans, legumes, and grains—the staples of a vegetarian diet—are high in a substance known as phylate. Phylates cause the elimination of zinc from the body.[40] Vegetarians forego one of the best sources of this mineral—meat.

Food sources: whole grains, nuts, seeds, oysters, shellfish, and pumpkin seeds. Supplements: zinc sulfate, found in many multivitamin/multimineral preparations, is not easily absorbed by the body. Other forms of zinc that are more readily absorbed are zinc picolinate, zinc citrate, and zinc monomethionine. Typical recommended dose: 25 mg of zinc per day, along with 3 mg of copper (zinc tends to deplete copper reserves). Precautions: With medical supervision, the dosage of zinc could be increased, if necessary. However, dosages should be increased with caution, as too much zinc can interfere with the functioning of the immune system. Toxicity of zinc is rarely reported, however prolonged use of over 150 mg a day can cause anemia.

Amino Acids

Amino acids are the building blocks of proteins; in fact, proteins are actually chains of amino acids linked together, each one having a specific function. Proteins are in turn the building blocks of the body. Twenty-two amino acids are vital to the body's growth, development, and maintenance. Some are manufactured in the body while others, called essential amino acids, must be obtained from the diet or nutritional supplements. Semi-essential amino acids can be made by the body in amounts that are adequate to maintain basic protein require-

A Guide to Taking Supplements

In addition to knowing what supplements to take, it is also important to know how to take them. Jeffrey Bland, Ph.D., and Lindsey Berkson, D.C., offer the following recommendations:

■ Nutritional supplements should be taken with meals to promote increased absorption. Fat-soluble nutrients (such as vitamins A and E, beta carotene, and the essential fatty acids linoleic and alpha-linolenic acid) should be taken during the day with the meal that contains the most fat.

■ Amino acid supplements should be taken on an empty stomach one hour before or after a meal and taken with fruit juice to help promote absorption. When taking an increased dosage of an isolated amino acid, be sure to supplement with an amino acid blend.

■ If you become nauseated when you take tablet supplements, consider taking a liquid form, diluted in a beverage.

■ If you become nauseated or ill within an hour after taking supplements, consider the need for a bowel cleanse or rejuvenation program prior to further supplementation.

■ If you are taking high doses, do not take the supplements all at one time, but divide them into smaller doses throughout the day.

■ Take digestive enzymes with meals to assist digestion. If you are taking pancreatic enzymes for other therapeutic reasons, be sure to take them on an empty stomach between meals.

■ Do not take mineral supplements with high-fiber meals, as fiber can decrease mineral absorption.

■ When taking an increased dosage of an isolated B vitamin, be sure to supplement with B complex.

■ When taking nutrients, be sure to drink adequate amounts of liquid to mix with digestive juices and prevent side effects.

ments; however, additional dietary sources are required during times of growth or stress.

Amino acid deficiency may be an underlying factor, often undetected, for many common disorders. Vegetarians and vegans (vegetarians who eat no dairy products) often have difficulty meeting dietary protein requirements, and should take an amino acid complex supplement. Amino acid supplementation is also valuable to athletes, bodybuilders, people in mentally or physically stressful professions, and dieters who are trying to prevent sugar or carbohydrate cravings.

Below, we discuss the amino acids that are particularly useful for people trying to lose weight.

■ Isoleucine aids in energy production, hemoglobin (carries oxygen in blood) formation, and in the regulation of energy from blood sugars. Since it assists in the metabolism and formation of muscles, isoleucine is a useful supplement for bodybuilders (weight-lifters), when taken with balanced proportions of leucine and valine.

- Leucine helps heal injured or weakened muscles, fractured or weakened bones, and skin conditions or injuries. Leucine can also be used as a nutritional support for post-surgery recovery. It reduces excessive blood sugar levels and is a good source of fuel during prolonged workouts or exercise. Leucine (with balanced proportions of isoleucine and valine) assists in the metabolism and formation of muscles.

- Lysine assists in the formation of antibodies (immune cells that inhibit viruses), enzymes, and hormones. Lysine helps develop bones by assisting in the metabolism of calcium from the intestinal tract. Lysine is also useful for building muscles and for recovering from surgery or muscular and sports injuries.

- Methionine is the source of organic sulfur (which must be constantly replaced) and is a potent antioxidant. It helps prevent excessive accumulation of fats in the liver and vascular system, detoxify heavy metals and toxins, and protect against the damaging effects of radiation on the body.

- Phenylalanine is a precursor of the neurotransmitters (chemical nerve messengers) dopamine and norepinephrine, which regulate mood, promote alertness, and enhance memory and cognitive function. It is used for certain types of depression, headaches (especially migraine), menstrual cramps, weight gain or obesity (phenylalanine acts as a natural appetite suppressant), and Parkinson's disease.

- Valine can be used by the body to produce energy and is important for the formation, metabolism, and repair of muscle tissue. It has a natural stimulating effect and can benefit bodybuilders if used in balanced proportions with leucine and isoleucine.

- Arginine is most needed during times of growth (childhood or pregnancy) and great stress. It stimulates the release of human growth hormone (HGH) and is important for muscle metabolism, increasing muscle mass while decreasing body fat. It also combats physical and mental fatigue and enhances immune function.

- Alanine promotes immunity and assists the body in metabolizing glucose, which serves as fuel for the brain, nervous system, and muscles, as well as energy. Hypoglycemia may be associated with low alanine levels. Alanine assists in the metabolism of organic acids in the body and is important for the formation of vitamin B5 (pantothenic acid).

- Glutamic acid is a neurotransmitter important for brain metabolism. It assists in transporting potassium across the blood-brain barrier and in detoxifying ammonia from the brain. Important for the metabolism of other amino acids, fats, and sugars, glutamic acid is useful for balancing hypoglycemia (low blood sugar) and overcoming fatigue.

■ Glutamine assists in improving mental alertness and memory. It can readily pass through the blood-brain barrier and be converted into glutamic acid (see above). It also increases GABA (gamma-aminobutyric acid), a central nervous system neurotransmitter important for brain function and mental ability. It has been used to treat alcoholism and alcohol poisoning, mental illness, and degenerative brain conditions. Glutamine helps stop alcohol and sugar cravings and aids in the absorption of minerals into the tissues. Glutamine also assists in the formation of muscles.

■ Glycine has a calming effect on the brain and is important for central nervous system function. It supports immune function, promotes the healing of wounds, and assists in the conversion of stored sugars into energy. Glycine is used as a sweetener and is also a building block for other amino acids.

■ Ornithine stimulates the release of growth hormone. When taken with arginine and carnitine, it has the effect of increasing muscle mass while decreasing body fat. Ornithine is needed for a healthy liver, as it detoxifies ammonia from the liver and is involved in liver regeneration. It supports immune function and tissue repair and healing.

■ Serine is a component of brain proteins and the fatty (myelin) sheaths that protect nerves. It is a source of stored energy for the liver and muscles and helps metabolize fats, oils, and fatty acids. It also is important for muscle growth and a healthy immune system (by improving antibody protection).

■ Taurine is the primary building block for other amino acids and is crucial for the proper assimilation of calcium, magnesium, potassium, and sodium. It is important in the formation of bile and is a component of white blood cells, skeletal and heart muscles, and the tissues of the central nervous system. Taurine supports normal brain function and has been used to help control hyperactivity, epilepsy, and nervous system imbalance caused by alcohol or drug abuse. It has also been used to treat atherosclerosis (fatty buildup in the arteries), heart disorders, high blood pressure, hypoglycemia (low blood sugar), and seizures.

■ Tyrosine is a building block of the neurotransmitters norepinephrine and dopamine, which help regulate mood, appetite, anxiety, and depression. It helps regulate the adrenal, pituitary, and thyroid glands and increases muscle growth while reducing body fat.

Supplements: The preferred amino acid supplements are labeled "USP pharmaceutical grade," L-crystalline, free-form amino acids. The term *USP* means that the product meets the standards of purity and potency set by the United States Pharmacopeia. The term *free-form* refers to the highest level of purity of the amino acid. The L refers to one of the two forms in which most amino acids come, designated D- and L- (as in D-lysine or L-lysine). The L-form amino acids are proper for human biochemistry, as proteins in the human body are made from this form. The exception is phenylalanine, which consists of a combination of the D- and L- forms (thus its full name DL-phenylalanine).

See *The Supplement Shopper* (Future Medicine Publishing, 1999; ISBN 1-887299-17-3); to order, call 800-333-HEAL.

Generally, it is not recommended for people to take individual amino acids for extended or indefinite periods as this can create an imbalance of other amino acids in the body and possibly cause other health conditions. If individual amino acids are going to be used to support specific health conditions, follow this course of treatment with a complex of free-form amino acids to ensure balanced nutrition. Please consult a qualified health-care professional before beginning such therapies. Individual amino acids often come with warnings or precautions for women who are pregnant or for people with certain health conditions.

Other Nutrients for Weight Loss

A number of other nutrients have proven to be helpful as part of a weight-loss program, including the "green" foods chlorella and spirulina, hydroxycitric acid (HCA), and fiber.

"Green" Foods—Green foods are rich in vitamins, minerals, and chlorophyll, the green pigment found in most plants. Chlorophyll has long been used as a healing agent and is well-known for its anti-aging properties. It helps heal wounds of the skin and internal membranes, stimulates the growth of new cells, and hinders the growth of bacteria. Important to detoxifying, chlorophyll also promotes regularity and is an excellent liver purifier and healer.

Chlorella, a freshwater single-celled green algae, is more popular than vitamin C in Japan. There are an estimated five million people taking this algae every day. Chlorella is approximately 60% protein, including all the essential amino acids, 20 different vitamins and minerals, and contains high levels of carotenoids and chlorophyll. It has very high levels of RNA and DNA, which support tissue repair and healing. An antioxidant, chlorella also helps remove heavy metals and pesticides from the body. Chlorella absorbs toxins from the intestines,

For information on
**"green" food
products**, contact:
Solar Greens,
Nutraceutical
Corporation, P.O. Box
681869, Park City, UT
84068; tel: 800-669-
8877. New Chapter, 22
High Street,
Brattleboro, VT 05301;
tel: 800-543-7279 or
802-257-9345.
Rainbow Light, P.O.
Box 600, Santa Cruz,
CA 95061; tel: 800-
635-1233 or 408-429-
9089.

helps relieve chronic constipation, and promotes the growth of healthy intestinal flora.[41] According to Bernard Jensen, Ph.D., author of *Chlorella: Jewel of the Far East*, chlorella is an excellent remedy for a toxic, mineral-deficient liver and can also normalize blood sugar imbalances, both important for weight loss.[42] Other green food sources of chlorophyll include sprouted barley grass and wheat grass (available at most health food stores).

Spirulina contains eight times more protein than tofu, five times more calcium than cow's milk (in a more easily absorbed form), and more of certain amino acids than any other vegetables. Spirulina is important in reversing adrenal and thyroid exhaustion, battling depression and mood swings, and is excellent for weight control because it acts as an appetite suppressor. It also is the highest vegetable source of vitamin B12, a necessity for vegetarians.[43] Spirulina chelates (binds with) heavy metals and helps remove them from the body.

Hydroxycitric Acid (HCA)—Hydroxycitric acid is derived from the dried rind of the tamarind fruit (*Garcinia cambogia*). It helps to clear fats from the liver, suppresses appetite, and slows the rate at which the body converts carbohydrates into fat. Studies show that HCA reduces food consumption by approximately 10%.[44] HCA has been found to be more effective when taken in combination with the mineral chromium (either the polynicotinate or picolinate form).

For **products contain-
ing HCA (*Garcinia
cambogia* extract)**,
contact: Nature's
Herbs, 600 East
Quality Drive, American
Fork, UT 84003; tel:
800-437-2257 or 801-
763-0700. Nutrition
Now, 501 Southeast
Columbia Shore Blvd.
#350, Vancouver, WA
98661; tel: 800-929-
0418 or 360-737-
6800. Natural Max,
Nutraceutical
Corporation, P.O. Box
681869, Park City, UT
84068; tel: 800-669-
8877.

Supplements: Dallas Cloutare, Ph.D., a nutritional consultant in Berkeley, California, recommends beginning with a minimum dose of 250 mg of HCA three times daily along with 100 mcg of chromium, taken 30-60 minutes before each meal. Dr. Cloutare also indicates that the dosage may be doubled after three weeks if results are unsatisfactory. If after another week you are still not satisfied, he recommends doubling the dosage again to 1,000 mg, three times daily (chromium should not be increased).

Fiber—Fiber helps flush wastes from the body, works to reduce blood sugar levels, and contributes to feelings of fullness. Fiber acts like a sponge, absorbing water as it goes through the stomach and the small intestine, and arrives in the colon full of moisture. Diets low in fiber cause fecal material to become dry and hard to expel, causing a buildup of toxins that can lead to weight gain.

Fiber consists of the cell walls of plants and certain indigestible food residues. Foods with a high fiber content include brown rice, broccoli, oatmeal, and almonds. There are two basic types of fiber, soluble and insoluble. The insoluble fibers, those that do not dissolve in water, are found in wheat and corn bran, whole grains, nuts, legumes, and some vegetables. They increase fecal size and weight and promote regular bowel movements. However, insoluble fibers can also irritate the bowel, especially if it is already sensitive or inflamed. Too much grain fiber, especially wheat bran, may interfere with the absorption of calcium, magnesium, iron, and zinc. Soluble fibers, found in fruits, vegetables, oats and oat bran, barley, beans, and peas, are not irritating to the bowel. Ingesting foods containing these fibers stimulates bowel movements, decreases appetite, and thus leads to weight loss.

Supplements: One excellent source of fiber is powdered psyllium husk, the form of fiber most often used for intestinal cleansing due to its superior ability to absorb moisture, lubricate the intestines, and "mop up" contaminants. Other good forms of soluble fiber are flaxseed, guar gum, and apple pectin. Fiber products mixed with water or juice produce a gelatinous mass that, when taken before a meal, creates a feeling of fullness and thus reduces appetite. This mixture also assists in controlling blood sugar, decreasing the number of calories absorbed, and cleaning out the intestinal tract. Supplementing with fiber compared to only reducing calories can result in 50% to 100% more weight loss.[45] Typical dose: start by taking 4-5 g per day of fiber and gradually increase intake as your body adjusts. Remember to drink 6-8 glasses of water per day to prevent constipation.

4 Enzymes for Healthy Digestion

MANY OVERWEIGHT individuals suffer from impaired digestion and a chronic deficiency of enzymes, the proteins necessary for digestion to take place. When your digestion is not functioning properly, your body weight will almost certainly be out of balance. If proteins, fats, and other foods aren't being digested properly in your stomach and intestines, they tend to get stored as fat throughout the body. Alternative medicine offers testing procedures that can determine if you have impaired digestion due to an enzyme deficiency. For many, enzyme and digestive support have helped them achieve permanent weight loss.

Success Story: Enzymes for Lasting Weight Loss

Edith, 73, weighed 250 pounds and suffered from severe indigestion; she was taking 35 antacid pills per day. Edith, a gourmet cook, generally ate a well-balanced and healthy diet, despite indulging too often in rich desserts. To treat her weight and digestive problems, Edith consulted enzyme therapist Lita Lee, Ph.D., of Lowell, Oregon.

Dr. Lee recommended that Edith take a multiple-digestive enzyme formula, which soothes stomach problems and indigestion by helping to heal the delicate lining of the intestines. After beginning the treatment, Edith quickly began to feel better. The enzymes in the formula also improved her digestion, helping her extract more nutrients from each mouthful of food. Consequently, her body adjusted to the greater nourishment by lowering its demand for food. With time, Edith noticed that she was eating smaller portions of food but still feeling satisfied and full. Her weight steadily dropped and, in less than a year, had stabilized at 170 pounds.

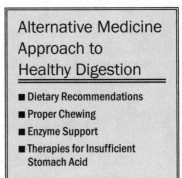

Alternative Medicine Approach to Healthy Digestion

■ Dietary Recommendations
■ Proper Chewing
■ Enzyme Support
■ Therapies for Insufficient Stomach Acid

Poor Digestion Puts on the Pounds

Edith's problems with digestion and weight gain were unusual because she ate such a healthy diet. But her diet was not able to compensate for the fact that she was 73 years old. As people age, they naturally lose their capacity to produce enough enzymes to digest food properly. This is why many older individuals notice they have a harder time with foods that they were able to easily handle in their youth. But enzyme deficiencies do not occur only with age—anyone who fails to maintain a diet that supports good digestion can experience the same symptoms and weight problems well before they reach their golden years.

When digestion is impaired, even a diet of the most wholesome foods will be of little value, because your body can't absorb the nutrients. "If your digestion is not functioning well, it doesn't matter how healthy the food is that you eat," says Maile Pouls, Ph.D., a clinical nutritionist in Santa Cruz, California. "The body becomes deficient, not to mention toxic, as a result of poor digestion."[1] Digestion can't happen without enzymes, the specialized living proteins that activate the millions of chemical reactions that take place in the body every day. Enzymes involved in digestion transform the complex molecules that make up the food we eat into simpler forms that our bodies need to stay alive. "Enzymes are substances that make life possible," says Edward Howell, M.D., a pioneer of enzyme therapy in the United States. "No mineral, vitamin, or hormone can do any work without enzymes."[2]

Howard F. Loomis, D.C., a chiropractor and enzyme expert based in Madison, Wisconsin, compares enzymes to a team of builders. "Foods are like the materials you'd use to build a house," he says. "It takes workers to make something out of them. You can have all the materials in the world sitting on your lot, but without the builders nothing happens. Digestive enzymes are our workers and their job is to reconstruct the body every day from the building blocks of food." Indeed, these "workers" are essential for building and maintaining the muscle, bone, and other tissues of our bodies. You can't breathe, eat, or even walk without enzymes being involved.

Many overweight individuals suffer from impaired digestion and chronic enzyme deficiency. When your digestion is poor, your body weight will almost surely increase. If proteins, fats, and other foods aren't being digested properly in your stomach and intestines, they tend to get stored as fat in the body, often in unwanted places. In addition, there can be serious health consequences to poor digestion—it can impair the functioning of your immune system, leaving you susceptible to infections (colds and flu) and chronic diseases (such as anemia, arthritis, and heart disease).[3]

In this chapter, we look at the importance of enzymes in digestion and explain how an enzyme deficiency can lead to weight gain. We also review the tests that are available to assess your digestive function and your need for enzymes, and guide you to the enzymes most suitable for your goals. Finally, we look at alternative and natural therapies, such as dietary and cooking recommendations, proper chewing of foods, and enzyme supplementation, that can help repair a weakened digestive system, restoring the body to health and helping you shed unwanted pounds.

Enzymes and Weight Gain

Forget about calories. That's the advice Dr. Lita Lee gives to people who want to lose weight. Dr. Lee is rarely concerned with either the calorie content or quantity of food her clients consume. Instead, she tries to make sure that, when they do eat, they thoroughly digest every mouthful. "If you digest the food you eat, you'll eat the right amount of food for you," says Dr. Lee. "Whatever you don't digest can make you fat." That's why Dr. Lee's approach to weight loss focuses not on calories but on the use of enzymes to improve digestion.

In the case above, Edith's indigestion included symptoms of gas and constipation. This was because the food, rather than being properly broken down (by enzymes) and absorbed, was putrefying (rotting) in her intestines. Dr. Pouls says that such putrefaction can contribute to numerous health problems, including headaches, fatigue, and even depression. It can also cause the colon to become toxic, which can lead to increases in body weight. If you have enzyme deficiencies and your digestion isn't working properly, nutrients will not be absorbed in the small intestine. The whole digestive system can malfunction as a result. In addition, when digestion is hampered, every bite of food provides fewer nutrients, leaving you feeling less satisfied, which can cause you to overeat. Digestion also stimulates the hypothalamus, the satiety center of the brain that gives you the feeling of fullness and satisfaction after eating. When digestion is impaired, you still feel hungry even though you are eating plenty of food, often leading to overeating, unwanted fat deposits, and weight gain.[4]

The Immune Connection–Poor digestion can also affect your immune system. "We're born with a 'bank account' of enzymes necessary for digestion," says Dr. Pouls, "but if over a lifetime we eat too many cooked and processed foods, this enzyme reserve gets depleted."[5] The pancreas then has to produce more enzymes at the expense of the immune system, making you more susceptible to illness.

> "If you digest the food you eat, you'll eat the right amount of food for you," says Dr. Lita Lee. "Whatever you don't digest can make you fat." Dr. Lee's approach to weight loss focuses not on calories but on the use of enzymes to improve digestion.

Poor digestion and enzyme deficiencies can lead to leaky gut syndrome, which further strains the immune system. This is a condition in which particles of partially digested or undigested food migrate into the bloodstream through the intestinal walls. Dr. Loomis explains the process in this way: "The body treats circulating particles of undigested food as 'foreign invaders,' and mobilizes its forces to handle what it perceives as an emergency. This taxes the immune system, and, over time, can lead to chronic degenerative diseases." Dr. Loomis indicates that many patients whose immune systems have been weakened through poor digestion are often overweight. "Overweight is a warning light," he says. "These people don't yet have a disease that conventional medicine can diagnose and treat, but they're not well and they know it." Dr. Loomis adds that enzymes are a way of restoring the body's immunological balance. "Over and over again I see that when patients are

What are Enzymes?

Enzymes are specialized proteins fundamental to all living processes in the body, needed for all the chemical reactions that take place during the normal activity of our organs, tissues, fluids, and cells. "Without enzymes, there would be no breathing, no digestion, no growth, no blood coagulation, no sense perception, and no reproduction," states Anthony C. Cichoke, D.C., author of *Enzymes and Enzyme Therapy.* Enzymes are specific biological catalysts, each one stimulating a particular chemical reaction in the body. Thousands of metabolic enzymes are made by the body and are involved in all body processes, including breathing, thinking, talking, moving, and immune function. The body also manufactures digestive enzymes (secreted mainly by the pancreas, but also in the mouth, stomach, and small intestine), which play a vital role in the digestion of food. Plant, or food, enzymes (present in all raw plants) are also essential in proper digestion.

The enzymes involved in digestion enable the body to assimilate the food we eat and to extract essential nutrients, such as vitamins and minerals, from that food. Think of them as chemical scissors, cutting apart the proteins, carbohydrates, and fats you eat into smaller units (such as amino acids or simple sugars) that can be absorbed and used by the body for energy. Other enzymes are involved in reassembling these smaller units for use by the body: for the formation of neurotransmitters (chemical messengers in the brain), hormones, antibodies, and myriad other structural components the body needs for healthy functioning.[6]

The Primary Enzymes in Digestion

No matter what specific foods we eat, our diets are composed of protein, fat, carbohydrates, sugars, and fiber, and we need the appropriate enzymes to break down each of these components in digestion. When a person is lacking in one or more of the primary digestive enzymes, the food associated with that enzyme does not get digested properly and that person is said to be "intolerant" to that food. If the enzyme deficiency is left untreated, health problems inevitably result.

Protease (digests protein)—Protease breaks down protein into smaller units called amino acids. This is not only protein from food, but also from organisms which are composed of protein, such as certain viruses, and harmful substances produced at sites of inflammation. Someone deficient in protease is protein-intolerant: their bodies can't digest any form of protein, including that found in vegetables.

Lipase (digests fats)—Lipase breaks down fats (triglycerides) into glycerol (an alcohol) and fatty acids. Before lipase can digest fat, bile (an emulsifier or degreaser secreted by the gallbladder) must break down the fat into smaller units. People who are low in hydrochloric acid (HCl; the primary acid in the stomach) cannot make adequate bile and will not be able to digest fats. There are two types of lipase-deficient people: those who are truly fat-intolerant and get sick when they eat fat—these people generally substitute sugar for fat; and those who are complex-carbohydrate intolerant—they compensate by eating excessive amounts of fat; both types of lipase deficiency can lead to weight gain.

Amylase (digests carbohydrates)—Amylase breaks down carbohydrates (polysaccharides) into smaller units called disaccharides, which are later converted into monosaccharides (simple sugars), such as glucose and fructose. As mentioned above, people who can't digest fats often eat large amounts of sugar; with excessive sugar intake, they may also develop an amylase deficiency.

Disaccharidases (digest sugar)—Disaccharidases (sometimes called carbohydrases) break down disaccharides into simple sugars. The three major disaccharides are sucrose (cane sugar), lactose (milk sugar), and maltose (grain sugar). The major cause of sugar intolerance is most likely excessive consumption of refined sugars. Just as an enzyme deficiency can produce intolerance to the food digested by that enzyme, eating too much of that food can result in intolerance because the body can't produce enough of the necessary enzyme. Eating too much sugar leads to a deficiency in disaccharidases and sugar intolerance develops.

Cellulase (digests soluble fiber)—Cellulase breaks down the soluble parts of fiber into smaller units, which are eventually converted to glucose. In this process, the soluble fibers beneficial to the body are released. The pancreas can make enzymes similar to those found in plants (including protease, amylase, lipase, and disaccharidases), with one exception—cellulase. Cellulase can be obtained only from foods (all raw fruits, vegetables, and whole grains) or enzyme supplements.

treated with enzyme therapy, their digestive problems are solved almost immediately. More importantly, I know this approach can prevent other problems before they happen."

What Causes Enzyme Deficiencies?

Now that we've outlined the link between poor digestion, enzyme deficiencies, and weight problems, what are some of the factors that can affect digestive function and lead to enzyme deficiencies?

Poor Diet—The body produces only a limited number of digestive enzymes, but it needs many more to stay healthy. We obtain the majority of the enzymes we need in the foods that we eat, specifically in fresh vegetables and fruits. But a steady diet of fast foods or highly processed foods will deplete our body of enzymes. Even a diet which includes ample portions of cooked or processed fruits and vegetables can result in enzyme deficiencies, as enzymes are easily damaged or destroyed by heat during cooking.

Enzyme Poisons—Certain substances act as enzyme poisons, inhibiting their activity in the body. These include heavy metals (lead, cadmium, mercury), pesticides, synthetic substances such as trans-fatty acids in margarine, and many common chemicals used by industry and agriculture. Enzyme poisons can interrupt important metabolic processes in the body, some of which control digestion, fat-burning, and appetite control. Some of the more common enzyme poisons are:

- Pesticides and chemicals
- Hybridization and genetic engineering
- Bovine growth hormone (BGH)
- Pasteurization
- Irradiated food
- Excess intake of unsaturated and hydrogenated fats
- Cooking at high temperatures
- Microwaving
- Radiation and electromagnetic fields
- Geopathic stress zones
- Fluoridated water
- Heavy metals
- Mercury amalgam dental fillings
- Root canals

Insufficient Stomach Acid—Many individuals suffering from an enzyme deficiency also prove to be deficient in hydrochloric acid (HCl), a condition called hypochlorhydria. Factors contributing to hydrochloric acid insufficiency include excess fat and sugar in the diet, overeating, bacterial (*Helicobacter pylori*) infections, weakened adrenal function, and stress. As is the case with enzymes, adequate HCl is absolutely essential for proper digestion. HCl is necessary to activate the stomach enzyme pepsin, which is needed for digesting proteins.

Pancreas Dysfunction—Since the pancreas produces most of the digestive enzymes manufactured by the body, any compromise in the function of this gland can cause serious enzyme deficiencies and problems in digestion. Overeating or eating too many processed, devitalized foods (lacking the vitamins and minerals needed by the pancreas) may exhaust the pancreas. Too little fiber or too much sugar in the diet can decrease pancreas output. Pancreatitis (inflammation of the pancreas) and pancreatic insufficiency (decreased production of enzymes) are side effects of alcoholism.[7]

A Primer on Digestion

Digestion begins in the mouth with digestive enzymes secreted by the salivary glands. These enzymes include amylase, lipase, and some protease. Also at work in the mouth are the enzymes (plant enzymes) present in foods being eaten.

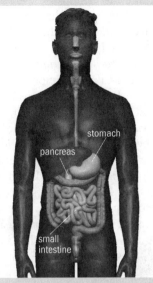

Salivary enzymes combined with the plant enzymes continue digestion in the upper (cardiac) portion of the stomach. Amylase will digest up to 60% of carbohydrates, protease up to 30% of protein, and lipase up to 10% of fat, before HCl (hydrochloric or stomach acid) and pepsin (a stomach enzyme) begin to work in the stomach.

After about an hour, stomach cells secrete enough HCl to further acidify the predigested food to a low pH. This acidic pH temporarily deactivates the plant enzymes and the predigested food passes to the lower portion of the stomach, where cells in the stomach lining secrete more pepsin; it is here that pepsin continues the digestion of protein. Adequate HCl is required to activate pepsin from its inactive enzyme form and to maintain the stomach pH below 3.0, the optimum level for pepsin to work.

In the next stage of digestion, the partially digested food and deactivated plant enzymes pass into the upper part of the small intestine (the duodenum). Here, digestion continues with the help of bile, pancreatic enzymes, and an alkalizing substance (bicarbonate) that reactivates the food enzymes by reducing acidity. Then digestion proceeds to the jejunum (the next section of the small intestine), where disaccharidases (sugar-digesting enzymes) are secreted. From the small intestine, the majority of nutrients from digested food are absorbed into the blood.

Success Story: The Enzyme Road Back to Health

Maria, 52, was a business consultant, a self-confessed "workaholic" in a high-stress job. Because of her busy life, her diet suffered: she typically drank 3-4 cups of coffee for breakfast, often skipped lunch, and ate a late dinner of red meats, fatty foods, and martinis. Maria was entering menopause and was experiencing some severe problems, particularly hot flashes and insomnia. As you might expect, Maria also had numerous other health complaints: a weight problem (she was 5'8" and weighed 185 pounds), high blood pressure (155/90), high cholesterol and triglycerides, digestive problems (heartburn, indigestion, and constipation), and no sex drive.

Maria was primarily interested in losing weight when she consulted Maile Pouls, Ph.D. Dr. Pouls immediately requested that Maria do a 24-hour urinalysis in order to assess her condition. The urinalysis evaluates a person's digestion—what they can or cannot digest as well as any nutritional deficiencies. The results provided the following information about Maria's condition:

■ Maria's kidneys were underfunctioning. This is indicated by the total urine output, which was very low in Maria's case (a condition called oliguria). Maria's heavy daily consumption of coffee and alcohol, plus a low intake of water, created this situation.

For more about **24-hour urinalysis**, see this chapter, pp. 109-112.

■ The urine test also revealed high levels of indican (see "A Glossary of 24-Hour Urine Analysis Terms," p. 111, for explanations of the terms used in this case), which indicated severe toxicity. This was due to her high intake of red meat and alcohol along with poor digestion, according to Dr. Pouls.

■ Maria's pH (SEE QUICK DEFINITION) was 5.1, indicating severe acidity. Again, Maria's diet of coffee, red meat, and alcohol was the main culprit, along with the putrefaction caused by enzyme deficiency and poor digestion.

■ The sediment analysis revealed low levels of calcium phosphate and high levels of uric acid and calcium oxalate, indicating that Maria was low in the enzyme amylase (for digesting carbohydrates), protease (for proteins), and lipase (for fats) and that her overall ability to extract nutrients from food was compromised. "She was basically nutrient deficient," says Dr. Pouls. "She was losing muscle, but was building fat."

■ Because of Maria's menopausal symptoms, Dr. Pouls also had her take a hormone (SEE QUICK DEFINITION) saliva test, which revealed deficiencies in DHEA and progesterone.

For Maria's therapy program, Dr. Pouls had to address not just a simple weight problem, but

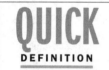

DEFINITION

The term **pH**, which means "potential hydrogen," represents a scale for the relative acidity or alkalinity of a solution. Acidity is measured as a pH of 0.1 to 6.9, alkalinity is 7.1 to 14, and neutral pH is 7.0. The numbers refer to how many hydrogen atoms are present compared to an ideal or standard solution. Normally, blood is slightly alkaline, at 7.35 to 7.45; urine pH can range from 4.8 to 8.0, but is usually somewhat acidic.

Hormones are the chemical messengers of the endocrine system that impose order through an intricate communication system among the body's estimated 50 trillion cells. Examples include the "male" sex hormone (testosterone), the "female" sex hormones (estrogen and progesterone), melatonin (pineal), growth hormone (pituitary), and DHEA (adrenal).

rather a complex set of issues—high toxicity and acid levels in the gastrointestinal tract, cardiovascular problems, and hormonal imbalance due to menopause. First, Dr. Pouls saw a direct correlation between Maria's low water intake and her weight problems. "The easiest way to gain weight is to drink insufficient amounts of water," explains Dr. Pouls. "Water is what flushes the toxins out of the body and helps break down fat and move it out of the system." She told Maria to increase her water intake to a minimum of eight 8-ounce glasses per day and to reduce her salt intake as well.

For Maria's high toxicity (indicated by elevated indican levels), Dr. Pouls recommended that Maria cut down on red meat and start eating more chicken and fish. She told Maria to quit skipping meals, because that can permanently lower the metabolic rate and intensify hunger and food cravings, leading to additional weight gain. Also, she advised Maria to reduce her use of artificial sweeteners, which, according to Dr. Pouls, can slow the digestive process and even cause some people to gain weight.

She also gave Maria an herbal liver support formula called Liv-52 (one capsule, three times daily) along with a fiber supplement. Both of these would help relieve Maria's constipation and restore normal bowel function, moving toxins and fats out of the body and lowering indican levels. Dr. Pouls recommended two enzyme formulas, Ness #5 and Ness #18, to address Maria's excess weight and high cholesterol and triglyceride levels. Both contain lipase (the enzyme that digests fat) and other enzymes to help the body process fat (including cholesterol deposits and triglycerides).

For digestive support, Dr. Pouls recommended a probiotic supplement, 401 Ness, which contains the "friendly" bacteria *Lactobacillus acidophilus* for intestinal support. She also suggested Gastritis Complex (two capsules, three times daily), containing enzymes, rice bran oil extract, marshmallow (*Althea officinalis*), and slippery elm (*Ulmus fulva*), for soothing Maria's heartburn and indigestion.

To reduce Maria's acidity, Dr. Pouls put her on a chlorophyll supplement (two capsules, twice per day). "The greener the vegetable, the more alkaline it is," says Dr. Pouls. "Chlorophyll is the most alkaline food you can get." It is also helpful for lowering cholesterol levels and coats and heals the lining of the intestinal tract. To help Maria's cardiovascular system (which was overtaxed because of her high blood pressure and elevated cholesterol), she recommended CardioProtector (one capsule, three times daily), which contains coenzyme Q10 and other nutrients to improve oxygenation of the heart.

**"The easiest way to gain weight is to drink insufficient amounts of water,"
explains Dr. Maile Pouls. "Water is what flushes the toxins out of the body and
helps break down fat and move it out of the system."**

For Maria's menopause symptoms, Dr. Pouls recommended a soy
protein powder, Nutra-Soy™, from Narula Research. Soy contains
phytoestrogens (substances with mild estrogenic activity), which can
decrease hot flashes and are helpful for preventing osteoporosis, the
bone loss that often accompanies menopause. She also added mineral
supplements—calcium, magnesium, and boron—as additional measures to prevent bone loss (magnesium also helps lower high blood
pressure). For the insomnia, she recommended a formula called
Tranquility and Sleep Support, containing enzymes, along with valer-
ian, passionflower, chamomile, GABA (gamma-aminobutyric acid),
and kava kava, which help ease stress and induce sleep.

After two months on this program, Maria had lost 15 pounds. Her
blood pressure, cholesterol, and triglycerides were all down, but not
yet to normal levels. Her constipation was gone, but she still had a
touch of indigestion. The hot flashes had decreased and she was sleeping better as well. Maria was drinking more water and had successfully adjusted her diet. This was revealed on a second urinalysis, which
showed that total urine output had increased, indican was down, pH
was up to a much less acidic 5.9, and sediment levels were reduced,
indicating better overall nutrient absorption. "She's no longer in a
state of anabolism [fat building]," states Dr. Pouls.

Dr. Pouls made a few adjustments to Maria's supplement program
at this point. She started her on a colon-cleansing program and
prescibed a topical progesterone cream (to help balance her hormones
and relieve the menopause symptoms). Dr. Pouls also added two supplements: Fat Burner, which contains enzymes and amino acids (such
as choline, carnitine, and inositol) that help the body convert fat into

Maile Pouls, Ph.D.: 517 Liberty Street, Santa Cruz, CA 95060; tel/fax: 831-425-2222. For **Ness enzymes**, contact: Ness, 100 NW Business Park Lane, Riverside, MO 64150; tel: 800-637-7893 or 816-746-6461. For **Liv-52** and **magnesium glycinate**, contact: Metagenics West, Inc., 12445 East 39th Avenue, Suite 402, Denver, CO 80239; tel: 800-321-META or 303-371-6848; fax: 303-371-9303. For **Gastritis Complex**, contact: Tyler Encapsulations, 2204-8 NW Birdsdale, Gresham, OR 97030; tel: 800-869-9705 or 503-661-5401; fax: 503-666-4913. For **Chlorophyll Complex Perles**, contact: Standard Process of Northern California, Inc., 1000 Atlantic Avenue, Suite 109, Alameda, CA 94501; tel: 800-662-9134 or 510-865-4322; fax: 510-865-4335. For **CardioProtector**, contact: Phyto-Therapy, Inc., Optimum Health, 483 West Middle Turnpike, Manchester, CT 06040; tel: 800-228-1507 or 860-647-9729. For **Nutra-Soy**, contact: Narula Research, 107 Boulder Bluff Trail, Chapel Hill, NC 27516. For **Tranquility and Sleep Support** and **Digestion and Stomach Upset Support**, contact: Healthy Alternatives, 2222 E. Cliff Drive, Suite 4B, Santa Cruz, CA 95062; tel: 800-962-4414 or 831-477-1040. For **Fat Burner**, contact: Health Plus Inc., 13837 Magnolia Avenue, Chino, CA 91710; tel: 800-822-6225 or 909-627-9393. For **Citrimax**, contact: Nature's Herbs, 600 East Quality Drive, American Fork, UT 84003; tel: 800-437-2257 or 801-763-0700; fax: 801-763-0789.

energy; and Citrimax, containing an herbal extract (*Garcinia cambogia*) that acts as a natural appetite suppressant.

After four months, Maria had lost a total of 32 pounds, her blood pressure (122/80) and cholesterol levels were normal, her digestive problems and constipation were gone, and she had no more hot flashes. Even her sex drive had returned. "She was incredibly pleased with the results," says Dr. Pouls. "Maria had completely shifted her diet, joined a gym, and she also had a new boyfriend."

How to Diagnose an Enzyme Deficiency

If you have been gaining weight and have suffered from symptoms of indigestion (such as gas, bloating, heartburn), your digestion may be impaired. Several diagnostic tools are available to assess both the function of your digestion and your potential need for additional enzymes: a 24-hour urine analysis, palpation test, and tests for stomach acidity.

Urine Analysis

Many alternative health-care professionals rely on urine analysis to assess a patient's digestive function and enzyme status. Dr. Pouls says that "it is crucial to look at as many issues involved in a health problem as possible and, for this, a 24-hour urine analysis is indispensable."[8] The urinalysis provides information on what a person cannot digest, absorb, or assimilate, along with any potential nutritional deficiencies one might have. This test is prognostic rather than diagnostic, except for the identification of substances, such as glucose, not normally found in the urine, which would indicate disease conditions (this is the focus of standard urine tests). In other words, it predicts what lies ahead if you do not clean up your diet and digestion.

Dr. Loomis emphasizes that an individual's total urine output over a 24-hour period must be collected, not just periodic samples. This enables a physician to see how the concentrations of various substances in the urine change over time.[9] The fluctuations are then averaged to give a complete picture of digestive problems. Looking at a 24-hour urinalysis is a way of peeking at the blood, explains Dr. Loomis. The health of the blood takes precedence in the body and cells will sacrifice nutrients in the service of maintaining the blood's relatively narrow pH range of 7.35 to 7.45 as well as its supply of electrolytes (SEE QUICK DEFINITION), protein, and other nutrients. Thus, the blood takes what it needs from the cells to achieve its necessary balance, or homeostasis.

QUICK

A Profile of Your Digestion—If a nutrient does not appear in the urine, it means the blood is using all there is. For example, there is a healthy threshold level of urinary calcium. If the level is lower in the urine test, it indicates that the blood has no calcium to spare and may even be taking calcium out of the cells and the bone, a condition that may lead to osteoporosis. On the other hand, levels of nutrients in the urine may be higher than what is considered normal, meaning the blood is dumping excess nutrients into the urine. For example, the urine test can show too much calcium or chloride (an electrolyte salt). High chloride levels can mean you are eating too much salt or have a lipase deficiency. (See "A Glossary of 24-Hour Urine Analysis Terms" for explanations of the terms used in this discussion.) An overly acidic urine pH means that the blood is dumping excess acid reserves into the urine in order to maintain its optimum pH. An overly alkaline urine pH means the reverse—the blood is dumping excess alkaline reserves into the urine.

The 24-hour urine test also shows whether a person has normal kidney function or if there is kidney-lymphatic stress. The lymphatic system becomes exhausted by working to neutralize allergens (substances which produce an allergic reaction) and environmental toxins. When this occurs, allergens and toxins build up in the bloodstream and the kidneys then become stressed from trying to cleanse the blood. Urine volume (the total output over the 24-hour period) in relationship to specific gravity (density of the urine) shows whether the person is suffering from kidney-lymphatic stress. A normal or low urine volume with a low specific gravity indicates a kidney-lymphatic stress pattern. If the urine volume is normal or high and the specific gravity is also high, it means there are substances in the urine which should not be there.

The urine test also determines what you cannot digest or are eating in excess. This is revealed by the total sediment analysis, which measures levels of calcium phosphate, calcium oxalate, and uric acid. Low phosphates indicate sugar intolerance or excessive consumption of sugar. High calcium oxalate indicates fat intolerance or excess. High uric acid indicates protein intolerance or excess.

Finally, the indican value indicates colon toxicity and the degree to which digestion is malfunctioning. Indican is a group of toxic com-

A Glossary of 24-Hour Urine Analysis Terms

The following are specific values measured in a 24-hour urine analysis:

Volume—The total urine output, either excessive (polyuria) or inadequate (oliguria), in relationship to the specific gravity indicates how well the kidneys are functioning.

Specific Gravity—This value measures the weight of total dis-

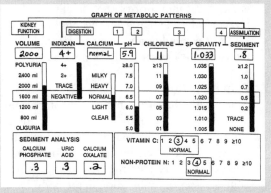

GRAPH OF METABOLIC PATTERNS

KIDNEY FUNCTION	DIGESTION 1 2		3		4 ASSIMILATION	
VOLUME	INDICAN	CALCIUM	pH	CHLORIDE	SP GRAVITY	SEDIMENT
2000	**4+**	**normal**	**5.9**	**11**	**1.033**	**.8**
POLYURIA	4+		≥8.0	≥13	1.035	≥1.2
2400 ml	2+	MILKY	7.5	11	1.030	1.0
2000 ml	TRACE	HEAVY	7.0	09	1.025	0.7
1600 ml	NEGATIVE	NORMAL	6.5	07	1.020	0.5
1200 ml		LIGHT	6.0	05	1.015	0.2
800 ml		CLEAR	5.5	03	1.010	TRACE
OLIGURIA			5.0	01	1.005	NONE

SEDIMENT ANALYSIS

CALCIUM PHOSPHATE	URIC ACID	CALCIUM OXALATE
.3	.3	.2

VITAMIN C: 1 2 ③ 4 5 6 7 8 9 ≥10
NORMAL

NON-PROTEIN N: 1 2 3 ④ 5 6 7 8 9 ≥10
NORMAL

URINALYSIS RESULTS.

solved substances in the urine against an equal amount of water, such that a normal reading of 1.020 means the urine is 2% heavier than water. Specific gravity shows the general water content (hydration) of the body. The optimum range for specific gravity is 1.018 to 1.022.

Indican—This indicates the degree of toxicity, putrefaction, gas, and fermentation in the intestines. Indican comes from putrefying undigested food in the large intestine that is kicked back into the blood and excreted through the kidneys. Indican is extremely toxic and causes many symptoms; the higher the level, the greater the intestinal toxemia or inflammation in the digestive tract. Readings as close to zero as possible are desirable.

pH—Based on hydrogen ion concentration, this value indicates the degree of urine acidity versus alkalinity on a scale of zero to 14, with optimum urine pH ranging from 6.3 to 6.7.

Chlorides—These are salt residues in the urine and the values provide information on salt intake and/or lipase adequacy.

Total Sediment Analysis—This indicates the amount of dissolved organic and mineral substances remaining in the urine after digestion; a normal reading for the three sediment categories (calcium phosphate, uric acid, and calcium oxalate) is 0.4-0.6.

■ Calcium phosphate—This indicates the status of carbohydrate digestion; a reading of 0.4-0.6 signifies normal carbohydrate processing.

■ Uric acid—Levels of uric acid signify the status of protein digestion; optimal digestion yields a reading of less than 0.1.

■ Calcium oxalate—This value indicates the status of fat digestion; a reading of less than 0.1 signifies optimal fat digestion.

Vitamin C—Levels of vitamin C indicate body reserves of this key nutrient; a reading of 1-5 is normal, over 5 deficient.

pounds which are formed when undigested protein is decomposed by pathogenic bacteria in the small intestine. The level of urinary indican is a general indicator of the inability to digest food—the higher the level of indican, the greater the digestive problem. There is one exception to this: undigested sugar interferes with the indican test, so zero indican indicates severe sugar intolerance.

Palpation Test

Along with the urine analysis, an important information-gathering procedure in enzyme therapy is the palpation test. Palpation means to elicit information by touch. Pain and internal organ dysfunction are always accompanied by muscle contraction. The enzyme therapist uses palpation to identify these places of muscle contraction to pinpoint stresses or dysfunction in the body. Dr. Loomis developed a palpation test in which each positive palpation point (meaning there is a muscle contraction) corresponds to a deviation in structure (vertebral subluxation), which, in turn, corresponds to an undernourished organ.[10] Each palpation point also corresponds to one of his enzyme formulations, so palpation serves as both diagnosis and guideline for treatment.

Thera-zyme Challenge Food Powder contains fig, psyllium seed husk, fennel seed, flaxseed, pumpkin seed, and guar gum, providing a balance of protein, carbohydrates, fat, and fiber. For more information about **Thera-zyme enzyme formulas,** see this chapter, pp. 119-120.

For the test, patients must fast for at least two hours. With the patient lying face-up on a chiropractic table, the practitioner first observes the position of the hips and feet. In most people, one hip is higher or lower than the other, and sometimes one leg is longer or shorter than the other. Then, the practitioner tests palpation points by touch and observes any shift in the position of the hips or leg lengths following palpation. Any observed shift (for example, the hips, which were uneven, become even) indicates a positive palpation, which means that the person may need the enzyme formulation corresponding to this palpation point. This phase of the test can also reveal nutritional deficiencies and acute conditions such as viral or bacterial infections. Then, the patient either eats a meal or consumes a tablespoon of Thera-zyme Challenge Food Powder (a nutritional supplement equal to a complete meal). After 45 minutes, the palpation test is repeated. Positive palpation points now indicate what the body cannot digest. They also indicate acute and chronic conditions, including inflammation, kidney or urinary tract problems, soft tissue trauma, allergies, and colon problems.

Testing Stomach Acidity

To determine if insufficient hydrochloric acid (HCl) is a contributing factor to digestive problems, the pH analysis performed as part of the

24-hour urinalysis can indirectly measure HCl levels in the stomach. In addition, a simple and inexpensive test used by many practitioners called the gastro test can also assesses the adequacy of HCl by measuring pH.[11]

Ralph Golan, M.D., a practitioner based in Seattle, Washington, describes the test procedure: "After an overnight fast, the gastro capsule is swallowed. This special weighted capsule has a string protruding from one end, which is held while the capsule is swallowed. The capsule carries the remaining string to the stomach, where the capsule melts and the highly absorbent cotton string soaks up gastric juices. Within fifteen minutes, the string is gently pulled out and tested for its pH." If the acid reading is normal, the patient takes a baking soda challenge (3 tsp in water) to see if the stomach can reacidify. The test is then repeated after 40 minutes. If after one or two challenge tests the stomach shows low acidity, this indicates that the patient may not be producing sufficient HCl.[12]

Another more expensive but also more accurate test is the Heidelberg gastrogram. This test, also called the "tubeless gastric analysis," is another way of showing abnormal conditions of acidity or alkalinity in the stomach or small intestine. The patient swallows a miniature electronic transmitter encased within a small capsule; once inside the stomach, the capsule transmits radio signals that show changing pH values after meals. When these fluctuations of pH are plotted on a graph, the resulting display is called a gastrogram. The testing capsule remains active for about 22 hours and is eventually eliminated.

For more about the **Heidelberg pH gastrogram**, contact: Heidelberg International, Inc., 933 Beasley Street, Blairsville, GA 30512; tel: 706-745-9698; fax: 706-781-6229.

For more about how an **underactive thyroid contributes to weight gain**, see Chapter 9: Overcome a Sluggish Thyroid, pp. 202-219. For more about **hormone imbalance and weight gain**, see Chapter 10: Restore Hormonal Balance, pp. 220-243.

Alternative Medicine Approach to Healthy Digestion

If your digestion is impaired, you may want to look into potential underlying factors, such as a toxic colon, an underactive thyroid, or food allergies (see the other chapters on these underlying factors for more information). There are also a number of therapy options available that can help you digest more efficiently and lose weight at the same time. Weight gain may be the result of not properly digesting the food you're eating: if you're not getting all the nutrients out of your meals, you may overeat to make up for it. The remedy may be as easy as choosing the right foods to eat or chewing your food more thoroughly. Enzyme supplements can help normalize your digestion and increase the absorption of nutrients. If your stomach acid is insufficient, dietary changes and supplements can alleviate this problem as well.

Dietary Recommendations

To ensure that your body gets the enzymes it needs for optimum digestion, the best approach is to go to the source—your diet. It should be enzyme-rich, with a variety of organic, whole, unprocessed foods. Foods in their whole, unaltered state have the ideal ratio of enzymes needed to digest them. For example, an apple, which is high in carbohydrates, contains more amylase than an avocado, which has a high concentration of fat and is high in lipase.

■ Eat plenty of organic, raw fruits and vegetables. While all fruits and vegetables contain enzymes, papayas and pineapples are two particularly good enzyme sources. Papaya contains the enzyme papain and pineapple contains the enzyme bromelain, both useful for helping you digest proteins. Other foods promoting protease (the enzyme that digests protein) activity include asparagus, ginger, and figs.[13]

■ Fermented foods, such as miso and raw sauerkraut, contain live enzymes that aid digestion. Soy sauce, a fermented brew of soy flour and barley, also contains highly active enzymes that help digest protein.

■ Freshly made vegetable juices are a good source of enzymes. However, they should be used to augment—not replace—whole, fresh vegetables in your diet. Fruit juices, while beneficial, should be ingested sparingly, since they contain high levels of fructose (a natural sugar). Carrots, also high in natural sugars, should be eaten in small amounts as well.

For more about **sugar and its effect on the body**, see Chapter 8: Strengthen Your Sugar Controls, pp. 184-201.

■ Aged garlic extract and "green" foods, such as green barley, wheat grass, and algae, can also contribute more enzymes to your diet. For example, green barley alone contains over 20 enzymes.[14]

Enzyme-Friendly Food Preparation—Enzymes in food are destroyed once heated above 118° F.[15] Pasteurization, canning, or microwaving are particularly destructive to food enzymes, due to the extreme heat involved in these methods of food preparation. So, it is best to avoid, if possible, foods processed in these ways, because they have probably been stripped of most of their nutrients, including enzymes. Foods should be eaten raw or, at the most, lightly steamed. There are a few exceptions: seeds, nuts, grains, and beans have enzyme inhibitors that must be deactivated by soaking, cooking, or sprouting. Cruciferous vegetables,

Success Story: Enzymes for Hidden Allergies and Weight Gain

Beatrice, 38, had a history of being overweight and had undergone a hysterectomy at the age of 24, but claimed she felt well otherwise. However, her health took a turn for the worse after she was exposed to chemicals in the workplace. "Around Christmas, I started a new job," she recalls. "There was extensive painting and varnishing of floors going on while I worked 10-hour days. Four days after I started, I began to feel sick and developed severe hives. After eight weeks, I had the following symptoms: severe swelling of my face, throat, tongue, hands, and feet; raised, rope-like hives over my entire body; pain between my shoulder blades, in my throat, and under my right rib cage; vomiting after meals; diarrhea; and weight gain of 50 pounds."

Beatrice sought the help of Dr. Lita Lee. Her conventional doctors had given Beatrice a cocktail of drugs for her problems: prednisone (a corticosteroid drug) for her hives, epinephrine (adrenaline), Prozac® for depression, Doxepin and Hismanal® (antihistamines), and Zantac® (an antacid required after taking prednisone). At one point, she was taking nine different antihistamines to stop the hives and swelling of her throat, but nothing worked. Her doctors had told Beatrice that they found no evidence of allergy problems (based on the results of standard allergy blood tests). But Dr. Lee had Beatrice do a urine test, which did reveal serious allergies, and Beatrice herself reported being allergic to cats, bee stings, and molds. Her allergy symptoms included swollen glands, headaches, nausea, and vomiting.

Beatrice's urine test also revealed severe fat and sugar intolerance, vitamin C deficiency, and excess acidity. A physical exam and palpation test revealed the need for 14 enzymes—a severe level of depletion. Dr. Lee put Beatrice on a multiple-enzyme program:

- Digestive enzymes and herbs to help fat and sugar digestion
- Enzymes plus the herb burdock root and bioflavonoids for her hives
- An enzyme formula with alfalfa juice, rosehips, echinacea, and other herbs for her allergies
- A fiber formula for colon cleansing

In addition, she gave Beatrice a thyroid extract (to boost her underfunctioning thyroid) and natural progesterone cream to balance her hormones. Both hypothyroidism and hormone imbalance can contribute to weight problems.

During the first three months on this program, Beatrice was able to stop taking all of her prescription drugs with no adverse side effects. First, the hives went away and then she experienced less vomiting; it stopped completely before the end of the third month. Enzymes were the key to normalizing her digestion and eliminating her allergy symptoms. At the end of three months, she had dropped 25 pounds.

Lita Lee, Ph.D.:
P.O. Box 516,
Lowell, OR 97452;
tel: 541-937-1123;
fax: 541-937-1132.

such as broccoli, cabbage, cauliflower, and Brussels sprouts, contain compounds that can inhibit the function of the thyroid gland and should not be eaten raw. In general, when cooking foods, advises Dr. Lee, choose low heat or slow cooking methods. Also, use salt sparingly, as it indirectly causes enzymes to become inactive.[16]

Chew Properly

It may sound simplistic, but one of the easiest ways to improve your digestion is by thorough chewing. "Chewing your food well is a great weight-loss technique, helping you get the most from every bite," says Dr. Loomis. Chewing is especially important when eating fresh fruits and vegetables, because the cells of a plant have rigid outer membranes (cell walls) that are composed of tough cellulose fibers. Chewing vegetables and fruits thoroughly helps to break down these cell walls and release the enzymes and other important nutrients contained inside the cells.[17]

Dr. Loomis points out that some people may have problems digesting uncooked food because they are deficient in cellulase, the enzyme which breaks down cellulose fibers. "People who rarely eat raw food can have problems when they finally eat uncooked fruits and vegetables because they don't chew their food thoroughly," he says. "Chewing liberates the cellulase from the food, but when you eat raw food and don't chew properly, the cellulase is never released." In addition, cellulase can be destroyed by pesticides and other chemical sprays used to treat vegetables. Dr. Loomis states that "some supermarket vegetables are missing cellulase because they have been sprayed with sulfites [a type of preservative], which can destroy these enzymes."[18]

Chewing also signals the digestive tract to begin releasing enzymes and other digestive juices. This helps to increase feelings of satiety and, in turn, reduces appetite. "When food is not properly chewed, there is a chain reaction: enzyme action is inhibited, digestion is hampered, and every bite provides less nutritional benefit," Dr. Cichoke explains. "This leaves you feeling less satisfied, so you are likely to eat more." Chewing actually stimulates the satiety center of the brain, the hypothalamus—the more you chew, the more the hypothalamus is activated, leading to a feeling of fullness. Without adequate chewing, you still feel hungry even though you are eating, because the brain is not getting the proper signals.

Researchers Mary Wagner, R.D., and Mark Hewitt, M.D., of the School of Public Health and Medicine at the University of Minnesota in Minneapolis, studied the relationship of chewing time to obesity.

They observed the chewing behavior of 31 adult patients in a local hospital. The researchers found that obese patients spent less time consuming their meals and chewed each mouthful of food for a shorter time than those who were not overweight; the obese subjects also ate all the food available to them. The researchers concluded that when food passes rapidly through the mouth, the body has less of a chance to respond to it. Individuals who eat quickly are therefore less likely to sense that they are full and continue eating.[19]

Counting Your Chews—So how do you know if you are chewing enough? Some health practitioners recommend counting each chew. If you're not chewing at least 20 times per mouthful, they say, you're not chewing enough and need to train yourself to slow down. One effective way to do this is with the Mayr Method, a procedure used to teach individuals proper chewing habits. The method involves eating dry bread rolls, each morning and before each meal, in order to stimulate salivary flow. When using this method, each mouthful of food is chewed at least 50 times, until the food becomes a paste. The breakfast meal consists of a dry roll, which should be eaten in small bites with no fluids consumed at all. When the bite of roll has become a paste, place one teaspoonful of yogurt (containing live cultures) into your mouth. Chew this mixture a few more times (adding up to a total of 50 chews) and then swallow. Continue following each mouthful of bread paste with teaspoons of yogurt until the entire roll is consumed.

Following this procedure should leave you satisfied and you will not need to eat anything else for breakfast. Thirty minutes after breakfast, you should have some herbal tea, such as pau d'arco (*Tabebuia impetiginosa*), lemon verbena (*Hippia citriodora*), linden blossom (*Tillia europaea*), fennel (*Foeniculum vulgare*), or sage (*Salvia officinalis*). Lunch consists of another dry roll (consumed as above), followed by lightly cooked vegetables along with a vegetarian, fish, or lean meat main course. Again, no liquid is consumed with the meal, but herbal tea should follow 30 minutes later. The evening meal should consist of another dry roll, followed with yogurt, lightly cooked vegetables, and herbal tea. While following this program, you should avoid all fruits, raw vegetables, fatty foods, alcohol, coffee, or sugar.[20] The Mayr Method can be used for as long as it takes to adjust your eating habits.

Enzyme Support
In addition to changing your diet to increase your enzyme intake, you may also need an enzyme supplement to help restore your digestive

function. Enzyme supplements come in two basic forms: pancreatic enzymes and plant enzymes. The pancreatic enzymes, also called pancreatins, are made from extracts of the pancreas glands of animals; plant enzymes are derived from natural food sources. Plant enzymes are prescribed primarily to enhance the body's vitality by strengthening the digestive system, while pancreatic enzymes have historically been used to benefit both the digestive system and immune system. For strict vegetarians (vegans) and individuals allergic to beef and pork, plant enzymes can be used to aid the immune system as well as to support food digestion.

"Conventional medicine's position is that all enzyme supplements are useless, because they are destroyed by the hydrochloric acid in the stomach," says Richard Shwery, O.M.D., Ac.Phys., an acupuncturist and nutritional consultant in Cary, North Carolina. "But this is simply not true. I've been using plant enzymes with my patients for more than five years, and I have seen for myself the important role they can play in restoring gastrointestinal health." HCl does not destroy the enzymes; rather, it merely deactivates them. They are reactivated later in the duodenum (upper segment of the small intestine), where the food is made less acidic by secretions from the pancreas and other organs.

In addition to their crucial role in digestion, enzymes directly assist the defense mechanisms of the immune system. Enzymes taken between meals act like "little Pac men" in the bloodstream, says Dr. Pouls, getting rid of unwanted material. With their ability to digest foreign proteins, enzymes are useful in clearing out infectious organisms, scar tissue, and the products of inflammation.

Enzymes in Your Genes

Your genes are one of the connections between enzymes and obesity. Lipase, an enzyme produced by the body, helps transport fat from the blood into storage in fat cells. The higher the lipase level, the more predisposed you are to store fat. Your inherent lipase level is partly determined by your heredity, which is one reason why, if your parents are obese, you probably have higher lipase levels than the children of thin parents, predisposing you to store more fat. Dieting will actually worsen this situation, because a low-calorie diet makes lipase more efficient at storing fat. According to a study published in the New England Journal of Medicine, this enzyme also causes some dieters to regain the weight they lost during a diet.[21]

When the body receives adequate enzymes from foods or supplements, the pancreas doesn't have to work as hard to manufacture enzymes for digestion. It is this easing of the body's enzyme workload that is thought to contribute substantially to the healing effects of enzyme therapy. When the body receives plentiful supplies of enzymes, according to Dr. Howell, "its internal enzyme supplies are preserved for the important work of maintaining metabolic harmony." As a result, immune function and many other body systems are strengthened.[22]

How to Take Enzymes—Depending on the situation, some enzymes are given with meals to facilitate the breakdown and assimilation of food, while some are given between meals to act as "scavengers" of abnormal protein found in the bloodstream. Enzymes that may be given with meals include protease, amylase, and lipase. Protease and lipase may also be given between meals to function as protein scavengers. As with all health problems, the proper enzyme therapy depends on the cause of the condition in the particular individual, but the following enzyme formulas (developed by Dr. Loomis and available from 21st Century Nutrition in Madison, Wisconsin) are ones that Dr. Lee commonly uses for clients with weight problems:

EDITOR'S NOTE

In the early 1980s, Howard Loomis, D.C., formulated his first line of enzymes called NESS (Nutritional Enzyme Support System), which was introduced in 1987. Over the past ten years, Loomis' continuing research has led to Thera-zyme, his second generation of enzymes. The Thera-zyme line is only available to professional health-care practitioners, but these formulas have a counterpart in a line of formulas called Enzyme Solutions, available to the consumer. For more information about Thera-zyme enzyme formulas or Enzyme Solutions, contact: 21st Century Nutrition, 6421 Enterprise Lane, Madison, WI 53719; tel: 800-662-2630 or 608-273-8100; fax: 608-273-8111.

■ Thera-zyme VSCLR (Vascular) or Enzyme & Herbal Formula #2—For people who have trouble losing weight (however, other digestive problems must also be addressed, such as sugar and protein intolerance). Contains the enzymes protease, amylase, and lipase, plus the following herbs: bilberry extract, fenugreek seeds, *Ginkgo biloba* leaf, and dandelion root.

■ Thera-zyme T9-L1 SmI (Small intestine)—For people whose weight problem is due to candidiasis (overgrowth of the yeast-like fungus *Candida albicans*). Contains a special form of cellulase that digests pathogenic yeast, disaccharidases, and beneficial bacteria (*L. casei*, *L. acidophilus*, *Bifidobacterium longum*, and others) for intestinal support.

■ Thera-zyme TRMA (Trauma) or Enzyme & Herbal Formula #28—To support a weak immune system; most effective when combined with SmI and a whole foods diet low in refined sugars. Contains the enzymes protease, amylase, lipase, and disaccharidases, calcium lactate, and kelp, a source of minerals.

See *The Enzyme Cure* by Lita Lee, Ph.D., and Lisa Turner, with Burton Goldberg (Future Medicine Publishing, 1998; ISBN 1-887299-22-X); to order, call 800-333-HEAL.

■ Thera-zyme C2-L5 IVD (Intervertebral disc) or Enzyme & Herbal Formula #5—For musculoskeletal support; can help decrease a big appetite. Contains the enzymes protease, amylase, lipase, and disaccharidases, plus nettle leaf, prickly ash bark, marshmallow root, and rose hips.

There is no doubt that enzymes are important for proper digestion and can help you to lose weight. Nevertheless, they should be considered as part of an overall program for health, not as a way to counterbalance an otherwise unhealthy lifestyle. Dr. Pouls makes sure that her patients understand that enzymes alone will not heal them. "I never tell my patients that enzymes are a magic bullet or that we're going to 'cure' anything," she says. "Rather, I say we will balance your chemistry, build up your enzyme and nutrient reserve, improve your digestion, and then watch many of the symptoms disappear as the body's innate wisdom takes charge."[23]

Therapies for Insufficient Stomach Acid

If insufficient hydrochloric acid (HCl), a conditon known as hypochlorhydria, is a factor in your poor digestive function, there are a number of steps you can take to remedy this situation:

■ Thoroughly chew your food.

■ Reduce your stress level at meal times.

■ Avoid excessive amounts of fat and sugar in your diet.

■ Have yourself tested for potential underlying problems, such as adrenal stress, hypothyroidism, or *Helicobacter pylori* infection.

■ Take bitter herbs, such as gentian, goldenseal, and Swedish bitters, to promote the secretion of digestive juices.

People who are taking nonsteroidal, anti-inflammatory drugs (like cortisone or aspirin) should not take additional betaine hydrochloride, as it could cause ulcers. Hydrochloric acid supplementation should be under medical supervision, as it is possible to take too much betaine hydrochloride without any immediately evident symptoms, which could lead to ulcers or serious bleeding in the stomach.

If these measures prove ineffective, you may want to consider (in consultation with a health-care provider) taking hydrochloric acid supplements. The most common form of supplement is betaine hydrochloride (an edible compound that forms hydrochloric acid in the stomach), available at most health food stores. Typically, physicians recommend taking one capsule (usually 5-10 grains) at the beginning of each meal. If after three days, this does not cause any adverse symptoms (heartburn, abdominal pain, nausea), the dose can be increased to two capsules, then three capsules, per meal. If symptoms do occur, reduce your dosage. (You can quickly neutralize any adverse effect by drinking milk, eating yogurt, or taking a bicarbonate like baking soda).[24]

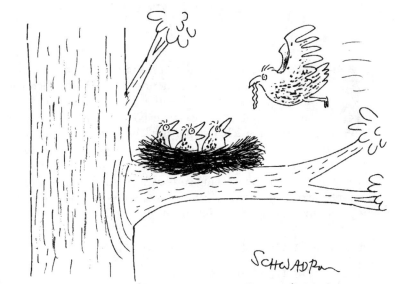

"WAIT A MINUTE! WHAT ABOUT THOSE REPORTS THAT WORMS ARE TERRIBLY HIGH IN CHOLESTEROL?"

5 Optimize Your Calorie Burning

THE BODY, when healthy, burns rather than stores excess calories in a process called thermogenesis. Even when you are asleep, you are still breathing, your heart is beating, your brain cells are active, your body temperature remains constant—these bodily functions burn calories. Your body also wastes a certain number of calories on a daily basis. Focusing exclusively on diet to control weight can fail if your normal calorie-burning processes aren't working correctly. A careful combination of nutrients, herbs, and exercise can get your calorie-burning fires on the job again and help you maintain a healthy body weight.

Success Story: Fat-Burning Herbs Help Shed Pounds

In This Chapter

Patrick, 35, had dieted many times to try to lose weight. Although he would usually succeed in losing a few pounds, he always gained it all back again. At one time, his weight reached as high as 400 pounds. His constant dieting and inability to lose weight caused him considerable grief. "I stopped going to the gym," he said, "because I was uncomfortable with how I looked and I was having so much trouble with my back, legs, and feet."

Patrick finally consulted chiropractor Roger Bond, D.C., of Salt Lake City, Utah, who put him on Thermogenics Plus™, an herbal formula used to stimulate thermogenesis, the process by which the body generates heat during normal metabolism. Thermogenics Plus contains the herb ephedra along with caffeine and aspirin, a combination that stimulates the body to burn calories faster, according to the manufacturer. "I used it three times a day, five days per week, and ate normally," said Patrick. "The only restrictions were to avoid high-fat foods and 'junk' foods, but I never went hungry, as I had on other diets." Because of his large size, Patrick's results were not immediately noticeable. "Although I was losing, I still looked huge for months," he said. Over the next several months, however, Patrick began to shed the pounds and the benefits included more than just a slimmer waistline. "I had more energy than I'd had in a long time. I even started walking and lifting weights again," he said. With the help of the thermogenic treatment, Patrick lost 200 pounds and has not gained it back.

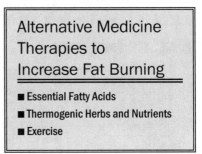

Alternative Medicine Therapies to Increase Fat Burning

- Essential Fatty Acids
- Thermogenic Herbs and Nutrients
- Exercise

For information about **Thermogenics Plus**, contact: Silver Sage, P.O. Box 1117, Draper, UT 84020; tel: 800-842-2742 or 801-571-6500; fax: 801-571-6545.

Dr. Bond has successfully treated many of his patients with thermogenic formulas. Dr. Bond admits, however, that he did not always prescribe thermogenic treatments. In fact, he had once been skeptical about using them. "As a rule, I'm suspicious, but the science behind thermogenesis was pretty impressive. I even decided to try it myself—after two months, I lost two inches from my waist and no longer had the impulse to snack during the day."

Increase Your Calorie-Burning and Lose Weight

Even though he dieted and exercised, Patrick still couldn't lose weight, but he was finally able to obtain significant and lasting weight reduction by boosting his body's ability to burn off calories (SEE QUICK DEFINITION). Weight loss can be boiled down to a simple concept: you have to use or burn off more calories than you take in through food. If your calorie intake matches your body's fuel needs, you will main-

"It's not simply a question of how much you eat or how little you exercise. It's a question of how effectively your body's systems use the calories that you ingest," says Daniel Mowrey, Ph.D.

tain a constant weight. But when you take in more calories than you burn off, weight gain is the result, as Patrick knew only too well.

Diets focus on reducing calorie intake, a sometimes difficult prospect for those troubled with excess weight. But you can also lose weight by increasing the number of calories that are burned off. Exercise is probably the method you think of most readily for this, but the body has more than one way to burn off excess calories. Even when you are asleep, you are still breathing, your heart is beating, and every cell is busy keeping you alive—all of these bodily functions burn calories. The body is also constantly using calories to maintain normal body temperature. As Daniel Mowrey, Ph.D., author of *Fat Management: The Thermogenic Factor*, says, "It's not simply a question of how much you eat or how little you exercise. It's a question of how effectively your body's systems use the calories that you ingest." Following a nutritious diet and regular exercise program is still important in achieving a healthy, permanent reduction in body weight, but there are also ways to boost your body's day-to-day calorie-burning (or thermogenic) ability.

In this chapter, we discuss the ways the body burns calories and how this can affect your ability to lose weight. Specifically, we examine how the body normally produces heat—thermogenesis—to carry on its normal functions. When this process is impaired, the calories don't get burned off as quickly and end up stored as fat. So, we'll look at the causes that may hinder the calorie-burning process. Finally, we offer natural therapies for boosting your thermogenesis and reducing unwanted weight, including nutritional supplements, herbal treatments, and exercise.

Thermogenesis: Turning Up the Heat

Stephen Langer, M.D., of Berkeley, California, author of *Solved: The Riddle of Weight Loss*, describes the different ways the body uses calories. "Energy output," he says, "actually breaks down into three parts: basal metabolism (how fast you burn up energy in your cells in a resting state); thermogenesis (energy, in the form of heat, given off above the metabolic resting rate); and, of course, physical exercise."[1] The first two ways of burning calories are unknown to most people. However, when metabolism (SEE QUICK DEFINITION) or thermogenesis is not functioning properly, weight gain often results. To illustrate how this happens, think of them as two streams that flow from a lake (the body's store of calories). Each has a certain rate of flow that helps keep the level of the lake constant—if either stream becomes blocked, the water in the lake will back up and flood the shores. Similarly, if either basal metabolism or thermogenesis is impaired, your body loses one of its outlets

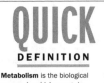

DEFINITION

Metabolism is the biological process by which energy is extracted from the foods consumed, producing carbon dioxide and water as by-products for elimination. Metabolism involves catabolic and anabolic activity. The catabolic function controls digestion, disassembling food into forms the body can use for energy, while the anabolic function produces substances for cell growth and repair.

for burning calories. These calories then accumulate in your body as fat, even if you are dieting and exercising.

"The underlying distinction between the fat and the thin person is not how well they 'use' calories, but how well they 'burn' them," says Dr. Mowrey. The average person uses about 85% of their calorie intake, although some might use up to 88%. The remaining 12% to 15% of calories must be either burned or stored. If this excess cannot be used up, it is stored as fat and you gain weight. This means that if your weight reduction plan focuses on reducing the 85% of essential or usable calories while ignoring what happens to the 15% of excess calories, you will most likely see no benefits.[2]

Lean individuals immediately convert 40% of the calories they consume into heat. In contrast, overweight individuals convert only 10% of the calories they ingest into heat. Daniel Ricquier, Ph.D., a researcher at the Centre National de la Recherche Scientifique in Meudon, France, indicates that a 1% to 2% decrease in an individual's heat-producing ability, which would not necessarily cause any change in body temperature, can result in significant weight gain.[3]

Metabolism—A central concept here is that of basal metabolism: the number of calories used by the body at complete rest to maintain basic life processes such as breathing and circulation. Basal metabolism is controlled by the thyroid gland (the largest endocrine gland, located near the front of the throat, just below the larynx) and keeps the body at a normal, healthy resting temperature of 98.6° F. The thyroid sends chemical messages using hormones to every cell in the body, directing the maintenance of body temperature, heart

For more about the **thyroid gland and how to detect and treat hypothyroidism**, see Chapter 9: Overcome a Sluggish Thyroid, pp. 202-219.

Obesity and Impaired Thermogenesis

A team of researchers in France observed a high correlation between obesity and poor thermogenic activity. The researchers fed glucose (sugar) to a group of women and then measured how their bodies burned off the calories. While the lean women exhibited high thermogenic activity, the overweight women in the group experienced little or no thermogenic response. The researchers also observed that the women who were just starting to become overweight already showed some signs of impaired thermogenesis.[4]

rate, and muscle movements. When the thyroid is dysfunctional or underactive—a condition called hypothyroidism—it sends out fewer hormones, causing basal metabolism to slow down. This slowing causes a number of problems, including general feelings of sluggishness and increases in body weight.

Thermogenesis—As with basal metabolism, the rate of thermogenesis will determine whether the body sheds or accumulates fat. Thermogenesis means, simply, to generate heat in the body during metabolism. The digestion of food, the movement of the muscles, and other metabolic processes all produce heat as a by-product. In certain metabolic activities, however, heat is the primary product. This type of pure thermogenesis is one of the body's key weight control mechanisms and serves as a kind of waste incinerator for excess calories. But when this mechanism does not burn fat as it should, weight gain is sure to follow. To understand how the process works, you need to know about a little-known fat in your body called brown adipose tissue, or brown fat, for short.

Brown Fat—The Body's Calorie-Burning Furnace

"Brown fat may well be the most important discovery to explain why some people can remain thin while eating everything in sight while others, no matter how restricted their caloric intake, still cannot lose weight," says nutritionist Ann Louise Gittleman, M.S., of Bozeman, Montana, author of *Beyond Pritikin*.[5] Why is brown fat so important? Unlike the more common white or yellow fat in the body, this type of fat is "metabolically active," meaning that brown fat cells actually burn calories.

This is possible because brown fat cells contain large numbers of mitochondria (SEE QUICK DEFINITION), cellular components that generate energy through a process called oxidation. Mitochondria are what impart the brownish hue to this type of fat. In comparison, yellow or white fat serves only as an insulator and a warehouse for unused or excess calories (which is why this is the type of fat most people want to shed). Here's a simple way to understand the difference between brown and yellow fat: brown fat is the body's furnace, yellow fat is the fuel.

In most areas of the body, energy loss is minimized, with the energy being conserved as fat. Brown fat, on the other hand, wastes energy by burning more fat and generating more heat.[6] "If your body is not efficient at wasting unneeded calories via brown fat activation, you can't help but gain weight, regardless of how few calories you consume," observes Carol Simontacchi, C.C.N., M.S., author of *Your Fat Is Not Your Fault*. For those who do not have weight problems, the brown fat is able to eliminate any excess calories they consume by burning them to produce body heat. In those who are overweight, however, the excess weight can shut down the mitochondria in brown fat, essentially turning it into yellow fat.[7]

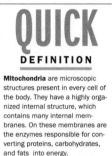

QUICK
DEFINITION

Mitochondria are microscopic structures present in every cell of the body. They have a highly organized internal structure, which contains many internal membranes. On these membranes are the enzymes responsible for converting proteins, carbohydrates, and fats into energy.

"Brown fat may explain why some people can remain thin while eating everything in sight while others, no matter how restricted their caloric intake, still cannot lose weight," says nutritionist Ann Louise Gittleman, M.S.

You can appreciate the importance of brown fat to healthy weight management by considering how much yellow fat you accumulate when brown fat is lost. Dr. Mowrey estimates that a mere 1% loss of brown fat leads to the accumulation of 20-30 pounds of body fat over a period of 10-15 years. When losses of brown fat are more severe, the impact on the body is much greater and can even cancel out the weight-loss effects of diet and exercise.[8]

Brown fat is located deep in the body, near the shoulder blades and extending down the back around the spine; it is also found adjacent to the heart (where it warms the blood), kidneys, and adrenal glands. These are areas of "intense metabolic activity," according to Dr. Mowrey, where "caloric energy is converted into heat energy." When it is healthy, brown fat accounts for approximately 25% of the heat generated in the body, a remarkable percentage given that this type of fat accounts for a mere 0.5%-5.0% of total body weight.[9]

Brown Fat and Your Set Point for Body Weight

One reason dieting often fails has to do with the body's natural set point. Nutritionists Elanor Noss Whitney, Ph.D., R.D., and Marie Anne Boyle, M.S., R.D., authors of *Nutrition and Health*, describe set point as "the body's tendency to settle at a weight plateau for long periods of time."[10] The set point is your equilibrium point for body weight, your physiologically ideal weight. The set point automatically controls your body weight the way a thermostat controls the temperature in your home.

When you gain weight, your body responds by increasing calorie-burning activity, the way the furnace in your home turns on when the room temperature falls below a set temperature. Similarly, when you start to lose weight, your body's calorie-burning furnaces slow down, thus carefully conserving calories. In this way, the body maintains its weight within a narrow range. One of the mechanisms for controlling set point is increasing or decreasing the calorie-burning activity in brown fat. Scientists believe that the set point is what enabled our agrarian ancestors to cope with annual cycles of food abundance and scarcity. Dr. Langer explains, "The basic purpose of the body's set point is survival: to store enough fat to keep us alive in the event of starvation."[11]

The problem for dieters is that the body cannot distinguish between a famine and a crash diet. Consequently, your body may fight to retain weight when it senses a decrease in calories. "The body reacts to what it perceives as a threat, quickly regaining weight to once again reach its natural set point," explains Elson Haas, M.D., director of the Preventative Medicine Center of Marin in San Rafael, California.[12] It is important to understand that the set point can be thrown out of balance, causing you to gradually gain weight. One of the ways this occurs is when your brown fat is deactivated.

Why You Lose Brown Fat

Unlike yellow fat, we do not gain brown fat by eating more food. In fact, we slowly lose brown fat as we grow older. It is also possible for brown fat to become inactive as a result of exposure to toxins in food, water, or air. According to Dr. Mowrey, a combination of factors (dietary, behavioral, age-related, and environmental) can shut down the activity of brown fat. Once brown fat has been deactivated, your body can no longer burn off excess fat as effectively—instead, it will store it.

■ Essential Fatty Acid Deficiencies—Nutritional deficiencies brought on by a poor diet can cause brown fat to become inactive.

One of the most important nutrients necessary to keep thermogenic processes healthy in brown fat cells are essential fatty acids (EFAs—SEE QUICK DEFINITION). These substances are the primary fuels that stoke the body's thermogenic furnace. When they are in short supply, brown fat turns "cold" and becomes inactive. An essential fatty acid deficiency is often the hidden reason for why individuals who try to lose weight by cutting all fat from their diet often gain weight. Dr. Mowrey warns that individuals who try crash diets can seriously impair their thermogenic capacity. "Dieting sends the body all the wrong signals when it comes to permanent weight loss," says Dr. Mowrey. If you want to know if you have an essential fatty acid deficiency, there are several test procedures available. Hair analysis and blood tests called lipid profiles are often used by health-care practitioners to determine an individual's essential fatty acid status.

For more about **essential fatty acids and lipid profile tests**, see Chapter 2: Healthy Eating, pp. 50-75.

QUICK DEFINITION

Essential fatty acids (EFAs) are unsaturated fats required in the diet. Omega-3 and omega-6 oils are the two principal types. Omega-3 oil is found in flaxseed, canola, pumpkin, walnut, and soybeans. Fish oils, such as salmon, cod, and mackerel, also contain important omega-3 oils. Omega-6 oil is found in most plant and vegetable oils, including safflower, corn, peanut, and sesame, as well as evening primrose, black currant, and borage oils.

■ Behavioral Factors—Excessive exercise and fasting can deplete your stores of brown fat. "Yo-yo" dieting may also make it more difficult to burn off excess calories, as your body will tend to store them as body fat.

■ Age and Genetics—You are born with a certain amount of brown fat and if this amount is inadequate, you may be prone to weight gain. In addition, as we age, we slowly lose or deactivate the brown fat in our body. Diabetes and hypothyroidism may also affect brown fat function.[13]

■ Toxins and Medications—Various medications, when taken daily, can have devastating effects on brown fat, eventually interfering in the mitochondria's ability to produce energy. A healthy liver can readily filter out the toxins that accumulate from a few days of medication or from brief environmental exposures to toxins, but over a prolonged period the body is no longer able to clean out these damaging chemicals.

Mitochondria produce energy in the cells by generating ATP (adenosine triphosphate), the primary cellular fuel. Damaged mitochondria often lose their ability to use fats to make ATP. When this occurs, the body may draw upon lean body tissue to fuel metabolism, which can cause serious weakness and fatigue. Individuals who have problems at this cellular level often have trouble exercising which, in turn, will make them more susceptible to weight gain.

Alternative Medicine Therapies to Increase Fat Burning

Fortunately, it is possible to reactivate your brown fat and its thermogenic activity with proper treatment. First, be sure to rule out any underlying problems, such as decreased thyroid function or adrenal stress. Dr. Mowrey asserts that regular stimulation of thermogenic (calorie-burning) processes can not only revive the activity of your existing brown fat, but actually increase the mass of brown fat cells in your body.[14] Essential fatty acids (EFAs), herbs and nutrients, and exercise can help boost your body's fat-burning capabilities.

Boosting Thermogenesis With Fatty Acids

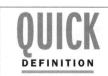

QUICK DEFINITION

Omega-3 and omega-6 oils are the two principle types of essential fatty acids, which are unsaturated fats required in the diet. A balance of these oils in the diet is required for good health. The primary omega-3 oil is alpha-linolenic acid (ALA), found in flaxseed, canola, pumpkin, walnut, and soybeans. Fish oils, such as salmon, cod, and mackerel, contain the other important omega-3 oils, DHA (docosahexaenoic acid) and EPA (eicosapentaenoic acid). Linoleic acid is the main omega-6 oil, found in most vegetable oils, including safflower, corn, peanut, and sesame. Another omega-6 oil, gamma-linolenic acid (GLA), is found in evening primrose, black currant, and borage oils.

Gamma-linolenic acid (GLA), an omega-6 (SEE QUICK DEFINITION) essential fatty acid, has been shown to be effective at reactivating brown fat and increasing thermogenesis.[15] Normally, the body can manufacture GLA from dietary sources of linoleic acid, another omega-6 oil; sources of linoleic acid include safflower, sunflower, corn, soybean, and flaxseed oils. However, a diet high in saturated fats combined with stress, alcohol, aging, or illness, can block this conversion, resulting in a GLA deficiency. In addition, many overweight people already suffer from chronic deficiencies in EFAs. Since GLA obtained directly from food sources may be insufficient, when a deficiency occurs, it should be taken as a dietary supplement. Evening primrose oil, black currant oil, and borage oil are good sources of GLA. The typical recommended dosage for GLA is 500 mg daily.

CAUTION

Diabetics and those with liver disorders should approach the use of MCTs with caution, as the fat tends to be burned very rapidly in the liver. Individuals with these conditions should avoid MCTs entirely or use them only under a doctor's supervision.

Medium-Chain Triglycerides (MCTs)—Medium-chain triglycerides are saturated fats that have been shown to promote weight loss. MCTs are a form of natural fat that tends to accelerate metabolism while lowering blood levels of cholesterol. Naturopath Michael T. Murray, N.D., says that MCTs, unlike other types of fat, tend to be rapidly burned up rather than stored as fat. In fact, one study found that those who added just 1-2 tablespoons of MCTs to their normal diet burned 5% more calories.[16]

Recently, researchers compared how individuals responded to meals that contained only MCTs and those that contained common long-chain triglycerides (LCTs), such as those found in animal fats. Seven male subjects were given either 48 grams of MCT oil or 45 grams of corn oil, an LCT oil. The researchers measured metabolic rates both prior to the meal and six hours after the meal. The results showed that, on average, the meal with MCTs caused a 12% increase in the resting metabolic rate compared to a 4% increase for LCTs. The researchers concluded that MCTs can produce weight loss through increased thermogenesis, without a reduction in calorie intake.[17]

Good sources of MCTs are grapeseed and coconut oils, available at most health food stores. MCT oil can be used on vegetables and in salad dressings and you can cook with it as with any other vegetable oil. Dr. Murray typically recommends 1-2 tablespoons of MCTs daily.[18]

For more about **adrenal stress and weight problems**, see Chapter 7: Heal Your Emotional Appetite, pp. 156-182.

For information on **Max-Omega Oil**, which contains black currant seed oil (high in GLA), linoleic acid, and alpha-linolenic acid, contact: Bio-Nutritional Formulas, 106 East Jericho Turnpike, Mineola, NY 11501; tel: 800-950-8484. For **MCT oil**, contact: Sound Nutrition, P.O. Box 555, Dover, ID 83825; tel: 800-844-6645 or 208-263-6183. For **grapeseed oil** (containing MCTs), contact: Spectrum Naturals, 133 Copeland Street, Petaluma, CA 94952; tel: 707-778-8900.

Ephedra-Based Herbal Treatment

Certain herbal formulas based on the Chinese herb ephedra (*Ephedra sinica*) may help you burn fat faster, increase your metabolic rate, and restore thermogenic activity in brown fat. However, they are not for everyone and can produce significant side effects if abused; but used carefully (under a qualified practitioner's guidance), these formulas can contribute to a weight-loss program.

These herbal formulas work primarily by prompting the release of norepinephrine, a brain chemical called a neurotransmitter (SEE QUICK DEFINITION) that stimulates brown fat cells.[19] Ephedra, also known as ma-huang in Chinese medicine, is a popular thermogenic herb; its active ingredient is a substance called ephedrine. According to Dr. Mowrey, ephedra is the most effective herbal stimulant for reactivating brown fat, but it must be used prudently. He points out that the whole herb is safer and preferable to the synthetic ephedrine alkaloid extract, which has been misused and over-prescribed and thereby castigated as dangerous by the media. Ephedra is generally safe and effective in stimulating thermogenesis, Dr. Mowrey states, but for some individuals (and depending on dose) it can

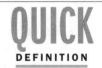

QUICK

DEFINITION

A **neurotransmitter** is a brain chemical with the specific function of enabling communications to happen between brain cells. Chief among the 100 identified to date are acetylcholine, gamma-aminobutyric acid (GABA), serotonin, dopamine, and norepinephrine. Acetylcholine is required for short-term memory and all muscle contractions; GABA works to stop excess nerve signals; serotonin does the same and helps produce sleep, regulate pain, and influence mood; norepinephrine is an excitatory neurotransmitter.

sometimes produce unwanted side effects, including hand tremors, heart palpitations, insomnia, and headaches. These side effects tend to occur when the herb is taken at too high a dose.[20]

Ephedra's thermogenic effect is helped when it is taken with methylxanthines, chemical compounds that include caffeine, according to Dr. Murray. The preferred sources of caffeine for thermogenic formulas are cola nut (*Cola nitida*) or guarana (*Paullinea cupana*), while the herb yerba maté (*Ilex paraguariensis*) contains a substance called mateine, which can be substituted for caffeine. Coffee and black tea, while containing caffeine, are considered to be less desirable sources by most practitioners. Aspirin may also help increase the effectiveness and reduce the side effects of ephedra, according to Dr. Mowrey.[22] Because ephedra and caffeine are stimulants and their prolonged use is considered controversial, it is best to have your dose tailored to your specific requirements. A trained practitioner will take into account your sensitivities and preexisting health conditions, such as an impaired thyroid or adrenal stress. Dennis Wright, D.C., a chiropractor from St. George, Utah, who has successfully treated many overweight patients with thermogenic formulas states, "It is my professional opinion that anyone using a thermogenic product should be following a doctor's instructions and be monitored closely."

Precautions When Taking Ephedra—Some individuals may experience mild dizziness, insomnia, increased perspiration, or a slight increase in blood pressure after starting a thermogenic treatment. Over time, however, all of the above symptoms should fade; if not, your doctor should lower your dosage. Dr. Wright notes that patients who drink large quantities of coffee or tea are the most likely to experience negative side effects—from the sheer excess of caffeine in their system. Cutting out all other sources of caffeine, taking the capsule with meals, and drinking plenty of water, can generally reduce these reactions, notes Dr. Wright. It is also prudent to avoid synthetic versions of ephedrine (dexfenfluramine and fenfluramine) that have been developed by the pharmaceutical industry, according to Dr. Mowrey, because they will have "a more pronounced tendency to elicit the more serious of the possible side effects."[23] Numerous studies have shown that the herbal combination not only has fewer side effects but also produces better results than the synthetic products.[24]

Other Thermogenic Herbs and Nutrients

Garlic—Garlic (*Allium sativum*) is probably the most well-recognized medicinal herb. It is used by traditional medicines worldwide and its applications are as varied as its geographical distribution. The chemistry and pharmacology of garlic is well studied—over 1,000 research papers have been published in the past 25 years. A recent study indicates that garlic may boost thermogenesis. Two groups of animals were fed identical high-fat diets, with one group given additional garlic powder. After 28 days, the body weights of the group given garlic were significantly lower.

Studies Demonstrate Effectiveness of Thermogenics

Numerous studies have demonstrated that the combination of ephedra with caffeine and aspirin increases thermogenesis and promotes weight loss. Researchers at Harvard University measured the weight-loss effects of the formula on a group of volunteers. Half of the study's participants took the formula, while the other half took a placebo. After two months, the patients on the thermogenic formula lost three times more weight than the patients on the placebo; they also experienced few side effects. Another study showed that patients taking the same combination formula three times daily for six weeks lost six times as much weight as the placebo group.[21]

Ephedra

Amounts of brown fat as well as levels of norepinephrine and mitochondrial protein were also greater in the garlic group—all indicators of increased metabolic and fat-burning activities.[25] Studies demonstrate general benefits from almost any type of garlic, be it raw garlic, dried garlic, garlic oil, or a prepared commercial product.

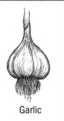

Garlic

Cayenne or red pepper (*Capsicum frutescens*) is a thermogenic food spice. Research indicates that cayenne induces fat burning and helps mobilize fat and sugar metabolism.[26] Other pungent food spices, particularly ginger (*Zingiber officinale*) and cinnamon, may also stimulate metabolism, but there is as yet little scientific evidence to verify their thermogenic properties.[27]

Ginseng—Ginseng has an ancient history and has accumulated much folklore about its actions and uses. Common varieties are Oriental ginseng (*Panax ginseng*), American ginseng (*Panax quinquefolius*), and Siberian ginseng (*Eleutherococcus senticosus*). In traditional Chinese medicine, ginseng is used as a general tonic to improve stamina during exercise, sharpen mental abilities, and relieve fatigue. Research indicates that ginseng may be able to raise basal metabolic rates as well. Ginseng should not be abused, however, as serious side effects can occur, including headaches, skin problems, and other reactions.[28]

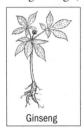
Ginseng

Green Tea—Green tea (*Camellia sinensis*) can increase the metabolic rate and stimulate thermogenesis. This is mainly due to its caffeine content, but it also contains two related compounds (not found in coffee), theophylline and theobromine, that boost thermogenic activity. Even modest doses of these compounds can increase basal metabolism by as much as 10%, an effect which lasts for several hours.[29]

Yerba maté (*Ilex paraguariensis*) is another tea, well-known in South America and now available in health food stores in the U.S., which also acts as a stimulant to boost thermogenesis. Yerba maté's stimulating effect comes primarily from a compound called mateine, a close relative of caffeine, plus small quantities of theophylline and theobromine. Mateine seems to have the stimulatory effects of caffeine without the side effects.[30]

For information on **products containing hydroxycitric acid (HCA)**, contact: AMNI, P.O. Box 5012, Hayward, CA 94540; tel: 800-356-4791 or 510-783-6969; fax: 510-783-8196. Futurebiotics, 145 Ricefield Lane, Hauppauge, NY 11788; tel: 800-845-1721 or 516-273-6300; fax: 516-273-1165; website: www.futurebiotics.com. Nature's Herbs, 600 East Quality Drive, American Fork, UT 84003; tel: 800-437-2257 or 801-763-0700; fax: 801-763-0789.

Hydroxycitric Acid (HCA)—HCA is an extract from the fruit of a tree called *Garcinia cambogia*, found throughout Asia and India. The fruit and rind are used in curries and other common foods of the region. Research indicates that HCA may promote fat burning indirectly by inhibiting the enzymes involved in the formation of fat, thus more fat is burned off instead of stored as body fat. HCA may also help to curb your appetite. The typical recommended dosage is 175-300 mg, three times daily, taken 30-60 minute before meals.[31]

Carnitine—Carnitine is a nutrient primarily found in meats and dairy products that can boost your metabolism by helping your body burn off fat more efficiently. "Carnitine is the forklift that takes fat to the fat incinerators in our cells—the mitochondria," says Robert Crayhon, M.S., author of *The Carnitine Miracle.* "Unless fat makes it into the mito-chondria, you can't burn it off no matter what you do or how well you diet." As part of a weight-loss program, Crayhon typically recommends 1,000-4,000 mg of carnitine daily.[32]

DHEA—DHEA (dehydroepiandrosterone), the most abundant hormone in the body, is naturally produced by the human adrenal glands and gonads and functions as an antioxidant and hormone regulator. You produce the optimal amount of DHEA in your twenties, then levels gradually decline with age. Animal studies indicate that DHEA may promote thermogenic activity and decrease body fat, however human clinical studies are needed to establish DHEA's effect on body weight. Also, DHEA seems to stimulate weight loss in men more than in women. No serious side effects have been reported with DHEA, although headaches, irritability, insomnia, and fatigue have been reported with high DHEA doses.[33]

Since DHEA can affect hormone levels in your body, it is best to take it under medical supervision.

For more about **exercise programs and weight loss**, see Chapter 6: Start Exercising, pp. 138-155.

Exercise to Maximize Thermogenesis

Proper exercise increases the body's thermogenic response, not only during the activity, but for long afterward. Exercising regularly increases your basal metabolism rate (BMR)—it's a bit like gasoline consumption while your car is idling. Even a moderate exercise schedule can raise your metabolism and the physiology is such that you burn additional calories for approximately 12 hours immediately after exercise because of your elevated BMR. This can amount to as much as 15% of the calories burned during your workout, a significant amount when you're trying to lose weight. Moderate physical activity, done in cool, non-humid environments, is ideal. Swimming and brisk walking, particularly in the early morning or evening hours, are highly recommended. Other activity choices may include aerobics, cycling, running, or jogging.

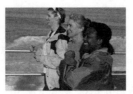

Starting to exercise is an absolute

necessity for any long-term weight loss program.

Watching what you eat and getting enough

physical activity to burn off excess calories is

the key to good health and maintaining

a healthy body weight.

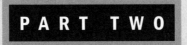

PART TWO

Change
Your Lifestyle

6 Start Exercising

BECAUSE OF OUR increasingly automated and push-button world, many people drive to work, breeze into an elevator just steps away from the office, and spend the day immobile, staring at a computer screen. With everything at our fingertips, we barely move anymore. At night, we go home and plop down in front of the TV for the evening, our only "exercise" is using the remote control to surf through the channels. In our day-to-day lives, we're simply not getting as much physical activity as our ancestors. It should not be surprising, then, that obesity and physical inactivity have reached what experts are calling "epidemic" levels.

Studies continue to show the dramatic health benefits of even moderate levels of exercise—for preventing heart disease, diabetes, osteoporosis, and many other health problems. But in spite of this growing body of evidence, many Americans are still ambivalent toward fitness. According to the American Medical Association (AMA), one in four adult Americans still spend their leisure time doing little or nothing—in other words, blissfully not exercising. And many are paying a high price for that blissful ignorance in extra weight. The AMA studied nearly 10,000 adults in the U.S. and found that 22% engaged in *no* physical activity during leisure time and 46% stated that they don't exercise regularly. A related study of 2,783 men and 5,018 women, age 65 and above, indicated that only 37% of men and 24% of women in this age group exercise at least three times weekly.[1]

Starting to exercise is an absolute necessity for any long-term weight loss program. Watching what you eat and get-

In This Chapter

- Changing Sedentary Habits
- Designing Your Own Exercise Program
- The Oxygen Priority
- Moderate Activity for Weight Loss
- A Muscular Advantage
- Exercise From the East

ting enough physical activity to burn off excess calories is the key to good health and maintaining a healthy body weight. And you don't have to be a marathon runner—even moderate exercise like walking the dog or gardening can produce health benefits. Exercise can help build muscle, boost your energy levels, improve your cardiovascular fitness, reduce stress, and promote weight loss.

Changing Sedentary Habits

While experts have always urged people to exercise regularly, they are now saying that low to moderate physical activity such as taking the stairs and walking the dog can help establish a basic level of fitness. Whereas a strenuous exercise program may be too daunting for many people to sustain, moderate activity may be a more realistic and attainable goal.

Exercise is important for long-term weight management because it speeds metabolism and preserves lean muscle. Muscles burn more calories and, in the absence of exercise, muscle mass can be lost during a restricted calorie diet. While dieters may lose weight, those who incorporate regular moderate exercise are building muscle that increases their metabolism and improves their overall health.

In a recent study, three groups of dieters were assessed on their weight management over the course of two years. The first group was assigned to a restricted-calorie diet, the second group was prescribed diet and exercise, and the third group assigned an exercise program only. A year later, the dieters lost an average of 15 pounds, the dieters who exercised lost 20 pounds, and the exercisers lost six pounds. During the second year, however, dieters regained about a pound, the dieters who exercised regained all of the weight they had lost, and the exercisers regained less than half a pound. "We were shocked," said researcher John Foreyt, Ph.D., of Baylor College in Waco, Texas. "We'd put our money on the diet-plus-exercise group, but apparently the negative effects of restrictive dieting—feelings of hunger and deprivation—eventually lead to overeating."[2] Striking a balance between a good diet that allows you to safely lose weight and also provides enough fuel for your body is important once you have begun a regular exercise program.

Designing Your Own Exercise Program

What does it mean to you to be physically fit? After the media bombardment with images of very slender models, superbly conditioned

For more on **detoxification**, see Chapter 12: Detoxify the Colon, pp. 272-293.

athletes, and other extreme examples, it may be difficult to define what fitness goals you have. The important thing is to decide what will be a realistic and attainable goal for you. This may mean developing a workout schedule to lose weight, lower your cholesterol levels, and improve general health or it may mean simply returning to regular participation in your favorite physical activity or sport.

Before beginning any exercise program, consult your physician and have a thorough exam to rule out any health conditions that may need attention. If you have heart disease, diabetes, or are at high risk for these or other serious illnesses, begin an exercise program only with your physician's approval. Inactive men over the age of 40 and women over 50 should also consult their physician. If you have been physically inactive for some time, it is important to determine if you may need to undergo an accelerated detoxification program before you begin exercising. The toxins we are exposed to in the air we breathe, water we drink, and food we eat accumulate in the liver, lymph, and colon. Nutritionists and other health-care professionals advise clients to avoid strenuous exercise until they have adequately cleansed the body of toxins. "Toxins released from the lymphatic system during exercise can circulate without being neutralized by the liver or removed from the body and resettle in the various tissues, causing damage wherever they go," explains Jack Tips, N.D., Ph.D., a nutritionist in Austin, Texas.[3]

According to the President's Council on Physical Fitness and Sports, a balanced physical fitness program incorporates the following elements:[4]

Warming Up—Begin gradually. Start with some basic warm up exercises, which can include gentle stretching or a short, slow walk for 5-10 minutes.

Cardiorespiratory Fitness—Endurance athletes, such as long-distance runners or swimmers, have the stamina for their physically demanding sports because they have good cardiorespiratory fitness. The heart and lungs are able to deliver oxygen and nutrients to the tissues and remove wastes over sustained periods of activity.

The main thing is to get moving, be it walking, running, cycling, or any other aerobic activity. After you have warmed up your muscles and you are breathing more deeply, begin your activity and gradually pick up the pace. This may mean moving from a slow walk to a brisker pace or increasing the speed on a treadmill. If it has been a long time since you have exercised regularly, begin slowly. Your first session may consist of five minutes of warming up and another 5-10 minutes of walking. Always be sure to cool down afterward—avoid stopping your exercise abruptly without giving your body a chance to slow down and cool off. If you have just walked a mile in 20 minutes, take another five minutes to bring your pace to a slower stroll and allow your body to gradually shift into low gear.

For more **fitness tips**, contact: The President's Council on Physical Fitness and Sports, 200 Independence Avenue SW, Room 738-H, Washington, DC 20201; tel: 202-690-9000; fax: 202-690-5211; website: www.surgeongeneral.gov/ophs/pcpfs.htm.

To see improvement, it is recommended that you exercise for 20 minutes at least three times a week. Again, some studies suggest you can break these workouts into shorter, more frequent sessions or add activities such as vigorous yard work to establish a baseline of fitness.

Muscular Strength—A muscle's capacity to exert force for a brief period of time can be developed by participating in sports or by specific weight-training exercises. By regularly working individual muscle groups, they increase in strength. Begin a weight resistance program—join your local gym and learn how to use the free weights or perform activities that require regular lifting, such as chopping wood and gardening. Be certain you are observing proper lifting stances to protect your back and joints from injury.

Strive for at least two sessions of 20 minutes of free weights a week. Weight training helps change your body composition, the amount of lean muscle mass and fat in your body. Exercise builds lean muscle, which helps your body to burn off more calories, thereby improving your metabolism.

Muscular Endurance—The muscle's ability to undergo repeated contractions or to continue applying force against a fixed object; performing 100 pushups requires this kind of endurance. Groups of muscles are recruited to perform a certain activity over a sustained period of time. Try to incorporate at least three 30-minute sessions of exercises such as pushups, sit-ups, and similar calisthenics for training of all the major muscle groups. Public parks often have an "obstacle course" that includes many of these exercises at designated stations. Again, other activities involving vigorous work around the house, such as washing the car, can provide similar benefits.

Flexibility—Flexibility is the ability to move your muscles freely through a full range of movement. Dancers rely on their excellent flexibility, but everyone can benefit from increased flexibility as it can help prevent injury. Try to incorporate 10-15 minutes of gentle, non-bouncing stretching exercises into your workouts. This can be done before you set off on a walk or bike ride and also at the end of the session. If you are familiar with yoga or *tai chi*, both are excellent for increasing flexibility.

The Oxygen Priority

Exercise is not the only way we burn calories. Even when you are asleep, your heart is beating, your lungs breathing, and every cell in your body is busy keeping you alive. All of these functions require calories. If the physiological processes that support these vital functions are impaired, you will gain weight, sometimes even if you exercise. The initial step in any weight-loss plan is thus to first identify and correct any physiological impairment or imbalance that is causing you to burn fewer calories.

Although we generally take it for granted, the oxygen we inhale is vital for burning fat and a key ingredient in metabolism (SEE QUICK DEFINITION). The body extracts most of the energy it needs from fat and glucose—the latter being a simple sugar that the body makes from carbohydrates and sugars. The energy in these substances is stored in the chemical bonds that hold the individual molecules together. Oxygen serves as a kind of chemical wedge that splits open the molecules, liberating their energy for use by the body. To illustrate this, think of the chemical bonds as stretched rubber bands—when a bond is broken, it releases stored energy similar to how a stretched rubber band snaps when you suddenly let go of one end.

When we are deficient in oxygen, our metabolism slows and we do not burn as much fat. Pam Grout, author of *Jumpstart Your Metabolism*, explains that a lack of oxygen causes the metabolic activity within each cell to begin shutting down. "When you don't get enough oxygen, you literally strangle your cells," she says. "As hard as they might try, they can't process food properly."[5]

Oxygen enters the body through the lungs, where it is absorbed by the blood and then transported to every cell. Over time, regular exercise helps to increase the oxygen supply to the body by strengthening the heart and increasing the quantity of blood vessels in the body, which improves blood flow (also called cardiovascular fitness). One of the measurable signs of a strong heart is how fast it beats when you are not exercising (called the resting heart rate). A strong heart beats fewer

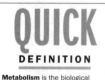

DEFINITION

Metabolism is the biological process by which energy is extracted from the foods consumed, producing carbon dioxide and water as by-products for elimination. There are two kinds of metabolism constantly underway in the cells: anabolic and catabolic. The anabolic function produces substances for cell growth and repair, while the catabolic function controls digestion, disassembling food into forms the body can use for energy.

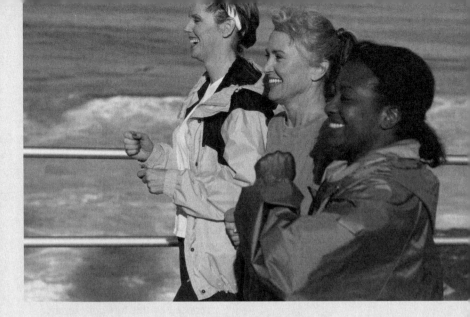

Calories Burned by Vigorous Exercise

According to a recent report by the Surgeon General, everyone should try to exercise at least 30 minutes daily. Here are some examples of the number of calories that are burned during vigorous exercise (the number of calories burned will vary according the weight of the individual):

Activity	Calories Burned/Hour
Bicycling 6 miles per hour (mph)	240
Bicycling 12 mph	410
Jogging 5.5 mph	740
Jogging 7 mph	920
Running 10 mph	1,280
Skiing cross country	700
Swimming 25 yards/minute	275
Swimming 50 yards/minute	500
Tennis (singles)	400
Walking 2 mph	240
Walking 4 mph	440

Source: *The American Council on Exercise, 5820 Oberlin Drive, Suite 102, San Diego, CA 92121-3787; tel: 619-535-8227; fax: 619-535-1778.*

times per minute than a weak heart. This is because it has a larger capacity to move blood, delivering a higher volume of blood with every beat. If a heart is very weak, it may have a hard time delivering enough blood to meet the body's oxygen demands even during sleep.

Aerobic exercise also increases red blood cell count, allowing faster oxygen transport through the body, and can help lower elevated blood pressure. Exercise helps dissolve blood clots and increases the amount of high-density lipoproteins (HDL, the so-called good cholesterol and a major factor in the prevention of atherosclerosis) in the blood, according to John A. Friedrich, M.D., of Duke University. The capacity of the lungs increases so that they can process more air and replenish oxygen in the cells of the body's tissues and organs more quickly. Metabolism is enhanced and you tend to absorb nutrients from your food more efficiently. Any tendency towards constipation, kidney stones, or diabetes is reduced by this form of exercise.

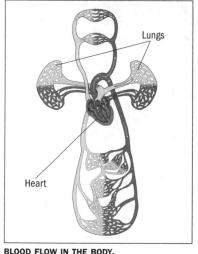

BLOOD FLOW IN THE BODY.

Researchers at the University of Colorado in Boulder demonstrated that a lower heart rate was among the measures highly correlated with increased activity levels in older adults. The researchers compared the heart rates of groups of active and sedentary women (average age 62) and a group of young active women (average age 29). Heart health was measured by heartbeats per minute, the amount of blood pumped with each beat, and the total blood volume pumped by the heart. The study showed the heart health of the active women to be the same regardless of age. In contrast, the heart health of the older sedentary women was significantly worse, with a heart rate that was, on average, six beats faster per minute. These women pumped 24% less blood with each heartbeat and had a 23% lower total blood volume. In addition, the sedentary women were 22 pounds heavier on average than the active women.[6]

The good news is that it doesn't take long to bring your resting heart rate down. In one study reported in the *British Journal of Sports Medicine*, a regular walking program was shown to decrease the heart rates of previously sedentary individuals within 18 weeks.[7] Ann Louise Gittleman, M.S., a nutritionist based in Bozeman, Montana, considers brisk walking the best weight-loss exercise. She recommends a vigorous 30-minute walk outdoors, at least three times per week.[8] Walking outdoors gives you the added benefit of sunlight, which helps to increase the body's production of the neurotransmitter serotonin, a brain chemical that helps to control appetite. Any activity that elevates your heart rate to your target heart rate (see "Identifying Your Exertion Cues," p. 150) is adequate. This could be brisk walking (include walking up small hills for increased difficulty), biking, walking or running on a treadmill, as well as other sports such as tennis or racquetball.

The key to starting and staying with a program of physical activity is finding one that you like and will continue to do. It is important not to choose an activity just because it is known to burn the most calories or promises quick results. Gittleman considers enjoyment as an essential ingredient for the long-term success of any exercise program. "Whenever you enjoy what you do, you are more likely to continue to do it," she says.[9] If you are having difficulty choosing an exercise and are not sure where to begin, consult your physician for further guidance.

Pedal Your Way to Health with Exercise Bikes

Always popular among home exercise equipment is the stationary bicycle—or exercise bike, as it's commonly known—because it is easy to use, can accommodate all fitness levels, takes up a small amount of space, and provides the exercise you need for good health. That stationary bicycles can be beneficial no matter what your fitness level is demonstrated by the fact that they are used in many physical rehabilitation programs. Stationary bicycles are gentle on the back and joints and, unlike running or walking, they provide a non-impact workout that is nonetheless effective in strengthening the heart and lungs.

A recent French study (*Archives des Maladies du Coeur et des Vaisseaux*, 1996) compared fitness tests of elderly patients (65 years and older) with a second group aged 65 and younger. Exercise tests were conducted on stationary bicycles during

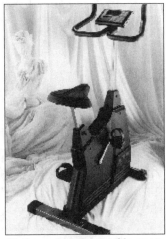

Stationary bicycles provide a non-impact workout for strengthening the heart and lungs.

For more on **basal metabolism**, see Chapter 1: Individualize Your Diet, pp. 34-39, and Chapter 5: Optimize Your Calorie Burning, pp. 122-135.

the patient's period of hospital admission for heart surgery. The results showed a 21% increase in power output and a 28% increase in duration of the elderly patients' exercise periods compared to 25% and 28%, respectively, in the younger group. In other words, the bikes helped both groups of heart patients exercise harder and longer. All patients showed significant improvements in fitness levels without any serious complications.

Using a stationary bike can assist weight loss by burning calories. As with other forms of aerobic exercise, there is an additional weight control benefit from exercising regularly: it increases your basal metabolism rate (BMR). This is the number of calories used by the body at complete rest to maintain basic life processes such as respiration and circulation. Even a moderate exercise schedule—30-40 minutes, three to four times per week—can raise your BMR. You burn additional calories for approximately 12 hours immediately after exercise because of having elevated your BMR (as much as 15% of the calories burned during your workout).

Get Fit While Running in Place on a Treadmill

A study by the Medical College of Wisconsin at Milwaukee compared the effectiveness of the most common exercise machines: a treadmill, exercise cycle, rowing machine, cross-country skier, stair stepper, and combination cycle/upper body machine. The researchers found that "the treadmill machine induced higher rates

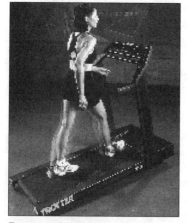

Even a moderate program on the treadmill can help you control your weight.

of energy expenditure [measured by number of calories burned] and aerobic demands than the other exercise machines." Specifically, the treadmill produced the "greatest cardiorespiratory training stimulus during a given duration of exercise" and burned 700 calories/hour compared to 625 calories/hour for the stair stepper, and 500 calories/hour for the exercise bicycle.

In addition, the study measured the "rate of perceived exertion" (RPE) on the treadmill compared to the other exercise machines. RPE means how strenuous the subject felt the exercise was compared to how much energy was used in terms of calories burned. The 13 subjects (eight men, five women) of the study were given a beginning fitness test then acclimated to the machines over a four-week period to establish their individual RPE values. The RPE value of an exercise turned out to be a major factor in how strenuously a person exercised. In other words, how hard you think you're exercising determines how many calories you actually burn during the exercise. Treadmills came out on top, with a 40% greater energy expenditure, burning more calories at all levels of perceived exertion than the other exercise equipment.[10]

Whatever your initial fitness level, treadmills can provide the kind of workout you need, from gentle to strenuous. Even a moderate program on the treadmill can help you control your weight, guard against heart disease, and reduce your cholesterol levels by providing a regular cardiovascular workout. It can also improve your muscle tone, reduce your stress level for greater emotional stability, and improve your mood and self-esteem.

Moderate Activity for Weight Loss

Although recommendations for exercise have changed throughout the years, experts continue to exhort us to keep moving. For many people, it is more realistic to include activities of moderate exertion, such as walking the dog or taking stairs instead of the elevator, to get their daily exercise. Including more physical activity throughout your day can help you maintain a basic level of fitness. Park your car a block away from your destination and walk. If you can perform certain errands, such as going to the post office or the grocery store, by walking or biking, do so. Walking more frequently and using less timesaving devices can burn additional calories and help keep you active.

Research conducted by the Cooper Institute for Aerobics Research in Dallas, Texas, found that if a number of tasks around the home and workplace were performed throughout the day, as much as 10,500 calories could be burned in a month by a person weighing 150-160 pounds. The activities included unloading groceries, walking a flight of stairs three times a day, and washing the car by hand.

Short Bouts of Exercise

For many years, the prescription for weight loss and health maintenance included three to five 30-minute sessions of exercise per week. Current recommendations from the American College of Sports Medicine and the U.S. Centers for Disease Control and Prevention state that nearly

Calories Burned by Moderate Activities

In the table below, the calories burned are indicated for a 150- to 160-pound person; a lighter person would burn fewer calories and a heavier person more.[11]

Activity	Calories Burned
Cooking and preparing food for 30 minutes	25
Walking the dog for 30 minutes	125
Raking leaves for 30 minutes	150
Washing and waxing the car for 60 minutes	300
Going up a flight of stairs three times a day	15
Walking 10 minutes to public transit, riding 30 minutes, walking 5 minutes to work	60
Walking at the mall for 60 minutes	240

everyone should strive for 30 minutes daily or alternately divide that amount into three eight- to 10-minute bouts per day.[12] Research has shown that people exercising in more frequent, shorter intervals reap the same health benefits as those participating in longer sessions of exertion.

In one study, 148 overweight and sedentary women were divided into three groups: one group exercised in long bouts of exercise, a second group exercised in short bursts, and the third did the same on treadmills at home. Eighteen months later, there was no significant difference in weight lost by those women who exercised in short bursts or those who went for a longer session.[13] Even if you are seriously short of time, set a minimum goal of three daily walking sessions of ten minutes each.

A Muscular Advantage

Preserving lean muscle tissue is important for those trying to lose weight because this speeds your metabolism. Dieters who exercise have a tremendous advantage because they are essentially stoking the internal furnace that will burn more calories. "While exercise alone does not appear to be as potent an initial weight-loss strategy as caloric restriction alone, when exercise is added to caloric restriction, initial weight loss is often much greater than diet alone," state Stanford University researchers Abby King and Diane Tribble.[14]

Dieting alone may lead to an actual loss of muscle tissue and this will only slow down your progress. One review of 55 medical reports on weight loss from exercise showed that, in 50 cases, there was less muscle loss than if the weight had been reduced by diet alone.[15] If you are cutting calories to lose weight and not exercising, you may lose up to 15% of your muscle mass. Curbing your calories signals your body to slow down your metabolism and, if you consume too few calories, your body begins to metabolize muscle tissue. In a sense, your body is cannibalizing itself to survive. This emphasizes the importance of maintaining an adequate, well-balanced diet while exercising to allow your body to drop weight safely and permanently.

In order to lose one pound, you must burn off 3,500 calories. This is not as impossible as it sounds. For most people that will mean a combination of reducing calories and increasing physical activity. In one study, dieters exercised an hour three times a week, bringing their total caloric expenditure to about 1,500 calories. This study found that as compared to a group who dieted to shed weight, dieters who exercised regularly were able to keep the weight off for more than three years after the initial loss.[16]

How Your Body Burns Calories—Intense, prolonged exertion, such as weight-lifting, is fueled primarily by glucose, a simple sugar that the body makes from dietary carbohydrates and sugars. Conversely, fats are the preferred fuel for fast movements, such as running or jumping. These different types of activities also involve different types of muscle fibers. Weight-lifting, for example, relies on "slow-twitch" fibers, while running relies on "fast-twitch" fibers.

The fact that fat is the preferred fuel of fast-twitch muscle fibers does not necessarily mean that quick-action exercises should be performed to the exclusion of strength-building exercises to lose weight. Strength-building exercise increases lean muscle mass, one of the best ways to increase how many calories your body burns. Muscle cells have high energy demands even at rest. Consequently, the more muscle you have, the more calories you will burn throughout the day.[17]

Exercise From the East

Moderate to strenuous exercises such as running or tennis are not the only way to increase your metabolism and boost your body's ability to burn off calories. Even more basic than exercise is proper breathing.

Identifying Your Exertion Cues

When starting an exercise program, you should not try to do too much too quickly. It is important to monitor your vital signs before, during, and throughout exercise sessions. Learn how to accurately measure and be aware of your body's exertion cues so that you can exercise safely.

■ Monitor your resting and target heart rates, which will enable you to adjust your level of activity. Resting heart rate can be measured by simply placing your fingers across your wrist and counting the number of beats for 15 seconds, then multiply by four; this is the number of beats per minute. To determine your target heart rate, use the following formula: maximum heart rate (220-your age) x 70%. For example, for a 50-year-old person, their maximum heart rate is determined by subtracting 50 from 220, which equals 170. Then, 170 is multiplied by 0.7 (70%) to reach the target heart rate of 119. Always take your heart rate before you begin your exercise, during the session, and after you have cooled down.[18]

Alternately, you could wear a heart monitor, a device worn directly on the chest to provide your heart rate as you exercise. Once primarily worn by people recovering from heart disease, heart monitors are available to anyone wanting to know if they are exercising safely.

■ Notice your breathing. If your breathing is short and labored, slow down. Once you have gained some stamina, your breathing during exertion should be steady and even.

■ Take the talking test. If you are able to carry on a conversation comfortably during exercise, you are probably moving at a good pace.

■ Watch for signs of physical pain. If you experience any short or sudden pain or are not able to breathe comfortably, discontinue your exercise by slowly coming to a stop.

■ Notice changes in body temperature. Experts recommend that you drink fluids before, during, and after exercise to keep your body temperature from rising too much and to prevent dehydration. If you find that you are overheating during exercise, slow your pace, drink water, or reduce the layers of clothing you are wearing.

■ Observe general energy levels. While starting an exercise program will not be comfortable if you have been inactive, you should be able to enjoy the activity. Begin with a modest level of movement and exertion and gradually increase the duration, frequency, and intensity of the activity. Don't throw yourself into a highly demanding physical conditioning program and risk the possibility of injury.

CAUTION

If you are recovering from heart disease, respiratory illness or any other serious illness, consult your physician for recommendations on a safe exercise schedule.

The lungs are capable of holding as much as two gallons of air, but most of us breathe only two to three pints per breath. Ordinarily air is very poorly exchanged at the base of the lungs, far down in the chest cavity. This is particularly true when we breathe by expanding the chest, rather than expanding the abdomen. Breathing with the abdomen, also called diaphragmatic breathing, involves first expanding the abdomen when you inhale, before expanding the chest. Using this technique empties the lower portions of the lung. Taking such deep, full breaths occasionally throughout the day is a good way to increase your oxygen intake, raise your energy level, and burn fat. Simple activities, such as focused breathing, not only burn calories, but have a balancing and harmonizing influence on every body system.

You can shed fat and become fit through a number of exercises that are not strictly vigorous or taxing. Many alternative health practitioners recommend exercises from the East, such as yoga, *qigong*, and *tai chi*, to their patients to improve their breathing. Besides learning how to breathe for increased metabolism, the practices can also develop strength, flexibility, and balance. Increasing flexibility, which is often overlooked in developing an activity or workout schedule, is vital for preventing injury.

Most Westerners who observe the practice of these ancient forms of exercise may have doubts as to their workout value. After all, when it comes to losing weight, how can meditating in a series of different poses compare with activities such as running or lifting weights? Paul Dunphy, a *tai chi* practitioner and health journalist, says that the exercises do look different to the uninitiated. "Anyone watching *tai chi* might consider that the movements are too ethereal to promote 'fitness' or too slow to qualify as 'exercise.' The more skillful the *tai chi*, the more effortless the motion appears," he says.[19]

Although they may appear effortless, yoga, *qigong*, and *tai chi* still deliver considerable physiological benefits. For example, they help to expand the lungs, increase muscle flexibility and relaxation, stimulate metabolism, and improve blood circulation. The effect on blood circulation is somewhat different from that of more vigorous forms of exercise, as they do not send a torrent of blood to the muscles. Instead, by focusing on breathing with the lower abdomen, blood flow is directed toward the vital organs. One study conducted at Emory University School of Medicine in Atlanta, Georgia, suggests that *tai chi* has multiple benefits for cardiovascular fitness, building muscular strength, and improving posture.[20]

Central to all these practices is the belief that by sustaining a steady breath not only increases oxygen intake, but the increased blood flow helps circulate *prana* or *qi* (SEE QUICK DEFINITION). This "life force" or "vital energy" is what can vitalize even a physically strong body but one that may be energetically zapped. While Western standards for

Qi (pronounced *CHEE*) is a Chinese word variously translated to mean "vital energy," "essence of life," and "living force." In Chinese medicine, the proper flow of *qi* along energy channels (meridians) within the body is crucial to a person's health and vitality. There are many types of *qi*, classified according to source, location, and function (such as activation, warming, defense, transformation, and containment). Within the body, *qi* and blood are closely linked, as each is considered to flow along with the other. *Qi* may be stagnant (non-moving), deficient (partially absent), or excessive (inappropriately abundant) from a given organ system. *Qi* has two essential qualities: yang (active, fiery, moving, bright, energizing) and yin (passive, watery, stationary, dark, calming).

physical fitness tend to focus solely on body weight and muscular development as the criteria for physical health, these Eastern healing arts can provide your body with other benefits that standard exercises may not provide.

Yoga

Yoga is one of the most ancient systems of self-healing practiced today. Yoga teaches a basic principle of mind/body unity: if the mind is chronically restless and agitated, the health of the body will be compromised. Similarly, if the body is in poor health, mental clarity will be adversely affected. The practice of yoga can help integrate mind, body, and spirit.

Classical *Ashtanga* (meaning "eight limbs") yoga is divided into eight branches that give guidance as to the proper diet, hygiene, detoxification regimes, and physical practices to help the individual integrate their personal, psychological, and spiritual awareness. The most well-known type of yoga is Hatha yoga, which teaches certain *asanas* (postures) and breathing techniques to create profound changes in the body and mind. One important aspect of yoga is to harness and increase the flow of *prana*, or life energy. The blockage of *prana*, through improper diet, lifestyle stressors, or imbalance in one's physical, emotional, or spiritual health, can lead to illness. Breathing techniques and duration of holding certain postures remove blockages to the flow of *prana* and can improve oxygen intake.

The safest and most reliable way to use yoga therapeutically is to follow a balanced program of postures to achieve an overall normalizing and health-inducing effect. It is best for the beginner to start with a simple program of basic postures. A structured course can teach the

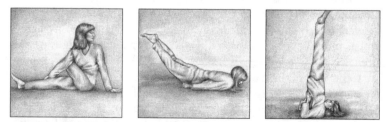

Yoga postures or *asanas*: half spinal twist, locust, and shoulder stand.

fundamental breathing techniques and postures for exercises later practiced on one's own.

Qigong

Qigong (also referred to as chi-kung) is an ancient exercise that stimulates and balances the flow of *qi* along acupuncture meridians (energy pathways). *Qigong* cultivates inner strength, calms the mind, and restores the body to its natural state of health. Although less artistic and dynamic than *tai chi*, *qigong* is much easier to learn and can be done by the severely disabled as well as the healthy. *Qigong* practice can range from simple calisthenics-type movements with breath coordination to complex exercises that direct brain-wave frequencies, deep relaxation, and breathing to improve strength and flexibility and reverse damage caused by prior injuries and disease.

Breathe with *Qigong*—Naturopathic physician and *qigong* instructor Michael Frost, Ph.D., of Cleveland, Ohio, offers the following breathing exercise to help expand the lungs and lose weight:

- Sit in a comfortable position.
- Place the palm of your hand over your navel and inhale normally, allowing your chest and abdomen to expand.
- As you slowly exhale, pull the navel in towards your spine as far as you can, completely expelling all the air as the abdomen and chest contract.
- Inhale again, gently pushing the abdomen out and keeping your chest and shoulders relaxed.
- Exhale as before.
- Listen to the sound of your breath; closing your eyes will help you concentrate.
- Repeat this procedure for five minutes.

Because it only takes five minutes, Dr. Frost recommends doing this exercise several times a day.

Tai Chi

Tai chi is a unique Chinese system of slow, continuous, flowing movements that create a sense of tranquillity and vitality. It is gentle, yet effective in stretching muscles and circulating the blood. Traditional Chinese medicine holds that *tai chi* stimulates and nourishes the body's internal

For more information about **yoga** and **qigong**, see *Alternative Medicine: The Definitive Guide* (Future Medicine Publishing, 1995; ISBN 1-887299-33-5); to order, call 800-333-HEAL.

For more information on **yoga**, contact: the International Association of Yoga Therapists, P.O. Box 1386, Lower Lake, CA 95457; tel: 707-928-9898. For more about **qigong**, contact: American Foundation of Traditional Chinese Medicine, 505 Beach Street, San Francisco, CA 94133; tel: 415-776-0502. For more about **qigong** and **tai chi**, contact: Michael Frost, Ph.D., American Association of Taoist Studies, 445 Richmond Park West, Suite 603-B, Richmond Heights, OH 44143; tel: 800-646-5731, ext. 4619 or 216-646-9129.

The Swimming Dragon Exercise

In Chinese medicine, the swimming dragon is a type of *qigong* exercise considered to be effective for weight loss. It helps burn fat by stimulating the physiological furnaces in the body, known as the "three burners," the primary regulators of metabolism. One burner directs breathing; the second affects digestion, sending energy to the stomach, spleen, liver, and pancreas; and the third manages the intestines, bladder, and kidneys, overseeing elimination. Philip Lansky, M.D., and Shen Yu, M.D., who specialize in Chinese medicine, explain that these burners are not part of the physical anatomy. "They are invisible organizing principles which keep the machinery of the body running smoothly."[22]

The swimming dragon involves tracing three circles in the air with your hands, following a continuous serpentine pattern. Each of the circles is traced at a level that corresponds to

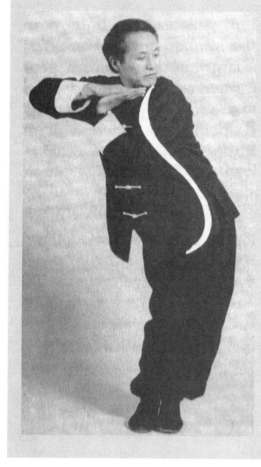

the location of each burner's region of influence. The top burner is traced near the head and chest, the middle burner is traced near the chest and waist, and the lower burner near the waist and knees. As you trace these circles, the motion of your hands should be smooth, moving from left to right, and tracing one-half of each circle as you descend from top to bottom. As you move your hands from left to right, your hips should move in the opposite direction. It is helpful to watch yourself in a mirror when you attempt this for the first time. If done correctly, your body should move just like a serpent in water. Here are the step-by-step instructions:

■ Stand erect but relaxed, with your hands at your sides.

- Bring your hands in front of your face, holding your fingers and palms together and pointed away from you.
  - Tilt your head and hands to the left, and begin tracing the first half of the first circle. As you do this, begin moving your hips to the right, keeping your thighs together.
  - Trace three connected half-circles in a smooth serpentine motion, slowly bending your knees and lowering your body.
  - When you reach the bottom of the third half circle—near the height of your knees when standing—complete the circle and move upward making another serpentine motion with your hands that is the mirror opposite of what you did on the way down. You have just traced the three circles.[23]

Each cycle of three circles should take one full minute. For beginners, one to three cycles should be adequate. Eventually, you should work up to 20 cycles.

An instructional video-cassette (*The Swimming Dragon: Ancient Chinese Exercise for Rapid Weight Loss*) and book (*The Swimming Dragon*) are available from: Chinese Healing Arts Center, P.O. Box 286, Glenford, NY 12433; tel: 914-657-8822; fax: 914-657-7759; website: www.qihealer.com.

organs by circulating *qi*, which also facilitates emotional and mental well-being. *Tai chi* also teaches the mind how to control the body.[21]

The meditative quality of yoga, *qigong*, and *tai chi* distinguishes them from conventional Western exercise techniques. Regular practice of any of these three practices helps to integrate the mind and body. Majid Ali, M.D., director of the Preventive Medicine Institute in Denville, New Jersey, recommends that yoga, *qigong*, or *tai chi* be performed in silence to allow individuals to become better attuned to the inner functioning of their bodies. This involves listening to the breath, feeling the pulse of the heart, and sensing the flow of inner energy. "Most of us are not connected to our own bodies," says naturopath Virender Sodhi, M.D., N.D., director of the American School of Ayurvedic Sciences in Bellevue, Washington. He explains that the experience of these Eastern healing arts helps us to better handle stress and maintain overall health.

Heal Your Emotional Appetite

AS EXPLAINED THROUGHOUT this book, weight gain is often the outcome of an underlying physiological problem, whether it be a toxic liver, blood sugar imbalance, food allergy, or other condition. At the same time, each of these physical causes also have a distinct emotional dimension. For example, anger tends to occur with a toxic liver, moodiness with a blood sugar imbalance, and anxiety with a food allergy. However, these emotions are not simply the effects of the physical illness, they can also be the cause—anger can make the liver become toxic, and a toxic liver may induce anger. Mainstream medical science has largely failed to appreciate the relationship of the emotions and health.

In contrast, alternative medicine therapies, particularly those based on centuries-old health traditions, have long recognized that emotional well-being is inextricably linked with physical health. Consequently, disease cannot be reduced to either a psychological or physiological problem; it is always a little of both. "In the practice of Oriental medicine, the psychological and the physiological are addressed at one and the same time," says Roger Jahnke, O.M.D., of Santa Barbara, California. "The idea is to enhance the body's own operating abilities at every level." Encouraging the body's ability to heal itself is at the core of alternative treatment programs that address the emotion-

In This Chapter

- Success Story: Emotional Gains and Weight Loss
- Feeding the Emotional Appetite
- Food Cravings and Stress
- Are You Stressed Out?
- Mind/Body Therapies for Weight Loss

al and physical aspects of illness and health. Combining the physical and emotional in a comprehensive approach to illness is considered by alternative medicine practitioners to come under the broad category of mind/body medicine.

Mind/body treatments enable you to examine what may be unconsciously driving you to gain weight and help raise your consciousness regarding what you choose to eat and why. They can relieve stress, alleviate depression, and, in turn, help you to lose weight permanently. In this chapter, we discuss ways that you can heal your body with the mind by examining the emotional components of your weight problems and exploring ways to alleviate stress.

Mind/Body Therapies for Weight Loss

- Develop Deliberate Eating Habits
- Cognitive Therapy
- Guided Imagery
- Neuro-Linguistic Programming
- Hypnotherapy
- Ultradian Rhythms
- Meditation
- Acupuncture and Therapeutic Touch
- Breathing Exercises
- Flower Essence Therapy
- Aromatherapy

Success Story: Emotional Gains and Weight Loss

Weight loss involves physical and emotional transformation, a process that must take place in every dimension of your life. "People who come to see me have tried to lose weight many times," says Paul Epstein, N.D., a naturopath from Norwalk, Connecticut. "They've either failed completely or lost only to gain it all back again. They have never understood how they use food and how food uses them. Instead, they substitute one obsession or compulsion for another and never get to the real source of what drives them." As an example of what "drives" people to gain weight, Dr. Epstein offers the following case study:

Clarissa tried every diet plan on the market, but with no success. She also suffered from high blood pressure and had been on medication for 25 years, with no improvement in her condition. When her weight reached 250 pounds (she was 5'6"), her doctor told her she was beginning to develop diabetes. He wanted to prescribe additional medications to help control the diabetes, but Clarissa was reluctant to become dependent on yet another drug. Consequently, she decided to seek out a second opinion and that's when she came to Dr. Epstein.

Paul Epstein, N.D.:
Center for Mind-Body
Medicine, Berkeley
Street, Norwalk, CT
06850; tel: 203-853-
6800.

He determined that Clarissa's condition stemmed from a nutritional deficiency and an addiction to sugary, greasy "junk" foods. He immediately started her on a recovery program that included nutritional supplements and mild exercise. While these remedies were important to help Clarissa break her sugar addiction, a key aspect of her treatment program involved exploring emotional issues. "Dr. Epstein helped me to understand that there was a real and concrete link between my health and some very painful emotional issues in my life," she said. "I discovered that I had been eating to comfort myself and that my fat was a way to cover up my feelings."

To help Clarissa with her psychological issues, Dr. Epstein used a technique called guided imagery. In guided imagery, a therapist suggests images to patients and instructs them to visualize the image in their mind. Patients are then asked to discuss what thoughts and feelings arise in response to the image. The expressed thoughts and feelings often become a means of drawing out buried emotional conflicts.

"I came to see that there were things in my life I needed to change, choices I had to make in order to be well," says Clarissa. "Improvements in diet and lifestyle were an important part of the process, but I couldn't make any of those changes until I became more sensitive to what was going on inside me. Once I did, it was easy to give up certain foods and adopt some new habits." The treatments helped Clarissa develop a new attitude towards food and a new outlook on life, which enabled her to control her food cravings and eat a healthier diet. Consequently, after three months of treatment, Clarissa's high blood pressure began to subside and her blood sugar problem disappeared. After nine months, she had lost 70 pounds. "For me, managing my weight continues to be a process of uncovering deeply buried feelings so that I can get in touch with what my body really wants and needs," she said.

Feeding the Emotional Appetite

Getting at the real sources that are driving you to gain weight may be one of the greatest challenges of achieving a healthy body weight. Like Clarissa, many individuals who look inside themselves for the answers discover that they have been struggling against a buried emotional conflict. Unresolved or unexpressed emotional issues may be driving you to food cravings and bingeing and any attempts at weight loss will prove unsuccessful until these issues are resolved.

"People that are overweight may be using food as a tranquilizer or a reward or a substitute for affection," says Douglas Ringrose, M.D., director of the Ringrose Wellness Institute in Edmonton, Alberta, Canada, which specializes in the treatment of eating disorders. "Others eat because it's something to do when they're bored or to turn themselves into a fortress against the world."

For more on **carbohydrate addictions and weight problems**, see Chapter 11: Break Food Allergies and Addictions, pp. 244-270.

Everybody has consumed foods for reasons other than that they were hungry. Occasional "emotional eating," to relieve anxiety or make you feel better, is perfectly normal. But when it leads to overeating, significant weight gain, and poor dietary choices, emotional eating can seriously affect your health. Food can become a substitute for or an escape from addressing the underlying psychological problems. These buried feelings can also be detrimental to your health: John P. Foreyt, Ph.D., of Baylor College in Waco, Texas, estimates that "two-thirds of all obese persons may be carbohydrate cravers who eat not for hunger but to combat tension, anxiety, mental fatigue, and depression."[1]

Researchers at Johnson State College in Vermont studied 112 undergraduate women divided into four groups: obese bingers, obese non-bingers, normal-weight bingers, and normal-weight non-bingers. What they found was that the bingers, regardless of whether they were obese or normal weight, suffered higher levels of depression and anxiety and lower self-esteem than the non-bingers.[2] Another study interviewed 100 significantly overweight patients enrolling in a dietary program regarding the onset of their weight problems. Compared to 100 normal-weight individuals, the obese patients had experienced a higher prevalence of childhood abuse, early loss of a parent, alcoholism in the family, depression, and marital problems. Many reported using overeating as a way to cope with emotional distress.[3] Other studies have found a clear correlation between emotions such as boredom, anxiety, hostility, and anger (particularly unexpressed anger) and the development of weight problems.[4]

"In situations such as boredom and loneliness, eating becomes a way to fill the emotional void," according to Elizabeth, Somer, M.A., R.D., author of *Food and Mood*. "While preventing boredom and developing meaningful relationships take time and effort, eating is easy and relatively effortless. Boredom, anxiety, anger, depression, jealousy, and other emotions are a normal part of life, but using food to treat them or to avoid resolving them is not a long-term solution for feeling better."[5]

Food Cravings and Stress

Although the concept of stress—being "stressed out" or "under constant stress"—may be commonly discussed today, its role as a contributing factor in many diseases is underappreciated. Estimates suggest that as many as 70% to 80% of all visits to physicians' offices are for stress-related problems.[6] Chronic stress directly affects the immune system, and if not effectively dealt with, can seriously compromise health. Stress is a pervasive problem among Americans, according to a 1996 poll of corporate executives. For example, 44% of employees polled said their work load is excessive compared to 37% in 1988; 43% are bothered by excessive job pressure; 55% worry considerably about their company's future; 25% of both men and women feel stressed out at work every day, another 12% feel it almost every day, and another 38% feel it once to several days a week.[7]

Stress can be defined as a reaction to any stimulus or interference that upsets normal functioning and disturbs mental or physical health. It can be brought on by internal conditions such as illness, pain, emotional conflict, or psychological problems, or by external circumstances, such as bereavement, financial problems, loss of job, relocation, food allergies, and electromagnetic fields. Stress, when it becomes chronic, is often unrecognized by the person whose body is experiencing it; one begins to accept it as a fact of life, without being aware of how it is actually compromising all bodily function and preparing the foundation for illness.

When we sense that we are "stressed," what we often feel is anxiety or even fear. On a physiological level, the adrenal glands (see "Stress and the Adrenal Glands," p. 161) begin releasing the hormones cortisol, adrenaline, and noradrenaline into the bloodstream. This so-called "adrenaline rush" rouses the body into action, causing an immediate increase in heart rate and breathing and a rise in blood pressure. Under severe stress, such as a life-threatening situation, the rush of adrenal hormones raises energy levels so that we can respond to the emergency. This "fight-or-flight" response has been programmed in our bodies by centuries of evolution. It is what gave our ancestors the strength to survive dangerous situations.

During a fight-or-flight response, the body channels all of its resources to the muscles. "You need every ounce of energy to supply the large muscles for instant, strenuous action," explains Stephen Langer, M.D., author of *Solved: The Riddle of Weight Loss*.[8] Under prolonged or high stress situations, the body will extract energy

Stress and the Adrenal Glands

The adrenal glands, part of the body's endocrine system, are located atop the kidneys. The glands are composed of two types of tissue: the adrenal medulla and the adrenal cortex. The adrenal medulla, comprising 10%-20% of the gland, is located in the interior portion and is responsible for the production of the hormones epinephrine (adrenaline) and norepinephrine (noradrenaline). These hormones are released in direct response to the sympathetic nervous system, which is responsible for the fight-or-flight response to stress or physical threats. The adrenal cortex, the outer layer, surrounds the medulla and accounts for 80%-90% of the gland. It is responsible for the production of corticosteroids (also called adrenal steroids). Over 30 different steroids have been isolated from the adrenal cortex, including cortisol and cortisone.

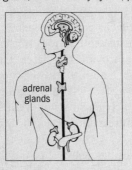

adrenal glands

Cortisol secretion (as well as the adrenal gland's other steroids, DHEA, adrenaline, and aldosterone) occurs in daily cycles, peaking in the morning and having the lowest values at night. Cortisol promotes protein building, regulates insulin and glycogen synthesis, and helps produce prostaglandins (hormone-like fatty acids involved in inflammatory processes). Under conditions of stress, high amounts of cortisol are released. Imbalances in cortisol secretion are linked with low energy, inflammation, muscle dysfunction, impaired bone repair, thyroid dysfunction, immune system depression, sleep disorders, and poor skin regeneration.

from protein and minerals cannibalized from the kidneys, liver, stomach, and bones. At the same time, the body will conserve energy in other areas by shutting down "non-emergency" functions, such as the digestion and absorption of nutrients.

Among the more serious impacts of chronic stress is impaired digestion, which causes nutritional deficiencies. Over time, the body will attempt to compensate for these nutritional deficiencies by demanding more food in the form of insatiable hunger and relentless food cravings. In response to these demands, we often eat far more than our systems can use or effectively handle. The net effect is that most of the food eaten in response to stress is converted into body fat.

Initially, many people experience a diminished appetite during stress and may even lose weight. However, as the body tries to recover, hunger returns with a vengence. Obesity specialist Maria

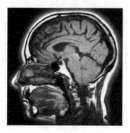

The production of cortisol, one of the hormones secreted by the adrenals during stress, stimulates the production of a brain chemical called neuropeptide Y. This chemical can set off an alarm within the body for sweet or starchy food.

Simonson, Ph.D., Sc.D., says that when people lose weight because they eat less during stressful periods of their lives, they tend to gain back even more from overeating later. Dr. Simonson, who directs the Health, Weight, and Stress Clinic at the Johns Hopkins University School of Medicine in Baltimore, Maryland, says that six to seven weeks following a stressful event, 40% of patients begin to eat excessively, often reaching a weight level that exceeds their original one.[9]

Stress also causes biochemical changes in the brain that induce sweet cravings. Sarah Leibowitz, Ph.D., of Rockefeller University, says that the production of cortisol, one of the hormones secreted by the adrenals during stress, stimulates the production of a brain chemical called neuropeptide Y. This chemical can set off an alarm within the body for sweet or starchy food. As we satisfy this desire by eating a candy bar or some other similar food, the neurochemical buzzer quiets down and we usually feel better. If the alarm goes off in the morning, however, it may stay "turned on" all day, causing a relentless craving for sweets.[10]

Other brain chemicals involved in appetite control, called neurotransmitters, may also be affected by stress. Neurotransmitters enable communications between brain cells or neurons—electrical thought impulses are changed into neurotransmitters at the dendrites, the branching tips of a nerve cell, then they are passed on to the next nerve cell. Serotonin helps produce sleep, regulate pain, and influence mood—it's called the "feel good" neurotransmitter—although too much serotonin can produce depression; low levels of serotonin may cause carbohydrate cravings. Dopamine regulates physical movements and muscular control, and it influences mood, sex drive, and memory retrieval; low levels are linked to depression and increased appetite. Norepinephrine causes the brain to be more alert; it helps carry memories from short-term to long-term "storage" and it enables one to maintain a positive mood; low levels are linked to mood disorders and increases in appetite.

Are You Stressed Out?

If you answer "yes" to more than five questions below, it indicates that you may have too much stress in your life. In parentheses after each question are some potential underlying causes for the problem.

- Do you often grind your teeth? (digestive dysfunction, parasites)
- Is your breath shallow and irregular? (low metabolic energy, food allergies) ✓
- Are your hands and feet cold? (hormonal imbalance, adrenal/thyroid weakness)
- Do you have trouble sleeping or tend to wake up tired? (liver dysfunction, food allergies) ✓
- Do you often have an upset stomach? (food allergies) ✓
- Do you get mad or irritated easily? (liver dysfunction) +
- Do you feel worthless? (low metabolic energy, chronic fatigue)
- Do you constantly worry? (hormonal imbalance)
- Do you have problems concentrating and articulating your thoughts? (low metabolic energy, digestive or hormonal imbalance)
- Do you frequently fidget, chew your fingers, or bite your nails? (food allergies, digestive disturbances)
- Do you have high blood pressure? (food allergies, digestive disturbances)
- Do you eat, drink, or smoke excessively? (low metabolic energy, poor diet)
- Do you sometimes turn to recreational drugs just to get away? (low metabolic energy, poor diet)

✓ ③
+ 1
• 2

Are Your Adrenal Glands Stressed?

The Adrenal Stress Index (ASI) can pinpoint whether an imbalance in the adrenal glands might be contributing to hormonal imbalance and weight gain. This test evaluates how well one's adrenal glands are functioning by tracking hormone levels over a 24-hour cycle (circadian rhythm). Four saliva samples taken at intervals throughout the day are used to reconstruct the adrenal rhythm in the laboratory. Saliva has been shown to closely mirror blood levels of hormones and a saliva test is also less invasive. These samples are used to determine whether two main stress hormones (cortisol and DHEA) are being secreted in proper proportion to each other and at the right times. Based on the results, a physician can prescribe the appropriate treatment to restore the balance of hormones and correct the circadian rhythm.

For the **Adrenal Stress Index test**, contact: Diagnos-Tech, Inc., 6620 South 192nd Place, J-2204, Kent, WA 96032; tel: 800-878-3787 or 425-251-0596; fax: 425-251-0637.

The Personal is
the Political

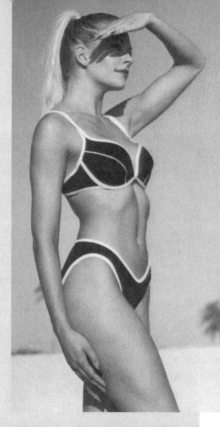

As you explore your emotional issues, it is important to keep in mind that your inner desires and feelings regarding body weight are shaped by what you see and hear everyday. Consequently, to really get at the source of what's driving you, you must be able to recognize how your inner desires are influenced by social factors. You need to distinguish between feelings that are you own and those that come from the outside in the form of social pressure. "Rapid weight loss at any price, so you can fit into a particular dress or feel comfortable in a swimsuit, is about image," says Jeremy Kaslow, M.D. "Weight management, however, is about the pursuit of lifelong health, and the two are very different."

Many individuals try to lose weight in pursuit of a sexier, slimmer image. While we are all entitled to pursue such an end, occasionally the yearning to "look good" is motivated by a need to conform to someone else's ideal of what you should look like. Ask yourself why you feel the need to reduce. It is important not to confuse the yearnings to satisfy someone else's demands with your own desire to be healthy and live at your peak physical level.

Psychologist Kathleen Pichola, Ph.D., tells her clients to carefully consider why they may be unhappy with their weight. She explains that the image of the perfect female body is a cultural construct and has changed many times in the past 150 years. "In the 1940s and 1950s, bigger, more ample women were considered most desirable," she says. Since the 1970s, however, the ideal woman has become increasingly thinner. As an example of the trend toward a super-thin standard of beauty, Dr. Pichola points to the fact that the weight of participants in the Miss America pageant has decreased by 16% over the past 20 years.

Dr. Pichola herself battled with weight for 35 years before she realized that it wasn't her body that was "wrong" but society's ideal of what is beautiful. That's when she decided to shift her focus from how much she weighed to how she felt, physically and emotionally. She decided to call a truce with her war on fat, and establish a peaceful relationship with food and her body. "Amazingly, befriending my body made me want to treat it well, feed it well, do whatever was necessary to feel healthy and balanced." Dr. Pichola emphasizes that women need to understand that today's idealized image of the super-thin model is not about anything real or beautiful. "Real beauty," she says, "is based on health, strength, and the visibility of our souls."

Because of the diet culture and the commercial interests that bombard us with images of ultra-thin models, we learn to hate our own bodies and, in turn, are led to destructive and self-defeating eating behaviors. The reality is that most of us can never attain the cultural ideal, no matter how hard we try. "The standard for a beautiful body, the movie-star magazine model body, is natural for only one-fifth of the population. This has created a whole generation of women who are dieting and exercising compulsively, and often uselessly, at the expense of their health, in pursuit of an unrealistic ideal," says Dr. Pichola.[11] Freeing yourself from such ideals may be the best thing you can do to restore your health.

Mind/Body Therapies for Weight Loss

Obviously, one way to prevent the weight-gaining effects of stress is to avoid stressful situations. However, since this is not always possible, it is important to be able to control how you react to a stressful situation. "With few exceptions, damage from stress results from a negative emotional response to stressors, rather that from the stressors themselves," says Dr. Langer.[12] Mind/body treatments, such as guided imagery, Neuro-Linguistic Programming, and hypnotherapy, can "reprogram" the negative psychological factors that may be contributing to weight gain, helping you gain greater control over your emotional responses. These therapies help you "stockpile positive emotions and sweep out negative thoughts," according to Dr. Ringrose. "You're programming your computer—the brain—for the emotions that you want, rather than any that are trying to intrude and sabotage your weight-loss efforts." Other therapies, including meditation, acupuncture, flower essences, and aromatherapy, can also be used to mitigate the effects of stress.

Douglas Ringrose, M.D.: Ringrose Wellness Institute, 8702 Meadowlark Road, Suite 380, Edmonton, Alberta, Canada T5R 5W4; tel: 403-484-8401.

Develop Deliberate Eating Habits

Much of the eating associated with emotional upset or stress is impulsive. When you reach for a candy bar or some other snack, you don't really think about why you are doing it. One way to control the weight-gaining effect of stress is to develop more deliberate eating habits. This requires focusing on the reasons why you are reaching for a snack or other food. It involves consciously exploring the many nuances of feeling that are associated with the desire to eat and distinguishing feelings of hunger from a desire to gratify an emotional need.

Nutrition expert Lita Lee, Ph.D., of Lowell, Oregon, recommends pausing before you reach for any food and asking yourself a series of questions. Are you really hungry? Do you feel upset? Is the food you desire nutritious or merely flavorful? Another way of becoming more conscious of your dietary habits is to keep a daily food diary. The diary should include notes about what you ate; how you felt before, during, and after eating; how many times you ate; the cravings you may have experienced; and whether you succumbed to them or not. Writing down this information will make you a more sensitive observer of your food choices and habits and allow you to assess long-term patterns in your behavior that may otherwise have been missed.

Cognitive Therapy

It has been estimated that the average human being has around 50,000 thoughts per day, according to Dr. Richard Carlson, author of *Don't Sweat The Small Stuff...And It's All Small Stuff*. Unfortunately, he reminds us, many of them are also going to be negative—angry, fearful, pessimistic, or worrisome. Up to 85% of the thinking we regularly engage in is negative and self-defeating.[13]

There are effective ways to reprogram your thinking for successful weight loss. The basis of cognitive therapy is to identify—through maintaining a journal and by introspection—the negative, self-defeating inner dialogue of thoughts (what cognitive therapists refer to as "automatic thoughts"). Positive, coping thoughts can then be used to counter the negative thoughts. The goal is to pull yourself out of reflexive self-destructive mental behavior that may be exacerbating your problem and to bolster the positive, self-reliant aspect of your personality. Cognitive therapy does not focus on the root causes of psychological problems, rather it seeks to support health by interrupting the flow of negative thoughts. Countering each negative thought with a list of positive responses to the same problem enables the mind to reframe the situation.

It is easy to feel overwhelmed during times of transition as you struggle to incorporate changes, such as new ways of eating, into your

---

For more on **cognitive therapy**, contact: University of Pennsylvania Center for Cognitive Therapy, 3600 Market Street, 8th Floor, Philadelphia, PA 19104; tel: 215-898-4100; fax: 215-898-1865; website: www.med.upenn.edu/psycct. American Institute for Cognitive Therapy, 136 E. 57th Street, Suite 1101, New York, NY 10022; tel: 212-308-2440; fax 212-308-9847; website: www.cognitivetherapynyc.com. For information about **support groups**, contact: National Self-Help Clearinghouse, 25 West 43rd Street, New York, NY 10036; tel: 212-817-1822; website: www.selfhelpweb.org. American Self-Help Clearinghouse, St. Clares-Riverside Medical Center, 25 Pocono Road, Denville, NJ 07834; tel: 201-625-7101; fax: 973-625-8848; website: www.njshc.org.

life. Resist the temptation to isolate yourself and remember why you are undergoing this process. As you continue to make choices for a healthier life, realize that any periods of discomfort are temporary. If you do not already have one, establish a support network of friends and family to help you get through the rough spots. You might also consider recruiting a "dieting buddy" or a workout partner to help you stay the course when your motivation begins to flag. Investigate joining a support group, where you may find that being in the company of like-minded people experiencing similar changes and difficulties may bolster your own progress and help keep things in perspective.

Guided Imagery

Many alternative health-care practitioners use guided imagery as a tool for healing. Jeanne Achterberg, Ph.D., president for the Association for Transpersonal Psychology, indicates that every mental image a person has can affect such important body processes as immune function, blood flow, and heart rate.[14] Studies have shown that guided imagery can decrease chronic nightmares, reduce substance abuse, and alleviate many other psychological and physiological problems.[15]

Five Healing Steps You Can Take Now

Christiane Northrup, M.D., of Yarmouth, Maine, honors the dictum "do unto yourself as you (usually) do unto others" in offering these five easy steps as a way to prevent emotional turmoil:

■ Say no: Draw boundaries and get rid of the "shoulds," guilt trips, and people-pleasing habits.

■ Listen to your body: Rest when you are tired, eat when you are hungry, and realize that your body has an innate, internal wisdom and always knows exactly what you need.

■ Let go of whatever is not working: To heal, you must be willing to let go of things that no longer serve you (bad relationships, old ideas and beliefs, a stressful job) and make room for healthy things (physical well-being, positive people, new opportunities).

■ Accept yourself "as is": Pat yourself on the back for coming as far as you have, and realize that healing only begins when you love yourself for who you are today, right this moment.

■ Say "yes" to feeling good: Believe you can feel better and take steps to make it so.[16]

Using the power of the mind and the imagination, guided imagery and visualization can elicit positive physiological responses. By directly accessing emotions, imagery can help an individual understand the needs that may be represented by an illness and can help develop ways to meet those needs. Imagery is also one of the quickest and most direct ways to become aware of emotions and their effects on health, both positive and negative.

For information on **guided imagery**, contact: Academy for Guided Imagery, P.O. Box 2070, Mill Valley, CA 94942; tel: 800-726-2070 or 415-389-9325; fax: 415-389-9342; website: www.healthy.net/agi.

Imagery is simply a flow of thoughts that one can see, hear, feel, smell, taste, or experience. According to Martin L. Rossman, M.D., of the Academy for Guided Imagery, in Mill Valley, California, while the sensory phenomenon that is being experienced in the mind may or may not represent external reality, it always depicts internal reality. What Dr. Rossman means is that the sensations in the body that imagery creates are very real phenomena that can be measured via laboratory devices. Research using brain scans indicates that imagery activates parts of the cerebral cortex and sensory centers of the brain. "If you are a good worrier," states Dr., Rossman, "and especially if you ever 'worry yourself sick', you may be an especially good candidate for learning how to positively affect your health with imagery, as the internal process involved in worrying yourself sick and 'imagining yourself well' are quite similar."[17]

Neuro-Linguistic Programming

Neuro-Linguistic Programming (NLP) helps people detect unconscious patterns of thought, behavior, and attitudes that contribute to their health problems. These unconscious patterns are then reprogrammed in order to alter psychological responses and facilitate the healing process. *Neuro* refers to the way the brain works and how thinking demonstrates consistent and detectable patterns; *linguistic* refers to the verbal and nonverbal expressions of thinking patterns; *programming* denotes how these patterns are recognized and understood by the mind and how they can be altered.

NLP was developed in the early 1970s by a professor of linguistics and a student of psychology and mathematics, both at the University of California at Santa Cruz. They studied the thinking processes, language patterns, and behavioral patterns of several accomplished individuals. They found that body cues—eye movement, posture, voice tone, and breathing patterns—coincided with certain unconscious patterns of a person's emotional state. Based on their findings, they developed the NLP technique to help people with emotional problems.

People who have difficulty recovering from physical illness or losing weight have often adopted negative beliefs about their recovery. They perceive themselves as helpless, hopeless, or worthless,

For information on **Neuro-Linguistic Programming**, contact: NLP University/Dynamic Learning Center, P.O. Box 1112, Ben Lomond, CA 95005; tel: 408-336-3457; fax: 408-336-5854; website: www.nlpu.com. NLP Comprehensive, 5695 Yukon Street, Arvada, CO 80002; tel: 800-233-1657 or 303-940-8888; fax 303-940-8889; website: www.nlpcomprehensive.com. NLP Seminars Group International, P.O. Box 424, Hopatcong, NJ 07843; tel: 201-770-1084; website: www.purenlp.com.

expressed in statements like "I can't get healthy" or "I'll never lose weight." NLP tries to move the person from their present state of discomfort to a desired state of health by helping reprogram these beliefs about healing.

NLP practitioners ask questions to discover how the person relates to issues of identity, personal beliefs, life goals, and their health, then observe the person's language patterns, eye movements, postures, muscle tension, and gestures. These relay information about how the person relates to their condition in both conscious and unconscious ways, revealing what limiting beliefs may exist. These belief structures can then be altered using NLP. The practitioner will ask the person to see herself in a state of health. By doing so, an outcome is set that facilitates the healing process. The brain's natural response is to duplicate whatever images or beliefs are created about getting better.[18] The brain then triggers the necessary immunological responses to guide the body toward health.

Hypnotherapy

Hypnosis can help change emotional attachments to a particular food. "If I truly, deeply believe that a big ice cream sundae is going to make me feel better," says Sharon Thorn, A.C.H.T., a hypnotherapist from Naples, Florida, "then there's no way that I can force myself not to think about it. We give energy to what we think about and even if I can resist the impulse for a short time, eventually I'll have to give in. That's why trying to control eating behaviors with willpower—'toughing out' our urges to eat certain foods—is useless in the long run."

Sharon Thorn, A.C.H.T., helps people deal with weight control issues. For more information, contact: Hypnosis Centers of Florida, 12781 World Plaza Lane, Fort Myers, FL 33907; tel: 941-278-5300. Hypnosis Centers of Florida, Detchess Centers Offices, 9853 North Tamiami Trail, Naples, FL 33963; tel: 941-594-7900. For more on **hypnotherapy**, contact: American Institute of Hypnotherapy, 1805 East Garry Avenue, Suite 100, Santa Ana, CA 92606; tel: 800-634-8766 or 949-261-6400. American Society of Clinical Hypnosis, 2200 East Devon Avenue, Suite 291, Des Plaines, IL 60018; tel: 708-297-3317.

Hypnosis works by helping you reach a state of consciousness where you are more receptive to suggestion. It adjusts your emotional programming, replacing one set of associations with another. "You have to actually replace the belief that the sundae will make you feel good with a different belief," says Thorn. "What happens with hypnosis is much like what happens with meditation: the body is relaxed, the chattering thoughts in the mind are stilled. The difference is that with meditation, you go to the edge of silence and find answers within yourself. With hypnosis, the suggestions come from the outside, from the hypnotherapist."

It is important to understand that hypnosis is controlled by the patient. Despite what you may have seen on televi-

SAD No More

Individuals who receive little natural light during the day often experience an imbalance in their serotonin and melatonin levels—specifically, a rise in melatonin and a corresponding decline in serotonin. When low-light exposure is chronic, it can lead to a specific type of illness called seasonal affective disorder or SAD. Often called "winter depression," SAD frequently occurs during the fall and winter months, when days grow shorter and natural light is limited.

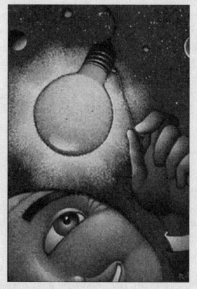

The symptoms of SAD's winter doldrums are no doubt familiar to many. In fact, it's estimated that over ten million Americans experience SAD every year, according to the National Institute of Mental Health (NIMH), and another 25 million get some milder depressive symptoms on a seasonal basis. What does SAD feel like? Typically, there is chronic depression and fatigue, which may leave you bedridden; hypersomnia (increased sleep by as much as four hours or more per night) and reduced quality of the sleep, leaving you feeling less refreshed; and cravings for carbohydrates and candy, which can lead to sometimes significant weight gain.

Individuals with SAD do experience elevated metabolism, which helps them burn more calories. Nevertheless, these increases are not sufficient to match corresponding increases in appetite. "If you had a higher metabolic rate in the winter, burning about 200 additional calories each day, you would expect to lose weight," says Russel J. Reiter, Ph.D., author of *Melatonin: Your Body's Natural Wonder Drug.* "But if you also had such a hearty appetite that you consumed 400 extra calories each day, you would have a net gain of 200 calories. Over the span of several months, you could easily gain five to ten pounds. We believe this is what causes many people with SAD to gain weight."

One way to restore serotonin levels is by stimulating the pineal gland, which produces serotonin and melatonin. One of the ways to stimulate the pineal gland is through light therapy. When light enters the eye, electrical impulses travel along the optic nerve to the brain where they trigger the pineal gland to secrete hormones. The levels of serotonin and melatonin seesaw according to the cycles of light and darkness. Light stimulates the pineal to produce serotonin, while darkness causes it to produce more melatonin. Dr. Reiter indicates that an increased appetite, particularly for carbohydrates, may be caused by low serotonin, while depression may be caused by too much melatonin.[19]

Light therapy is a technique used to counteract the effects of winter depression and assist in weight loss by helping to maintain healthy levels of serotonin and melatonin. The oldest form of light therapy is natural sunlight: the sun is the ultimate source of full-spectrum light, which means it contains all possible wavelengths of light, from infrared to ultraviolet (UV). Obviously, one solution is to spend the winter in the tropics and leave your SADness in New York or Ottawa. But if that isn't an option, why not simulate sunlight to get more summer into you. Seventh Generation, Inc., a producer of environmentally safe household products, based in Burlington, Vermont, offers a line of full spectrum light bulbs, which provide a "warmer," more natural light that closely resembles sunlight, according to the manufacturer. You can also cozy up to an artificial "sun" while you work. The Happylite is a portable light box (made by Verilux, Inc., of Stamford, Connecticut) which provides 10,000 lux light through a lens that blocks ultraviolet light and electromagnetic radiation.

Light therapy has been shown to be particularly effective in controlling appetite. In one study, ten patients treated with light therapy lost an average of nine pounds.[20] In anoth-

For more on **the role of hormones in weight gain**, see Chapter 10: Restore Hormonal Balance, pp. 220-243.

For more on **light therapy** contact: Society for Light Treatment and Biological Rhythms, Inc., 10200 West 44th Avenue, Suite 304, Wheat Ridge, CO 80033-2840; tel: 303-422-7905; fax: 303-422-8894. College of Syntonic Optometry, 1200 Robeson Street, Fall River, MA 02720-5508; tel: 508-673-1251. For sources of **full spectrum lighting**, contact: Seventh Generation, One Mill Street, Box A-26, Burlington, VT 05401-1530; tel: 800-456-1191 or 802-658-3773; fax: 802-658-1771. Verilux Inc., 9 Viaduct Road, Stamford, CT 06907; tel: 800-786-6850 or 203-921-2430; fax: 203-921-2427; website: www.ergolight.com.

er study, bright light therapy has proven helpful in cases of bulimia—an eating disorder that consists of a pattern of bingeing on large amounts of food followed by vomiting. Raymond W. Lam, M.D., assistant professor of psychiatry at the University of British Colombia in Vancouver, Canada, says, "During two weeks of bright-light therapy, 17 women, 20 to 45 years old, experienced a 50% reduction in the number of binges and purges, as well as in their feelings of depression."

In addition to light therapy, you can also increase serotonin levels by taking 5-HTP, short for 5-hydroxytryptophan. 5-HTP is a natural building block the body uses to make serotonin. A 1992 Italian study with obese subjects found that 5-HTP produced "significant weight loss." Specifically, 5-HTP helped patients reduce their carbohydrate intake and gave them a feeling of "early satiety"—that they'd eaten enough and felt calorically satisfied. This led to a reduced food intake and weight loss. Even without special diets, those in the group taking 5-HTP lost an average 3.1 to 3.7 pounds during the six-week study; those in the placebo group averaged only a 1.1-pound loss. "These findings together with the good tolerance observed suggest that 5-HTP may safely be used to treat obesity," concluded the researchers.

5-HTP is found naturally in several foods, particularly continued on next page

SAD No More (cont.)

proteins like cow's milk, eggs, poultry, and some nuts and seeds. Tryptophan obtained through the diet is usually converted in the brain into 5-HTP, which is then turned into serotonin. 5-HTP augments, rather than alters, the body's natural ability to produce serotonin. In contrast, Prozac, Zoloft, and other antidepressant drugs work by influencing serotonin levels. Specifically, they belong to a class of drugs known as selective serotonin reuptake inhibitors (or SSRIs), which increase the serotonin level indirectly by blocking its inactivation. The tryptophan in 5-HTP (an extract from *Griffonia simplicifolia*, a West African plant) provides brain cells with the necessary materials to make more serotonin, without blocking any normal metabolic processes and without the serious side effects of SSRIs, which include dry mouth, reduced libido, heart palpitations, tremors, and anxiety.

For more about **5-HTP**, contact: NutriCology, 400 Preda Street, San Leandro, CA 94577; tel: 800-545-9960 or 510-639-4572; fax: 510-635-6730. Vitamin Research Products Inc.; 3579 Highway 50 East, Carson City, NV 89701; tel: 800-877-2447 or 702-884-1300; fax: 800-877-3292 or 702-884-1331.

The typical recommended dosage of 5-HTP is 25-50 mg daily.

Precautions: Higher daily dosages (over 100 mg) could cause some side effects, including mild nausea. Consult a qualified health practitioner before taking 5-HTP, particularly if you are taking any prescription medications. 5-HTP can amplify the effects of many mood-altering or weight-loss drugs. People with heart conditions or asthma should proceed with caution, as elevated serotonin levels could affect these conditions. 5-HTP (or tryptophan) should only be taken under the supervision of a physician if you have Parkinson's, cancer, autoimmune conditions, lung or liver diseases, anorexia, allergies, nausea or diarrhea, sickle cell anemia, or hemophilia. Pregnant women should not supplement with 5-HTP or L-tryptophan. Vitamin B6 should also be taken on the same day as 5-HTP, because it is necessary for converting 5-HTP into serotonin.[21]

---

sion, a hypnotist cannot make you do anything against your will. "All hypnosis is self-hypnosis," states A. M. Krasner, Ph.D., founder and director of the American Institute of Hypnotherapy in Santa Ana, California. "The hypnotherapist is a facilitator. The fact is that there can be no hypnosis unless the client is willing to participate in the process. The client always enters hypnosis in a natural way, of his or her own accord, simply by following the suggestions of the hypnotherapist."

Hypnosis can be either superficial or somnambulistic. In the superficial hypnotic state, the patient accepts suggestions but does not necessarily carry them out. Patients who reach the deep, or somnambulistic, state benefit most from hypnotherapy. It is in this state that post-hypnotic suggestions (suggestions that take effect after the patient awakens from the trance) are most successful. According to the World Health Organization, 90% of the general population can be hypnotized, with 20% to 30% having a high enough susceptibility to enter the somnambulistic state, making them highly receptive to treatment.[22] Three conditions are essential to successful hypnotherapy: 1) good rapport between hypnotist and subject; 2) a comfortable environment, free of distraction; and 3) a willingness and desire by the subject to be hypnotized. People who benefit most from hypnotherapy are those who understand that hypnosis is not a surrender of control; it is only an advanced form of relaxation.

Many individuals have used hypnosis to successfully lose weight. "Once you're relaxed, I help you focus on your aim," explains Thorn. "Say your goal weight is 130 pounds but your actual weight is 170 pounds. Under hypnosis, I might suggest that you see yourself already at 130. I would ask you to feel all the good feelings that come with being that weight." Thorn generally makes a live recording of the sessions with her clients that they then play repeatedly at home. By repeating the taped session, the suggestions can penetrate to a deeper level of consciousness.

Ultradian Rhythms

The ultradian rhythm method is a technique related to hypnosis that can help you develop healthier eating patterns. Rather than actively inducing a state of unconsciousness, ultradian rhythms take advantage of the natural ebb and flow of consciousness that you experience throughout the day. Scientists know that humans run on an internal, biological clock. They've charted these rhythms, discovering that there are day-long cycles (circadian) and other cycles that repeat many times within a day (ultradian). Ultradian rhythms generally occur in 90-120 minute cycles. Although these cycles are commonly thought of in physical terms (such as changes in heart rate), they also have a psychological dimension.

Ernest Rossi, Ph.D., a Malibu, California, researcher specializing in psychobiology (the science of the interrelationships that exist between mind and body), says that within each ultradian cycle there are 20-minute "windows" when we are naturally receptive to change. These windows were first recognized by the late Milton Erickson, M.D., a pioneer in therapeutic hypnosis, who described the windows as "common everyday trances." It is a time when the individual's mind/body state shifts, for reasons that are unknown, from activity to quietness. According to Dr. Rossi, these 20-minute periods are really a mild form of spontaneous self-hypnosis, when the unconscious and conscious parts of the mind overlap a little. During these times, it is possible to obtain insights about troubling problems and resolve inner conflicts.

Signs that you are approaching a window include stretching, yawning, and sighing. You may also experience an urge to snack, go to the bathroom, doodle, or daydream. When you begin to notice yourself in need of such distractions, it is a good time to intentionally relax, breathe more deeply, and allow yourself to shift your focus inward. You should also momentarily disengage from your work or other activities. Although this is understandably difficult for many people to do, the consequences of ignoring your body's natural call to disengage can be harmful. According to Dr. Rossi, it can ultimately lead to illness.

Dr. Rossi recommends that if you want to control your eating habits and lose weight, you should use the signals from your ultradian rhythms to tell you when to eat. This generally means that, rather than eating two or three large meals a day, you should eat more frequently, generally every 3-4 hours. To prevent overeating, Dr. Rossi recommends that you prepare these "minimeals," dividing your total daily food intake into six separate portions.

Meditation

Meditation is a safe and simple way to balance a person's physical, emotional, and mental states. Meditation, in the broadest sense, is any activity that keeps the attention focused in the present. When the mind is calm and focused in the present, it is neither reacting to past events or preoccupied with future plans, two major sources of chronic stress. There are many forms of meditation, but they can be categorized into two main approaches, concentration meditation and mindfulness meditation.

Concentration meditation focuses the "lens of the mind" on one object, sound (mantra), the breath, an image, or thought, to still the mind and allow greater awareness or clarity to emerge. The breath is one of the most popular objects of focus in this type of meditation. As the person focuses on the ebb and flow of their breath, the mind is absorbed in the rhythm and becomes more tranquil. Mindfulness-based meditation entails tuning out the world and bringing the mind to a halt as much as possible. Mindfulness meditation helps us practice non-judgment. The meditator sits quietly and simply witnesses whatever goes through the mind, not reacting or becoming involved with

A Glossary of Traditional Chinese Medicine Terms

Traditional Chinese medicine (TCM) originated in China over 5,000 years ago and is a comprehensive system of medical practice that heals the body according to the principles of nature and balance. A Chinese medicine physician considers the flow of vital energy (*qi*) in a patient through close examination of the patient's pulse, tongue, body odor, voice tone and strength, and general demeanor, among other elements. Underlying imbalances and disharmony in the body are described in terminology analogous to the natural world (heat, cold, dryness, or dampness). The concept of balance, or the interrelationship of organs, is central to TCM. In TCM, imbalances are corrected through the use of acupuncture, moxibustion, herbal medicine, dietary therapy, massage, and therapeutic exercise.

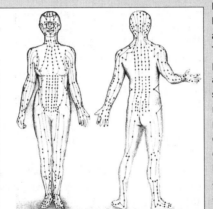

Acupuncture is an integrated healing system developed by the Chinese and introduced in the United States in the mid-1800s. The treatment is administered by an acupuncturist using hair-thin, stainless-steel needles, generally presterilized and disposable; these are lightly inserted into the skin at any of over 1,000 locations on the body's surface, known as acupoints. Acupoints are places where *qi* can be accessed by acupuncturists to reduce, enhance, or redirect its flow.

Acupuncture meridians are specific pathways in the human body for the flow of *qi*. In most cases, these energy pathways run up and down both sides of the body, and correspond to individual organs or organ systems, designated as Lung, Small Intestine, Heart, and others. There are 12 principal meridians and eight secondary channels. Numerous points of heightened energy, or *qi*, exist on the body's surface along the meridians and are called acupoints.

In **moxibustion**, a dried herb called moxa (usually mugwort) is burned over the skin at a specific acupuncture point. The moxa may be attached to a special acupuncture needle or in a free-standing cone set on a slice of ginger; its slow burning provides a penetrating heat. The purpose is to warm the blood and *qi*, particularly when a patient's energy picture is cold or damp.

thoughts, memories, worries, or images. This helps the person gain a more calm, clear, and non-reactive state of mind.

Transcendental Meditation™ (TM), a popular form of concentration meditation, is the most well-documented regarding the physiological effects of meditation, with over 500 clinical studies conducted to date.[23] Research shows that during TM practice, the body gains a deeper state of relaxation than during ordinary rest or sleep.[24] Brain wave changes indicate a state of enhanced awareness and coherence and TM has been found to increase intelligence, creativity, and perceptual ability and reduce blood pressure and rates of illness by 50%.[25] TM also causes decreased blood levels of cortisol, a hormone responsible for many of the deleterious physiological changes seen with stress.[26]

Acupuncture and Therapeutic Touch

To help patients cope with stress, as well as correct other imbalances that may be contributing to weight gain, practitioners of mind/body medicine often adjust a patient's energy fields. These fields, generally ignored by mainstream practitioners, link the emotions, consciousness, and physical body. "Other cultures recognize that there is a kind of energy that animates us," says Kristy Fassler, N.D., of Portsmouth, New Hampshire, a practitioner of both homeopathy and naturopathy. "It's called *qi* in China, *prana* in India."

In the Chinese model, *qi* is considered to be the life force that flows along specific pathways, called meridians, throughout the body (see "A Glossary of Traditional Chinese Medicine Terms," p. 175). Points of heightened energy along the meridians are called acupoints. Sometimes the flow of *qi* in the body can become blocked, causing illnesses to develop. An acupuncturist uses the acupoints to stimulate the flow of *qi* and thus restore health to the body. In addition to its physical effects, acupuncture has a positive psychological effect as well. Acupuncture is equivalent to the effect of drug-based therapies in cases of depression, insomnia, and other nervous disorders, and its action is swift and lasting without the side effects of drugs.[27]

Acupuncture is also a proven means of combating food cravings and controlling weight. "Acupuncture points, especially on the ear, can be used to help a person control carbohydrate cravings and regulate appetite so they feel full from less food," says Richard Shwery, O.M.D., L.Ac., director of the Acupuncture Center of Cary in Cary, North Carolina. Chinese researchers have demonstrated the effectiveness of acupuncture as a weight-loss technique. In a study conducted by researchers from the Guangxi College of Traditional Chinese Medicine, 42 patients lost an average of 19 pounds after three therapeutic courses of acupuncture. The technique used in the study included both traditional acupuncture and the use of microelectric current.[28]

Therapeutic touch is another method used in manipulating the body's energy fields to promote relaxation and, in turn, induce weight loss. The technique was first developed in 1972 by Dolores Krieger, Ph.D., R.N., a former professor of nursing at New York University, and is based on the idea that the therapist exudes a healing force that can affect the patient's recovery and cure. According to Dr. Krieger, therapeutic touch "is a contemporary interpretation of ancient healing practices in which the practitioner consciously directs or sensitively modulates human energies."

Despite the name, therapeutic touch generally involves no physical contact between patient and practitioner. Instead, the practitioner places his or her hands two to six inches away from the patient and, with slow and rhythmic hand motions, determines where the blockages in the patient's energy field lie. The practitioner then works to replenish the energy flow where necessary, release any congestion, and remove obstructions. Therapeutic touch has been shown to alter enzyme activity, increase the healing of surgical wounds, increase the manufacture of blood in the body, and reduce anxiety.[29]

Breathing Exercises

Breathing patterns often reflect the body's emotional state. For example, shallow chest breathing and hyperventilation are part of the body's natural response to stress. Individuals who suppress unpleasant feelings and thoughts may also unknowingly restrict their breathing. Proper breathing can help facilitate an emotional release and breathing techniques are utilized in most forms of meditation, as well as yoga and *qigong*.

Yoga is a form of stretching and movement that focuses on breathing techniques. Through a series of postures (called *asanas*), yoga

---

How to Breathe Using *Ujjayi*

Beryl Bender Birch offers the following step-by-step instructions for *ujjayi* breathing:[30]

1. Begin by whispering an "ahh" or " urr" sound with the mouth open on an exhalation. Completely empty the lungs as you make the sound.

2. Inhale by making the same "ahh" or "urr" sound. Completely fill the lungs.

3. Repeat this process with the mouth closed. You will notice a soft aspirant sound on the inhale, and a throaty sibilant sound on the exhale—much like a closed-mouth whisper. Continue to breathe with the mouth closed and inhaling and exhaling through the nose only. You should feel your diaphragm rising and falling and notice an increasing sensation of relaxation as you continue to breathe this way.

relaxes the mind and body and stimulates the body's endocrine glands. "Yoga is about learning to pay attention. Yoga means to unite—it's about joining the mind and body," says Beryl Bender Birch, director of the Hard and Soft Astanga Yoga Institute in New York City and author of *Power Yoga*. Birch adds that one of the benefits of yoga is that it trains you to pay attention to your breathing.[31] "As long as you can stay focused on your breath, you're in the present moment," says Birch. "You can't be with your breath and also be worried about a fight you had this morning—you can learn to use yoga breathing techniques to loosen that stranglehold, that stress." She specifically recommends a yoga breathing technique called *ujjayi*, a form of deep-chest breathing that lengthens the breath (see "How to Breathe Using *Ujjayi*," p. 177). According to yoga teacher Joel Kramer of Bolinas, California, *ujjayi* breathing makes yoga postures easier to perform and increases their relaxing effect.[32]

Qigong, which literally means "breath mastery exercise," is an ancient Chinese exercise technique that also integrates breathing exercise with movement and meditation. Similar to yoga, *qigong* helps to calm the mind and maintain the optimum functioning of the body's self-regulating systems. *Qigong* exercise can range from simple calisthenic-type movements with breath coordination to complex exercises where brain wave frequency, heart rate, and other organ functions are altered intentionally by the practitioner. It also stimulates and balances the flow of *qi*, the vital life energy that courses through the body. "The overall benefit of *qigong* is to mobilize and harmonize the body's naturally occurring healing resource," says Roger Jahnke, O.M.D., of Santa Barbara, California.

Flower Essence Therapy

Flower essence therapy is used to treat a variety of illnesses, including weight gain, by calming the emotions. The treatments consist of subtle liquid preparations made from the fresh blossoms of flowers, shrubs, and trees. The approach was pioneered by British physician Edward Bach in the 1930s, when he introduced the 38 Bach Flower Remedies, all based on English plants. Flower essences are made by floating fresh blossoms in spring water and letting them sit in the morning sun for a few hours. The blossoms are removed, leaving the mother essence of the flower, which is then diluted to a dosage level. Drops of the essences can be placed under the tongue, ingested in a tonic, or diluted in a bath.

"Flower essences precisely address the interface between body and mind," says Patricia Kaminski, of the Flower Essence Society in Nevada City, California. "Their impact is not weak but subtle, and when you take them they prompt a shift in view from within, engendering recognition of feelings that exist below the level of our ordinary awareness." Flower essences can help alleviate emotions such as apprehension, worry, loneliness, depression, and fear. They can also act as a catalyst for calmness and mental clarity; this is how they enhance our ability to recognize and understand what's driving our behaviors. As flower essences can help patients gain greater control over their unconscious food habits, Kaminski strongly recommends the therapy for those trying to lose weight. She describes the therapy as "the link between body and mind that is especially lacking in the standard psychotherapeutic and medical responses to weight control."

Flower essences are especially effective in treating addictive behaviors. Kaminski identifies a variety of flower preparations used to treat addictions (see "Flower Essences for Weight Loss," p. 180).[33] Although you can administer a flower essence treatment yourself, a trained flower essence practitioner can help tailor a treatment program specific to your needs and offer counseling as you work through emotional issues.

Success Story: The Power of Flower Essences—Flower essences can help you cope with tension and support your efforts to explore the psychological and emotional sources that contribute to your anxieties. Wendy, 39, who was 5'5" and weighed 155 pounds, suffered from allergies, fatigue, constipation, and feelings of low self-esteem, especially related to her body. To cope with her tiredness and constipation, she drank eight to ten cups of strong coffee every day. She'd been on many diets and her weight had fluc-

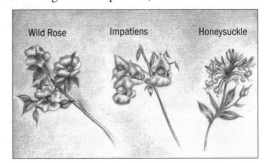

Wild Rose   Impatiens   Honeysuckle

Flower Essences for Weight Loss

Here are a few suggestions for how to therapeutically match flower essences with conditions that impact weight:[34]

Flower Essence	Effective For
Agrimony	Eating habits that stem from frustration
Black-Eyed Susan	Denial of gluttonous behaviors
Chestnut Bud	Breaking unhealthy and repetitive eating patterns
Impatiens	Tendency to gulp and swallow food
Iris	Cravings for sweets
Milkweed	Bingeing
Morning Glory	Addiction to junk food, bingeing, desire for stimulants such as caffeine
Pink Monkey Flower	Eating habits motivated by low self-esteem and shame
Pink Yarrow	Overeating to dull painful emotions
Rosemary	Stagnant digestion
Snapdragon	Oral fixations—continuous biting, crunching, and chewing as a sublimation for feelings of misplaced libido or unexpressed anger
Tansy	Sluggishness and lethargy

tuated between 110 and 160 pounds since high school.

Wendy sought the advice of Patricia Kaminski after hearing about the benefits of the therapy from friends. "I wanted to use the essences to support a complete program of change for her," says Kaminski, "so I suggested she also get a nutritional work-up. Her evaluation revealed that her adrenal glands were completely exhausted." Kaminski recommended a program of nutritional supplements to rebuild Wendy's adrenal function. She used a combination of flower essences, including Morning Glory, Walnut, California Wild Rose, and Nasturtium, to help wean her from coffee. In addition, Kaminski recommended baths in Lavender and Chamomile oil, Lavender flower essence, and Five Flower Formula.

The Flower Essence Society is a nonprofit educational organization, representing more than 60,000 flower essence practitioners worldwide. For more on **flower essence therapy** or help finding a practitioner, contact: Flower Essence Society, P.O. Box 459, Nevada City, CA 95959; tel: 800-548-0075 or 916-265-9163; fax: 916-265-6467. To order specific flower essences, contact: Flower Visions Research, 244 Madison Avenue, Suite 6H, New York, NY 10016; tel: 212-949-1973.

Wendy says that the flower essence therapy helped her realize a different source of energy—one that made her more sensitive to the nuances in her body. Kaminski also helped Wendy work through some emotional issues. As they delved into these difficult subjects, Kaminski used Manzanita and Mariposa Lily. After about a year of nutritional supplements and flower essence therapy, Wendy lost 25 pounds. Ultimately she reached her ideal weight of 120 pounds and stayed within a five-pound range of this weight for the next five years. "She felt this was a very different experience from her past attempts to lose weight," says Kaminski. "The process gave her more energy, a new outlook, and an increased sensitivity to her own body and its signals. In her words, 'it was a slow, gradual change from the inside out'."

Aromatherapy

Aromatherapy can be an effective technique to calm the emotions, achieve mental clarity, and control appetite. Like flower essence therapy, aromatherapy involves inhaling fragrances; however, instead of water-based essences, aromatherapy relies on oils extracted from the leaves, flowers, branches, or roots of plants. Due to the tiny size of their constituent molecules, essential oils can easily penetrate bodily tissues (either through the surface of the skin or by inhalation); this particularly effective absorption of the oils is the reason why aromatherapy can influence central nervous system activity.[35]

Jeanne Rose, author of *The Aromatherapy Book: Applications and Inhalations*, recommends oils of birch bark, fennel, juniper berry, myrrh, oregano, and tangerine as useful agents for weight loss.[36] Similarly, William Lee, D.Sc., R.Ph., and Lynn Lee, C.N., authors of *The Book of Practical Aromatherapy*, suggest bergamot to quell the urge for sweets or caffeine; cajeput for intestinal parasites; chamomile to stimulate the immune system and calm jangled nerves; juniper to promote lymph drainage; and lime for digestive and liver problems.[37]

For information about **aromatherapy**, contact: National Association for Holistic Aromatherapy, P.O. Box 17622, Boulder, CO 80308-0622; tel: 303-258-3791.

How to Administer an Aromatherapy Treatment—The benefits of essential oils can be obtained through inhalation, external application, or ingestion.

- Diffusers disperse microparticles of the essential oil into the air. They can be used to help respiratory conditions or to simply change the air with the mood-lifting or calming qualities of the fragrance.
- Oils applied externally are absorbed through the skin. Convenient applications of oils include baths, massages, hot and cold compresses, or topical application of diluted oils. Essential oils in a hot bath can stimulate the skin, induce relaxation, and energize the body. According to Debra Nuzzi St. Claire, M.H., an aromatherapist and herbalist from Boulder, Colorado, using certain essential oils such as rosemary in the bath can stimulate the elimination of toxins through the skin. In massage, the oils are worked into the skin and, depending on the oil and the massage technique, can be used either to calm or to stimulate an individual.
- Floral waters can be sprayed into the air or sprayed on skin that is too sensitive to the touch.
- Internal use is advantageous for certain organ disorders. It is essential, however, to receive proper medical guidance for internal use of oils.

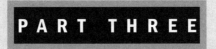

PART THREE

Correct
Imbalances

Strengthen Your Sugar Controls

THE HORMONE insulin is responsible for managing how our bodies use the sugars and starches we eat. When the body's insulin balance is disrupted, starches and sugars are turned into fat rather than being burned as a fuel. If left unchecked, the condition can result in serious illnesses, including diabetes and heart disease. Proper diet, nutritional supplements, and other alternative therapies can help to restore insulin health. That, in turn, will keep your blood sugar levels in check, control your appetite, and help you shed pounds.

Success Story: Balancing Insulin Reverses Weight Gain

Lucy, 42, was tired, lethargic, and about 40 pounds overweight when she came to see naturopath Willow Moore, D.C., N.D., of Owings Mills, Maryland. Even though she exercised regularly and thought she was eating a healthy diet, Lucy still couldn't seem to lose weight.

Upon questioning Lucy, Dr. Moore found that she had greatly reduced her dietary intake of meat and protein, believing that they were unhealthy for her (particularly the fat content), and was eating a high-carbohydrate (starches and sugars) diet. The first thing that Dr. Moore did was check Lucy's fasting serum (blood) insulin level. This is a simple blood test, performed after the person has fasted for 12-18 hours, to determine the amount of insulin (not produced in reaction to eating food) circulating in the bloodstream.

"Your body produces insulin based on what you ate during your last meal," explains Dr. Moore. "If you consistently eat meals with too many carbohydrates, your body keeps trying to produce more and more insulin. Finally, you get to a point where, even if you eat a meal without a lot of carbohydrates, you're still producing too much insulin so that you don't feel good after the meal. That makes you want to eat more sugar and perpetuates the cycle." If this cycle continues, the pancreas may have trouble producing enough insulin, leading to adult-onset diabetes.

The normal range for insulin on the blood test is up to 20, but Dr. Moore feels that the level should be under 10. Lucy's level was 26, two-and-a-half times the insulin she needed, according to Dr. Moore. Because of this insulin imbalance, Lucy had low blood sugar (hypoglycemia—SEE QUICK DEFINITION) and had to eat carbohydrates every two to three hours or she didn't feel good.

Dr. Moore also wanted to look at Lucy's thyroid function. An underactive thyroid (hypothyroidism) can be a factor in weight gain by slowing down the body's metabolism, the rate that the body converts food into energy. Dr. Moore used a blood test and the basal body temperature test (a self-test involving measuring underarm temperature first thing in the morning on consecutive days) to assess thyroid function. Lucy's basal body temperatures were low at 96.1° F, 96.5° F, and 96.1° F (normal body temperature is 98.6° F), which indicated an underactive thyroid.

The first step in treating Lucy's insulin imbalance was to change her diet. "You have to go on a very low carbohydrate diet for at least a month," says Dr. Moore. "The first three days are the hardest as the

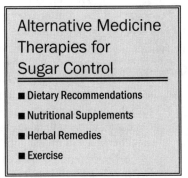

Alternative Medicine Therapies for Sugar Control

- Dietary Recommendations
- Nutritional Supplements
- Herbal Remedies
- Exercise

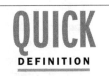

QUICK

DEFINITION

Hypoglycemia, or low blood sugar (glucose), is a condition often associated with diabetes. Glucose is the primary source of fuel for the brain. In healthy people, the release of insulin acts to keep blood sugar levels fairly constant; when the pancreas produces too much insulin, however, blood glucose levels drop suddenly. Symptoms of hypoglycemia include anxiety, weakness, and sweating.

For more about the **thyroid and how to take the basal body temperature test**, see Chapter 9: Overcome a Sluggish Thyroid, pp. 202-219.

Willow Moore, D.C., N.D.: 10806 Reisterstown Road, Suite 1E, Owings Mills, MD 21117; tel: 410-356-4600; fax: 410-654-8995.

body shifts from getting energy from carbohydrate intake to getting energy from protein intake. In the first three days, your body is still producing high amounts of insulin, so you're tired and generally don't feel good." She limited Lucy to less than 40 grams of carbohydrates a day (as a comparison, ½ cup of rice is about 22 grams). Lucy was allowed to eat animal proteins (beef, chicken, seafood) or tofu, leafy vegetables, cucumbers, onions, and celery.

Lucy, understandably, had difficulty sticking with this restricted diet the first month. She did somewhat better the second month and when Dr. Moore rechecked her insulin level, it had dropped to 20. Because Lucy's compliance to the diet was inconsistent, it took about nine months to get her insulin level down to a relatively normal reading of 12. At the end of one year, she had lost 30 pounds.

Dr. Moore also recommended a natural thyroid supplement (made from desiccated animal glands) to bolster Lucy's thyroid function. Dr. Moore's other recommendations to support the thyroid included: eat enough protein, which provides adequate levels of the amino acid tyrosine, an essential nutrient for the production of thyroid hormones (L-tyrosine can also be taken as a nutritional supplement); and make sure to get enough iodine in the diet (kelp is a good source). With these therapies in place, Lucy's basal body temperature slowly increased to 97.1° F.

Lucy now feels "tons better" than she did before, has a lot more energy, and she's complying with her diet. She's really changed the way she eats, says Dr. Moore. "The most important thing about weight loss is to look at all the contributing factors and remember that it's going to involve a lifestyle change as well as how you eat," says Dr. Moore. "Your goal should be a body that's healthy, one that's able to do what you like to do and that you're comfortable with."

Insulin, Appetite, and Your Weight

You probably know that sugar is high in calories and may contribute to weight gain. But did you know that excessive consumption of foods high in sugar or starch can permanently damage your ability to utilize these substances as energy sources? As the body loses its capacity to process sugar or starch, it resorts to converting and storing these substances as body fat. The net result is that whenever you eat sugar, you gain weight, even if you cut down on the calories you eat.

At the core of your body's ability to use sugar is the hormone insulin. Insulin is the body's chief sugar regulator and a key appetite hormone, affecting your choice of what, when, and how much you eat. In healthy people, insulin controls appetite by keeping sugar (glucose) levels in the blood fairly constant. However, the physiological mechanism that regulates insulin can be thrown off balance when it is forced to work overtime on processing excess sugars and starches, causing too much insulin to enter the blood. Studies have shown a clear connection between chronic obesity and high insulin levels. One study estimates that 10%-25% of adults suffer from some degree of insulin imbalance, but the proportion appears to be much higher in those who are obese.[1]

In this chapter, we examine the role of insulin and sugar imbalance in weight gain and what may be the potential causes of this problem. We also outline the tests available for assessing your sugar controls and provide alternative medicine therapies to help you regain your sugar and insulin balance and control your weight.

How Sugar Becomes Fat

All sugars and starches (called carbohydrates) and some of the proteins we eat are transformed into glucose, which is one of the body's key energy sources. Immediately after a meal, glucose levels rise in the bloodstream and the pancreas (the gland where insulin is manufactured) releases insulin to match the rise in glucose. The insulin reduces the levels of the circulating sugar by helping transfer it into the body's cells, where it is broken down and used as a fuel. Insulin acts like a chemical key that opens up the cell membranes, allowing glucose to

Obesity Statistics Rise Despite Decline in Calories Consumed

During the period 1976 to 1991, the percentage of obese Americans increased from 25% to 33%. This increase occurred despite the fact that the intake of calories had declined by about 3% in women and 6% in men. Fat consumption had also decreased during this period, from 41% of total calories to about 37%. The rise in obesity and decline in calorie and fat consumption have puzzled some researchers, as many would have expected corresponding decreases in obesity.

So what's behind these seemingly paradoxical trends? The answer, in part, is sugar. In 1970, Americans consumed an average of 121 pounds of sugar and corn sweeteners per person per year. As of 1992, the amount had increased to 142 pounds per year. Medical journalist Michael Fumento, author of *The Fat of the Land*, says this increase occurred "even though artificial sweetener use quadrupled in the same period."[2]

enter. As glucose is absorbed by the cells, the blood levels experience a corresponding decline. When the levels become low, we feel hungry and eat, thus beginning the cycle all over again. In a healthy individual, glucose and insulin rise and fall gradually in the blood.

Glucose that is not burned as a fuel is converted into glycogen, a type of starch that is stored in the liver and muscles. Some of it is also converted into fat (specifically triglycerides). Under normal circumstances, glucose is burned as fuel so that only minimal quantities are converted into body fat. However, this mechanism can be thrown out of balance, causing most of the glucose in the blood to be converted into fat. When such disruptions occur, changes in glucose and insulin levels are much more sudden and extreme. "Your blood sugar leaps high, and you feel all is right with the world. Then comes the big insulin surge, your blood sugar drops, and you plunge from the mountain tops to the pits," says Stephen Langer, M.D., of Berkeley, California.[3]

The rapid rise in insulin not only brings about a glucose "crash," but also keeps the sugar at a low level by preventing glycogen from being converted back into glucose; at the same time, the triglycerides cannot be reconverted into glucose. The resultant low blood sugar level, called hypoglycemia, leaves you feeling fatigued, light-headed, irritable or nervous, and depressed. You then crave sugar in order to feel good again.

With time, high blood levels of insulin lead to insulin resistance, a condition that occurs when the cells no longer react to the hormone, making it difficult to absorb glucose. The pancreas responds by releasing even more insulin into the blood, which only worsens the problem, as the rising insulin simply increases the cells' resistance. Over time, the body loses its ability to burn sugar, causing energy levels to spiral downward.[4] Controlling weight then becomes increasingly difficult, as insulin, unable to get glucose into the cells, converts more and more sugar into fat.

High insulin levels not only lead to fat accumulation but also salt and water retention (making you feel bloated and adding pounds); this condition also increases the appetite. "Usually insulin will signal the body to stop eating, but if a person has chronically elevated glucose levels due to inefficient insulin, he may eat more," says David K. Shefrin, N.D., of Beaverton, Oregon. As your cells become

QUICK

DEFINITION

Diabetes mellitus is a degenerative illness that centers around the hormone insulin and the pancreas. In Type I diabetes, also called juvenile diabetes, the pancreas is unable to manufacture insulin. Type II diabetes, or non-insulin-dependent adult-onset diabetes, develops in middle-age. Here, the pancreas produces insulin, but the body's cells do not respond to it and can't absorb the glucose from food. As blood glucose levels continue to rise, the pancreas releases more insulin to deal with the excess blood sugar. The result is both a state of low blood sugar and too much insulin (hyperinsulinism).

increasingly starved of glucose, you get trapped in a cycle of carbohydrate cravings. Once set in motion, the seesawing of glucose and insulin in the blood can cause sugar and carbohydrate urges as often as every two to three hours.[5]

Barry Sears, Ph.D., a research biochemist and co-author of *The Zone*, describes the experience of these recurrent cravings as "carbohydrate hell." Indeed, the periodic temptation to gorge on starchy, sugary foods can be overwhelming. Under these conditions, typical efforts at weight loss may prove to be useless. If left untreated, the swing of glucose and insulin becomes progressively worse, leading to dangerous and debilitating ailments, including heart disease and diabetes (SEE QUICK DEFINITION).

The Road to Carbohydrate Hell

Although genetics may predispose some people to sugar imbalances and insulin resistance, a number of other factors can contribute to this condition, including dietary choices, food allergies, an underactive thyroid, and stress and other emotional influences.

Too Many Carbohydrates—A diet high in certain types of carbohydrates is one of the principal causes of these disorders. Carbohydrates, which consist of both sugars and starches, come from plant sources and are an excellent energy source because they can be completely converted into glucose in the body. In contrast, only 10% of dietary fats and 50% of proteins get converted into glucose. Carbohydrates come in either simple or complex forms. Complex carbohydrates, found in vegetables, beans, and whole grains, are sugar molecules attached to protein, fats, vitamins, or minerals. These molecules break down slowly in the digestive tract and are gradually absorbed into the bloodstream. The result is a prolonged feeling of fullness and a sustained energy level. In contrast, simple carbohydrates (such as table sugar, honey, sugars from fruit, and corn syrup) break down immediately and are quickly absorbed by the blood.

Physicians and nutritionists are particularly concerned with "processed carbohydrates," a subgroup of simple carbohydrates. "Processed, denatured carbohydrates are the main ingredient in junk foods and sweets," says Gus Prosch, M.D., of Birmingham, Alabama. "They're in the pizza, the packaged white bread, the donuts, the soda, the ice cream, and the candy bars we learn to love when we're young. Foods like these go almost directly into the bloodstream, requiring very little digestive activity."

When you eat simple carbohydrates, the pancreas is faced with a sudden flood of glucose and often cannot gauge how much insulin is needed. It goes into high gear, over-responding in order to cope with what it interprets as a sugar emergency. "Sugary foods provoke a strong insulin response, so eating a lot of them eventually turns the pancreas into a 'hair trigger'; that is, it chronically overreacts to the amount of glucose in the blood. This is very destructive to health and definitely affects weight," says Michael Phillips, D.C., a chiropractor, based in Cleveland, Ohio, who specializes in treating diabetic disorders.

When sugary foods are eaten alone rather than in combination with other nutrients, such as protein, the situation is worsened. "Insulin secretion is 70% greater after eating a candy bar than after consuming the same number of calories from a [healthy] snack," according to Michael Murray, N.D., and Joseph Pizzorno, Jr., N.D., authors of *A Textbook of Natural Medicine*.[6]

Food Allergies—Food allergies can also disrupt blood sugar balance. The body's first reaction to an allergenic food is often hypoglycemia and insulin imbalance.[7] The connection between sugar disorders (such as hypoglycemia) and food allergies is often ignored and so remains undiagnosed and untreated. Ralph Golan, M.D., of Seattle, Washington, author of *Optimal Wellness*, explains that allergic reactions to some foods "produces symptoms identical to those of hypoglycemia." Dr. Golan cites wheat, milk, eggs, corn, beef, peanuts, and orange juice as foods that often cause such allergic reactions.[8]

For more about **food allergies**, see Chapter 11: Break Food Allergies and Addictions, pp. 244-270. For more on the **thyroid**, see Chapter 9: Overcome a Sluggish Thyroid, pp. 202-219. For more on **stress and weight gain**, see Chapter 7: Heal Your Emotional Appetite, pp. 156-182.

Hormones and the Thyroid—Hormone imbalances, particularly in women during perimenopause and menopause, may affect insulin levels and the function of the thyroid, potentially leading to weight gain. In this menopausal period, bursts of the female hormone estrogen are released, leading to a condition called estrogen dominance. These bursts of excess estrogen cause insulin to be released, causing more sugar to be turned into fat. Estrogen dominance also depresses the function of the thyroid, which slows the rate that you burn off fat, leading to additional weight gain.

"Women who are going through menopause often end up feeling hungrier because they have too much insulin and then they're not burning off fat as quickly because the thyroid is depressed," says Serafina Corsello, M.D., director of the Corsello Centers for Nutritional Complementary Medicine in New York City and

Huntington, New York. "It becomes a fuel-inefficient system, like an old car. It uses a lot of fuel, yet rather than producing energy, it produces wastes and smog, namely fat."

Stress—Stress and sugar imbalances are closely interrelated. Normally, a stressful situation triggers a "fight-or-flight" response in our bodies that helps increase our energy level to handle the emergency. The response begins with the adrenals (the endocrine glands located atop the kidneys), which release the hormones cortisol, adrenaline, and noradrenaline into the bloodstream. This "adrenaline rush" rouses the body into action, causing an immediate increase in heart rate, respiration, and blood pressure. The liver reacts by releasing stored sugars (glycogen) to provide the needed energy.

This is all well and good for an emergency situation. But when your blood sugar levels are moving violently up and down several times every day because of chronic levels of stress, the adrenals respond and can become exhausted. Blood sugar levels will then spike both higher and lower, meaning you will crave more sugar more often.[9] And you end up retaining more water in response to stress as well. "With the fight-or-flight response, you get a 'fat and flabby syndrome' as the cells fill up with water to deal with too many stress hormones," says nutritionist Colette Heimowitz, C.N., of New York City.

Analyze Your Insulin Function

Diagnosing problems with insulin function and sugar imbalances takes several steps. First, you need to evaluate what you eat, how various foods make you feel, and what these eating patterns may reveal about your insulin function. Tests are also available to measure blood glucose levels and to evaluate your insulin response.

Do You Have a Problem With Sugar?

If you are unable to manage your weight and think it could be related to an insulin or sugar imbalance, Dr. Phillips suggests asking yourself the following questions:

■ Do I eat when nervous?
■ Am I intensely hungry between meals?
■ Am I irritable before meals?
■ Do I feel a little shaky when hungry?
■ Does my fatigue disappear after eating?

Sugar On the Brain

Although we generally feel satisfaction or relief after eating a sugary snack, the sensation does not come directly from the glucose that enters our bloodstream, but rather from the corresponding surge in insulin. This is because, in addition to managing glucose, insulin is used by the body to transport the amino acid tryptophan, a building block of the neurotransmitter (SEE QUICK DEFINITION) serotonin, to the brain. Serotonin is sometimes referred to as the "happiness chemical" due to its influence on mood. High levels of serotonin in the brain produce feelings of self-confidence, calm, satisfaction, and composure. However, when levels start to decline, we feel anxious, cannot concentrate, and become depressed.

When tryptophan is scarce, serotonin is in similarly short supply. This creates an intolerable condition for the brain, which demands immediate action, hence our cravings for sugar. Sugar causes quick satisfaction by initiating the release of insulin, which delivers tryptophan to the brain and restores serotonin levels.[10] In effect,

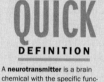

QUICK DEFINITION

A **neurotransmitter** is a brain chemical with the specific function of enabling communications to happen between brain cells. Chief among the 100 identified to date are acetylcholine, gamma-aminobutyric acid (GABA), serotonin, dopamine, and norepinephrine. Acetylcholine is required for short-term memory and muscle contractions. GABA works to stop excess nerve signals; serotonin helps produce sleep, regulate pain, and influence mood. Norepinephrine is an excitatory neurotransmitter.

sugar works like an antidepressant. "If serotonin levels are depressed, you're depressed," says Michael Phillips, D.C., who compares sugar's action to that of the drug Prozac. "Prozac, so commonly prescribed for depression, works by elevating levels of serotonin. The emotional aspects of blood sugar imbalances are rooted in a [similar] physiological response."

Because of this, you can get addicted to sugar as if it were a drug, becoming dependent on it to elevate your mood. Unfortunately, individuals who experience violent swings in their glucose levels frequently experience sudden and extreme changes in temperament. After giving in to a food craving, they feel a fleeting sensation of bliss that is often followed by a black mood. They become angry at others or themselves for no apparent reason and often punish themselves for failing to stick to their diet. Although such emotional responses may often be perceived as psychological in origin, for those suffering from a blood sugar imbalance, the problem has a distinct biochemical basis.

- Do I faint or have heart palpitations if meals are delayed?
- Do I get afternoon headaches?
- Do I crave coffee or candy in the afternoon?
- Do I regularly have intense cravings for sweets or snack foods?

If your answer is "yes" to any of these questions, sugar imbalances may be a factor in your weight problems.

Examining Your Eating Patterns—The next step is to start carefully monitoring your eating behavior. Write down everything you eat, when you eat it, and how you feel physically and emotionally before and after eating. Dr. Prosch asks patients to rate their degree of hunger throughout the day using a scale of 0-2, with zero meaning not hungry. He also tells them to try to distinguish appetite, which has to do with a particular food's appeal, from hunger, which is a more acute need felt within the body.

After a week of keeping this food journal, examine it with the following questions in mind:

■ Do you eat at regular mealtimes or at different times each day? Rather than set meals, do you graze throughout the day? Do you snack between meals?

■ What kinds of foods do you eat at meals or as snacks? Do you consume lots of carbohydrates (breads and pasta)? Fruits? Are you getting adequate protein (meat, chicken, fish, beans, eggs, dairy)? Do you consume fatty foods at every meal? Do you drink caffeinated beverages (coffee, tea, or sodas) every day?

■ Do you eat sweets every day? Try experimenting by consciously not eating any sugar at all for 24 hours. What happens? Were you more irritable or anxious than usual? Do you regularly binge on sweets?[11]

Looking carefully at your eating patterns in this way should give you an idea of your relationship to sugar and whether or not it is a factor in your weight problems.

Measure Your Blood Glucose

There are several testing methods available that measure how your blood sugar level changes over time. Normal glucose metabolism should reflect a gradual increase and an equally gradual decline in both glucose and insulin over time.

Glucose Tolerance Test—Conventional physicians generally use a glucose tolerance test to diagnose sugar imbalances. This test involves first measuring a patient's blood sugar level in the morning after an overnight fast. Then, pure glucose is fed intravenously to the patient and blood sugar is periodically measured over the following five to six hours. Although common among mainstream practitioners, many alternative health-care physicians consider the test to be a poor diagnostic tool, as it does not reflect what actually happens in the body in response to real food eaten in real time. Part of the problem is that different foods and food combinations have very different effects on blood sugar in each person. Dr.

Langer explains that many hypoglycemic patients also suffer from sensitivities and allergies to different foods, including corn, which happens to be the food used to make the glucose solution used for the test. "Is the patient reacting to glucose or corn (its food source) or both?" he asks. Cola flavoring, sometimes added to the solution for taste, may contain caffeine, which can also affect test results.[12]

Total Body Modification—Interpreting the results of a blood glucose test is often tricky. William Mauer, D.O., director of the Kingsley Medical Center in Arlington Heights, Illinois, says that each individual is likely to have their own range of normal blood glucose levels. He warns that doctors too often use arbitrary values to distinguish normal from abnormal glucose responses. "If a physician suggests that you do not have low blood sugar unless your blood sugar falls to 40-60 mg/dl, yet you have symptoms and reactions during the glucose test, then he is not taking into consideration the physiologic requirements of the brain and body," says Dr. Mauer.[13]

Dr. Phillips agrees that glucose tests are limited. "The standard blood glucose test is a roughly drawn picture of only one period in time," he says. "What's needed when diagnosing blood sugar imbalances is something more comprehensive and more subtle." Dr. Phillips uses a muscle testing technique called Total Body Modification (TBM), first devised 20 years ago by Victor Frank, D.C. It assesses muscle response to the application of pressure at certain reflex points on the body to evaluate blood sugar response and also to gauge overall endocrine gland function. Dr. Phillips says that, along with a patient's symptoms, TBM shows him "not only that there's a blood sugar imbalance, but where in the body the source of the problem is located."

Taking the Glucose Challenge—An alternative to the glucose test is the glucose challenge. This test of insulin function relies on slightly more realistic test conditions; it is also less expensive and easier to administer. The test can be performed at home with the purchase of a glucometer, a device commonly used by diabetics and available at most pharmacies. To take the test, you must follow these steps:

1) Do not eat for eight hours and then measure your blood sugar level. Place a drop of blood on the test strip (provided with the glucometer) and insert the strip into the glucometer. A normal reading should be 75-85 milligrams per deciliter of blood (mg/dl).

2) Ingest carbohydrates. Eat a meal of simple carbohydrates, such as pancakes or waffles with no butter but plenty of syrup, or any popular breakfast cereal, which contains up to 40 grams of sugar.

3) Test your blood sugar a second time. Measure your blood glucose 60-90 minutes after eating. At this point, the level in a normal individual should be either at its peak (175-185 mg/dl) or already descending (120-130 mg/dl). In a person who has hypoglycemia, however, the initial measure will be relatively low (50-70 mg/dl). In some cases, sugar levels may still be climbing, even this long after consuming a sugar-rich meal. It is important to observe how you react to the test—signs of disorientation, confusion, and muscle weakness suggest a blood sugar problem.

Success Story: Correcting Sugar Imbalances Leads to Weight Loss

Miriam, 27, was suffering from chronic fatigue, emotional stress and depression, PMS (pre-menstrual syndrome) symptoms, and obesity. She was five feet tall and weighed 180 pounds. Miriam consulted nutritionist Colette Heimowitz, M.S., of New York City.

Heimowitz suggested that Miriam get a glucose tolerance test to determine if she had sugar imbalances. This test helps the practitioner get an idea of how the patient's body processes the sugars in food. Miriam's response was so weak that Heimowitz considered her "prediabetic." Miriam was insulin-resistant, meaning that her body didn't respond normally to the hormone insulin and the sugar in her blood, rather than being burned off, was stored as fat.

"Someone who is insulin-resistant stores most of their weight around the middle of their body, the buttocks and belly," says Heimowitz. "They also crave sugar, are addicted to carbohydrates, and they're hungry all the time with a ravenous appetite." Miriam demonstrated all of these signs. Tests revealed that Miriam also had high levels of cholesterol and triglycerides.

Heimowitz put Miriam on Gluco Formula, a sugar-regulating formula developed by Serafina Corsello, M.D. Gluco Formula contains vanadyl sulfate, a dietary form of vanadium, and chromium picolinate (both minerals that regulate glucose), essential fatty acids and the amino acid carnitine (which help burn fat), and the herbs bilberry and *Gymnema sylvestre* (to reduce blood sugar).

Heimowitz also started Miriam on a high-protein, low-carbohydrate diet. "Carbohydrates, unlike protein and fat, are the only food source that raises glucose levels and requires an insulin response," explains Heimowitz. By limiting the amount of carbohydrates, this dietary plan

To reach **Colette Heimowitz, M.S.**, or for more information about **Gluco Formula**, contact: The Corsello Centers for Nutritional Complementary Medicine, 200 West 57th Street, New York, NY 10019; tel: 888-461-0949 or 212-399-0222; fax: 212-399-3817. She can also be consulted at: The Atkins Center Weight Management Program, 152 E. 55th Street, New York, NY 10022; tel: 212-758-2110.

helps stabilize levels of both glucose and insulin. Miriam could eat three meals a day consisting of proteins and vegetables, with limits on the high-carbohydrate vegetables like peas, carrots, turnip, and squash. She eliminated sugar, grains, dairy products, beans, and potatoes. Because she was pre-diabetic, Miriam was also allowed three between-meal snacks to keep her blood sugar levels stable. The snacks consisted of moderate amounts of nuts and fruit.

After six months on this program, Miriam lost 30 pounds and her cholesterol and triglyceride levels both dropped to normal readings. And Miriam's energy levels and outlook are both on the upswing.

Alternative Medicine Therapies for Sugar Control

A number of therapies can help stabilize your blood sugar levels and normalize insulin function, both of which can be an integral part of losing unwanted weight. Diet is the primary way to control blood sugar fluctuations, but additional therapies may also be helpful, including nutrients, herbs, and exercise.

Dietary Recommendations

Maintaining a healthy, sensible diet is crucial for restoring blood sugar balance. Many diet programs suggest ways you can cut calories; however, simply reducing your caloric intake can be self-defeating and cause greater harm to your sugar-regulating mechanisms, especially if you cheat. For example, as your system adjusts to a lower-calorie diet, it becomes more sensitive to change. If you have been dieting and suddenly give in to the temptation of a slice of chocolate cake, your system will overreact, releasing double and triple doses of insulin and converting the additional calories quickly into fat. The rebound weight gain that follows this response, sometimes called the "yo-yo effect," will leave you fatter than before you started to diet.

Rather than being concerned about calories, you should always try to eat foods low on the glycemic index (see below). Here are some other basic dietary rules for blood sugar health:

- Eat whole, fresh, and unprocessed foods as much as possible.
- Avoid simple or refined carbohydrates and sugar products (see "Watch Out for Hidden Sugars," p. 198) and replace them with

complex carbohydrates, such as whole grains, beans, and vegetables; complex carbohydrates are easier on the pancreas and promote insulin balance.

■ Eat at least three regular meals per day or, alternatively, eat five or six smaller meals throughout the day; this helps stabilize the release of blood sugar.

■ Eat adequate amounts of protein (meat, chicken, fish, eggs, dairy, beans, tofu, nuts) at each meal; proteins take longer to break down in the body, thus stabilizing blood sugar levels.

■ Avoid foods made with hydrogenated oils and be sure to incorporate adequate amounts of healthy fats, such as olive, sesame, or flaxseed oils; healthy fats extend the release time for sugar into the bloodstream.

■ Reduce your intake of fruit juices and dried fruits and drink vegetable juices (except carrot) and herbal teas instead; fruit sugars can cause a rapid rise in blood sugar levels.

■ Reduce your intake of caffeinated beverages, which stimulate blood sugar and insulin, and alcohol.

■ Avoid artificial sweeteners and products containing them.[14]

The Glycemic Index—Although pure sugar will cause the greatest insulin response in our bodies, many other foods have a similar insulinogenic (insulin stimulating) effect. To evaluate foods based on their insulin impact, a scientific rating system called the glycemic index was developed by diabetes researchers at the University of Toronto. The index offers a comparison of the insulin effect of different foods, measuring their real-life effect on blood sugar levels. Those foods with a high rating on the glycemic index cause a higher insulin response than those with a low rating.

"The glycemic index ranks foods according to how fast they are absorbed into the blood as sugar," says Ann Louise Gittleman, M.S., C.N.S., author of *Get the Sugar Out*. "A diet based on high glycemic index foods (those absorbed most quickly) usually leads to a condition of chronic low blood sugar because you have rapid rises followed by sharp dips in blood sugar levels."[15]

Richard Podell, M.D., medical director of the Overlook Center for Weight Management in Springfield, New Jersey, indicates that choosing foods with a low glycemic index is "the secret to keeping blood sugar stable, insulin low, and hunger in check." Dr. Podell has simplified the index into basic categories, which he presents in his book *The G-Index Diet*.[16] He makes the following general observations:

■ Foods with a higher rating, causing a greater insulin response, include white bread, bagels, English muffins, packaged flaked cereals, instant hot cereals, low-fat frozen desserts, raisins and other dried fruits, whole milk and whole-milk cheeses, peanuts and peanut butter, hot dogs, and luncheon meats.

■ Foods with a low rating, not causing a high insulin spike, include most fresh vegetables, leafy greens, pitted fruits and melons, coarse 100% whole-grain breads and minimally processed whole-grain cereals, sweet potatoes and yams, skim milk, buttermilk, poultry, lean cuts of beef, pork, veal, shellfish, white-fleshed fish, most legumes, and most nuts.

■ Cooked foods rank higher on the index than raw foods. Similarly, fruits and vegetables that have been juiced or puréed are higher on the index than when eaten whole.

Nutritional Supplements

The following nutritional supplements can help control your appetite and strengthen your body's natural glucose-regulating mechanisms.

Chromium—Chromium is a mineral that the body requires in minute amounts in order to be able to regulate insulin production and stabilize blood sugar. The biologically active form of chromium, commonly referred to as GTF (glucose tolerance factor) chromium, helps insulin bind to the receptor sites on each cell membrane.

It is estimated that up to 50% of Americans may not be getting enough chromium in their diet to sustain healthy insulin activity. Americans are likely to be deficient in chromium because it is not readily available through food sources. Nutritionist Betty Kamen, Ph.D., of Novato, California, author of *The Chromium Connection*, adds that uri-

---

Watch Out for Hidden Sugars

Finding out whether a food product contains sugar requires more sleuthing today than it once did. Only a few manufacturers currently include the word *sugar* in the list of ingredients of their sugar-containing products. Instead, wanting to avoid the sugar stigma that could negatively impact sales, many food producers hide the sugars in their products behind a host of chemical synonyms. Take note that any product listing any of the following ingredients really does contain sugar:

- dextrose
- glucose
- fructose
- corn sweetener
- maltodextrin
- malt
- sorghum
- modified cornstarch
- high-fructose corn syrup
- fruit juice concentrates

- sucrose
- sorbitol
- dextrin
- lactose
- maltose
- mannitol
- xylitol

Although all of these are sugars, fructose does stand apart from the rest. Of all the sugars, fructose has the least severe insulin reaction.[17]

Dietary Nutrients for Controlling Blood Sugar

Certain nutrients are required by the body for glucose metabolism, specifically chromium, manganese, zinc, B-complex vitamins (particularly pantothenic acid or B5), inositol, and vitamin C. The following are dietary sources of these nutrients (foods are listed in descending order of importance):

- Chromium—brewer's yeast, whole wheat and rye breads, beef liver, potatoes, green peppers, eggs, chicken, apples, butter, parsnips, and cornmeal

- Manganese—pecans, Brazil nuts, almonds, barley, rye, buckwheat, split peas, whole wheat, walnuts, spinach, oats, raisins, beet greens, Brussels sprouts, cheese, carrots, broccoli, brown rice, corn, cabbage, peaches, and butter

- Zinc—fresh oysters, ginger root, lamb chops, pecans, split peas, beef liver, egg yolk, whole wheat, rye, oats, lima beans, almonds, walnuts, sardines, chicken, and buckwheat

- B-complex vitamins—brewer's yeast, beef and chicken liver, mushrooms, split peas, blue cheese, pecans, eggs, lobster, oats, buckwheat, rye, broccoli, turkey and chicken (dark meat), brown rice, whole wheat, red chili peppers, sardines, avocado, and kale

- Inositol—navy beans, barley, wheat germ, brewer's yeast, oats, blackeyed peas, oranges, lima beans, green peas, molasses, split peas, grapefruit, raisins, cantaloupe, brown rice, peaches, cabbage, cauliflower, onions, sweet potatoes, watermelon, strawberries, lettuce, tomatoes, and eggs

- Vitamin C—acerola cherries, red chili peppers, guava, red sweet peppers, kale, parsley, collard and turnip greens, green peppers, broccoli, Brussels sprouts, mustard greens, cauliflower, red cabbage, strawberries, papayas, spinach, oranges, lemons, grapefruit, turnips, mangoes, asparagus, cantaloupe, Swiss chard, green onions, and tangerines

nary excretion of chromium can increase as much as fifty-fold under stress.[18] Eating sugar also substantially increases chromium loss from the body.[19]

Studies have repeatedly demonstrated the essential role of chromium in balancing blood sugar, improving insulin performance, and losing weight. In one study, patients were given three daily doses of chromium for nearly three months. Those given 200 mcg lost 3.3 pounds of fat and gained 1.5 pounds of muscle, resulting in a net weight loss of 1.8 pounds. Those who received 400 mcg lost 4.6 pounds of fat and gained 1.1 pounds of muscle, resulting in a net weight loss of 3.5 pounds.[20]

There are several forms of chromium supplements and chromium polynicotinate is one that recently has been receiving positive reviews.

In this form, chromium is chemically bound to niacin, a B-complex vitamin. According to Dr. Kamen and others, this form of chromium is superior to both chromium chloride and chromium picolinate. Kamen recommends a minimum daily dosage of 200 mcg.[21] In addition to taking a supplement, an excellent source of chromium is brewer's yeast, available in powder form from most health food stores.

Alpha-Lipoic Acid—Alpha-lipoic acid has been prescribed by German physicians for over 30 years to help patients with adult-onset diabetes. Researchers have shown that when administered intravenously at a dose of 1,000 mg, alpha-lipoic acid can help lower insulin resistance and increase the cellular utilization of glucose by more than 50%. That is, it helps turn more glucose into energy to be burned rather than fat to be stored. Nevertheless, taking supplements at this dosage is not recommended for everyone and should be done under a doctor's supervision. Julian Whitaker, M.D., who practices in Newport Beach, California, suggests that daily dosages above 50 mg are "only for people who are under treatment for diabetes, heart disease, AIDS, and any form of serious liver disorder." Dosages up to 50 mg generally do not require supervision.[22]

Vitamins and Minerals—Vitamins that help to both restore and maintain insulin potency are zinc (20-30 mg daily), manganese (5-10 mg daily), and vitamin C (3,000 mg daily). For maximum benefit, take these supplements once per day. A B-complex vitamin (50 mg, three times daily) is also useful for controlling blood sugar levels; deficiencies of vitamin B1 tend to mimic and aggravate hypoglycemia, B5 helps support the adrenal glands, and biotin enhances glucose utilization and reduces sugar cravings.[23] The trace mineral vanadium also helps regulate blood sugar levels. It is present in small amounts in unsaturated vegetable oils and grains and is also available in supplement form as vanadyl sulfate; typical dosage is 10-20 mg daily.[24]

Fiber—As mentioned earlier, complex carbohydrates do not result in a blood glucose surge and are thus preferable to simple or highly refined carbohydrates. Foods that contain complex carbohydrates often contain high quantities of fiber, which acts to lower blood glucose levels and diminish hunger. In addition, a high-fiber diet increases the number of insulin receptor sites on the cells, making them more sensitive to insulin. This allows the pancreas to produce less insulin to achieve the same glucose-lowering effect. Fiber supplements produce the same result, though they shouldn't be used as a substitute for a healthy, balanced diet.

Dietary fibers such as pectin and guar gum are especially effective in controlling blood sugar levels, because they reduce the biochemical demand on the pancreas. Evidence suggests that dietary fibers slow the rate of food passage through the intestines (called transit time), creating a more gradual rise in blood sugar levels after a meal. A good source of pectin is fresh fruits, especially apples. Guar gum, a dietary gum classified as a fiber, is not found in most food sources, although it is a component in many of the fiber blends available at health food stores.

Herbal Remedies

■ *Gymnema sylvestre*: an Ayurvedic herb often used to treat diabetes. *Gymnema sylvestre* inhibits the taste of sugar and also blocks the absorption of sugar by as much as 50%, making this herb useful for blood sugar control. In addition, some evidence suggests that it can enhance the activity of insulin in the body. Typical dosage is 150 mg of extract, three times daily.[25]

■ *Stevia rebaudiana*: a South American herbal sweetener that helps stabilize blood sugar while not requiring insulin for its metabolism. Stevia is over ten times sweeter than sugar and contains only one calorie per ten leaves. Available in powder or liquid forms, stevia can safely be used as a sugar substitute in cooking.[26]

■ Green Tea (*Camellia sinensis*): ingredients in green tea may influence the way sugars are absorbed and processed by the body. It is thought that green tea slows the release of carbohydrates, which prevents an insulin surge, and stimulates fat burning rather than fat storage. A typical recommended dose is two cups of green tea daily.[27]

Exercise

Although exercise is primarily regarded as a way to burn off fat, it is also effective in stabilizing blood sugar. "Regular exercise reduces the body's tendency to overreact to sugar intake with insulin surges," says Dr. Podell.[28] When you use your muscles vigorously, glucose is absorbed by the cells as an energy fuel without the help of insulin, so the body is less likely to react to sugar intake with surges in insulin.[29] Balancing your sugar level by exercising will also help reduce food cravings and addictive behaviors. Any program designed to restore healthy blood sugar levels should include daily sessions of light exercise, such as walking, swimming, or cycling.

For more on **supplements**, see Chapter 3: Supplements for Weight Loss, pp. 76-97. For more on **exercise**, see Chapter 6: Start Exercising, pp. 138-155.

9

Overcome a Sluggish Thyroid

THE THYROID GLAND plays a key role in weight problems because it controls the body's overall metabolic rate. However, the thyroid is possibly the most overlooked organ in the body. When it's not working properly, this gland can produce an astonishing number of health problems, as divergent as weight gain and arthritis, depression and cold feet, high cholesterol and hair loss. Many doctors, both conventional and alternative, do not pay the thyroid the attention it requires. The American Association of Clinical Endocrinologists (AACE) estimates that at least 6-7 million Americans suffer from hypothyroidism and that only half of those with thyroid problems have been diagnosed with the disease.

Why is such a common condition overlooked? One reason is that doctors confuse the symptoms with those of other conditions. For example, nutritionist Ann Louise Gittleman, M.S., says that because

In This Chapter

- Success Story: Tending the Thyroid Reverses Weight Gain
- Weight Gain and Your Thyroid
- What Causes Hypothyroidism?
- Detecting Hypothyroidism
- Alternative Medicine Therapies for a Healthy Thyroid

hypothyroidism tends to occur in women with the onset of menopause, doctors simply attribute the symptoms to "the change of life." Consequently, they often ignore and never treat the hypothyroidism, a condition which is four to seven times more common in women than in men.

In its early stages, hypothyroidism is difficult to detect because its symptoms are so diverse (see "Symptoms of an Underactive Thyroid," p. 205). "If a person comes in complaining about their high weight and low energy," says Steve Spiddell, N.D., a naturopath practicing in

Washington state, "I start asking questions—Are they constipated? Are they bothered by very dry skin? Are they extremely sensitive to cold? If they answer 'yes,' I have reason to suspect low thyroid function." However, as it advances, symptoms become more pronounced, with every system in the body becoming dulled and sluggish, from circulation to libido. While the list of associated symptoms is long, one of the most common is weight gain.

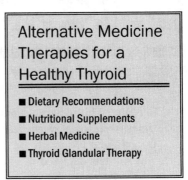

Alternative Medicine Therapies for a Healthy Thyroid

- Dietary Recommendations
- Nutritional Supplements
- Herbal Medicine
- Thyroid Glandular Therapy

In this chapter, we look at the relationship between the thyroid and weight gain. We examine the symptoms and causes of hypothyroidism and tests that determine if you have an underactive thyroid. Finally, we offer effective alternative therapies for correcting this problem.

Success Story: Tending the Thyroid Reverses Weight Gain

In his 18 years as a physician, John Dommisse, M.D., who practices nutritional and metabolic medicine as well as psychiatry in Tuscon, Arizona, has helped many obese people lose weight and regain their health. He has treated his patients mainly by correcting biochemical abnormalities and deficiencies with vitamins, minerals, and hormones. "All the traditional approaches for dealing with obesity, including psychotherapy, have only a 5% success rate," says Dr. Dommisse. "They simply don't address the underlying metabolic factors that are the real source of the problem, and I have found that one of the most common is low thyroid function." Dr. Dommisse reports that many patients come to him already taking a synthetic thyroid drug, such as Synthroid®. However, he says, "even though these people are on thyroid medication, they still have low thyroid that's not being treated and struggle with [their] weight."

John V. Dommisse, M.D.: Nutritional, Metabolic, and Psychiatric Medicine, 1840 E. River Road, Suite 210, Tucson, AZ 85718; tel: 520-577-1940; fax: 520-577-1743. For the **Complete Thyroid Panel test**, contact: Meridian Valley Clinical Laboratory, 515 West Harrison Street, Suite 9, Kent, WA 98032; tel: 800-234-6825 or 253-859-8700; fax: 253-859-1135. For more information on **thyroid-related health problems**, contact: Thyroid Foundation of Canada, 1040 Gardiners Road, Suite C, Kingston, Ontario, Canada K7P 1R7; tel: 613-634-3426; fax: 613-634-3483.

"The traditional approaches for dealing with obesity have only a 5% success rate," says John Dommisse, M.D. "They simply don't address the underlying metabolic factors that are the real source of the problem, and one of the most common is low thyroid function."

One of his patients, Maude, 47, ate a low-fat diet and exercised six times weekly. Nevertheless, her weight remained steady at 188 pounds—far too much for her height—and her feet were always sore and she felt depleted in energy. When Maude received the routine TSH test for underactive thyroid, the results came back "normal." Around this time, a physician suggested she try Weight Watchers and put her on a conventional weight-loss drug, but the drug dropped her blood pressure dangerously to 78/57. Her body temperature was also subnormal at 95°-96° F in the morning, and she felt "very tired."

Dr. Dommisse set Maude on a different course. He recommended three thyroid tests—T3, T4, and TSH—to more accurately pinpoint thyroid problems. While her T4 and TSH results were in the normal range, Maude's T3 was below normal (see "The Thyroid and Its Hormones," pp. 206-207). "I would never use the TSH blood level as the sole test for hypothyroidism or monitoring its treatment," says Dr. Dommisse. Maude's supposedly normal report gave her endocrinologist the false confidence to conclude that Maude's problem was excessive calorie intake and that a Weight Watchers program might be her best therapy.

Dr. Dommisse says that he usually treats for hypothyroidism even if the TSH results are in the middle of the normal range and that, provided the thyroid treatment is not excessive, he "always sees a definite clinical advantage to this approach." To correct Maude's underactive thyroid, Dr. Dommisse gave her combinations of T4, T3, and Armour® Thyroid (desiccated animal gland), which he regards as "a perfectly good T3/T4 combination product." He finds it especially effective when a patient's T3 level is lower than their T4.

On the basis of test results for vitamin and mineral status, Dr. Dommisse learned that Maude was deficient in zinc, manganese, vitamin B12, and chromium, and that her copper levels were too high. He gave her nutrients to rebalance these levels. Maude discontinued use of the weight-loss drug and, within a few months of starting Dr. Dommisse's program, she lost 50 pounds. As a result, a long-term infection disappeared, her energy levels rebounded, her depression lifted, and her feet no longer hurt.

Weight Gain and Your Thyroid

The thyroid, located in the neck, is the largest of the body's endocrine glands. This butterfly-shaped gland secretes hormones that affect the operation of virtually all body processes. It is the body's metabolic thermostat, controlling body temperature, energy use, and, in children, the body's growth rate. The thyroid controls the rate at which organs function and the speed with which the body uses food. When the thyroid is dysfunctional, there are a number of ways that it can seriously impact your weight.

Thyroid hormones control the activity of your organs and the speed of metabolism. Metabolism is the number of calories used by the body to maintain basic life processes, such as breathing and circulation. Metabolism also helps keep the body at a normal, resting temperature of 98.6° F. The thyroid sends chemical messages via hormones to every cell in the body, directing the maintenance of body temperature, heart rate, and muscle movements. When the thyroid is dysfunctional or underactive (hypothyroidism), it sends out fewer hormones, causing metabolism to slow down. This slowing leads to a number of problems, including general feelings of sluggishness and increases in body weight. Metabolism has an inverse relationship to body weight. When metabolism slows, the body will store rather than burn calories, causing an accumulation of fat.

Insufficient thyroid hormones and the consequent slowing of metabolism affects nearly every function in the body and several of these have a direct connection to weight problems:

Symptoms of an Underactive Thyroid

Hypothyroidism is a condition of low or underactive thyroid gland function that can produce numerous symptoms, including mental, emotional, and physical symptoms.

Mental/Emotional Symptoms— Depression, poor memory and concentration difficulties, mood swings, dual personality, paranoia, irritability, inappropriate crying, excessive worry, insomnia, slow reaction time and mental sluggishness, and attention deficit hyperactivity disorder (ADHD).

Physical Symptoms—Weight fluctuations, difficulty losing (or gaining) weight, edema, hypoglycemia, skin problems, chronic infections (respiratory, viral, or bacterial), chronic fatigue syndrome, lethargy or weakness, constipation, low body temperature and cold extremities, slow pulse, hair loss, headaches, infertility, rheumatic pain, muscle aches and weakness, burning/prickling sensations, anemia, labored breathing, brittle nails, poor vision, hearing impairment, menstrual disorders (excessive flow or cramps), heart disease, cancer, hypertension, high cholesterol, and multiple sclerosis.

The Thyroid and Its Hormones

The thyroid gland, one of the body's seven endocrine glands, is located just below the larynx in the throat with interconnecting lobes on either side of the trachea. The thyroid controls the rate at which organs function and the speed with which the body uses food; it affects the operation of all body processes and organs. The thyroid has four principal hormones: T1, T2, T3, and T4. Thyroid hormones are stored in the thyroid and released to the body as needed. T1 (mono-iodothyronine) and T2 (di-iodothyronine) are not considered especially active. T4 (thyroxine) contains iodine, is produced exclusively in the thyroid gland, and accounts for almost 93% of the thyroid's hormones; its chief function is to increase the speed of cell metabolism, or energy conversion.

Iodine and the amino acid tyrosine are essential to forming normal amounts of T4. When the body requires more T3 (tri-iodothyronine), T4 can give up its iodine to form T3 which, while representing only about 7% of the thyroid hormone complement, has a greater biological activity by a factor of three to four times. About 80% of the body's T3 comes from converting T4, typically in the liver and kidneys. When T4 conversion runs smoothly—that is, the enzyme cascade (sequencing of enzymes in chemical reactions) is correct—normal body temperature and metabolic rates are maintained.

If the thyroid is functioning poorly, however, T4 breaks down to form reverse tri-iodothyronine, or rT3 (a different chemical version of T3). Stress, fasting, illness, or elevated cortisol (from the adrenal glands) can contribute to the occurrence of this faulty conversion. As rT3 levels increase, metabolism and body temperature decrease and various enzymes fail to

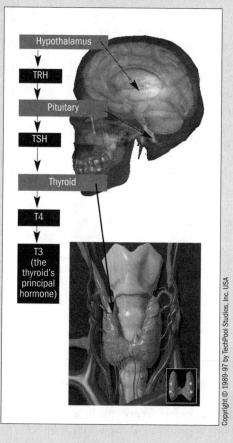

Hypothalamus

TRH

Pituitary

TSH

Thyroid

T4

T3 (the thyroid's principal hormone)

function properly. In addition, as rT3 levels build, levels of T3 decrease, leading to low T3 syndrome and thyroid dysfunction.

Total blood levels of T3 and T4 consist of only 1% biologically active components (called the free levels), while 99% is the metabolically inactive portion bound to proteins. In a healthy person, total T4 levels as indicated in a blood test (or thyroid panel) are 4.5-12.5, but for someone with hypothyroidism, those values will be less than 4.5. For free T4, the normal range is 0.9-2.0; hypothyroid, less than 0.9. For free T3, normal is 80-220; hypothyroid, less than 80. TSH is normally 0.3-6.0; for hypothyroid, greater than 6.0.

The formation and secretion of T3 and T4 are regulated by thyroid-stimulating hormone, or TSH (thyrotropin), secreted by the pituitary gland in the brain. TSH, in turn, is directed by another hormone called thyrotropin-releasing hormone (TRH) which is secreted by the brain's hypothalamus gland. When TSH reaches the thyroid gland, it signals it to secrete more hormones (both T4 and T3). The hormones released by the thyroid not only speed up metabolism, but also send a feedback message to the brain, telling it to stop secreting TSH and TRH. TSH blood levels are conventionally taken as the best index for thyroid dysfunction, both hypo and hyper (overactive). When thyroid function is low, TSH levels normally go up.

Subclinical hypothyroidism, the early stage of the disease, is particularly difficult to diagnose because of the action of TSH. During this phase, the pituitary gland recognizes that the thyroid isn't producing enough hormones, so it releases more TSH. The extra TSH causes the thyroid to work overtime to secrete more T4 and T3. A weak thyroid is thus often "propped up" by high levels of TSH during the early stage of the disease, and this masks the symptoms of the condition. Without adequate treatment, the thyroid will continue to deteriorate.

■ Many people with low thyroid function have puffy, thick skin and retain fluid throughout their bodies. This is because of an accumulation of hyalouronic acid, a sugar that binds with water in the body, causing swelling and an increase in weight.[1]

■ Hypothyroidism leads to a sluggish digestive system, often resulting in a number of gastrointestinal problems, including constipation, gas and bloating, abdominal pain, and decreased absorption of nutrients. Decreased digestive efficiency may lead to a condition called leaky gut syndrome, in which undigested food particles enter the bloodstream causing allergic reactions and depleting the immune system. Weight gain is one of the potential results of these digestive disturbances.[2]

■ Hypothyroidism is linked to pancreatitis, a decrease in insulin production by the pancreas. Insulin is the hormone which controls how the body processes sugars. When insulin imbalances occur, blood sugars, rather than being burned off, are turned into fat.[3]

- Imbalances in the levels of thyroid hormones reduce the body's thermogenic or fat-burning capacity, leading to increased fat storage.[4]
- Because low thyroid function causes fatigue and lack of stamina as well as muscle aches or weakness, people with this condition often get an insufficient amount of exercise or other physical activity, which is another factor in weight problems.[5]

What Causes Hypothyroidism?

Thyroid problems may be due to a number of factors, including environmental pollutants, dietary excesses or insufficiencies, certain drugs, stress, and yeast infections.

Toxic Environment

Thyroid problems have been on the rise due to the increasingly toxic environment in which we live. Exposure to radiation, fluoride (in water and toothpaste), mercury from silver amalgam dental fillings, pollutants (thyocyanide) in cigarette smoke, and chlorinated compounds (found in wood and leather preservatives) are just a few of the many causes of hypothyroidism.[6] Radiation is probably the greatest environmental cause of hypothyroidism and other thyroid problems, including thyroid cancer, states Lita Lee, Ph.D., an enzyme therapist based in Lowell, Oregon. John Gofman, M.D., Ph.D., director of the Committee for Nuclear Responsibility, agrees that increased radiation exposure has impacted the human thyroid. He studied the effects of the Chernobyl disaster—a nuclear reactor explosion that occurred in the mid-1980s in what is now the Ukraine—on human health. He found that individuals exposed to the radiation from Chernobyl had symptoms virtually identical to that of hypothyroidism.[7]

High levels of heavy metals, particularly mercury (a toxic heavy metal which comprises up to 50% of silver amalgam fillings), lead, and cadmium, depress thyroid function. Heavy metals poison an enzyme critical in converting the inactive form of thyroid hormone (T4) into the active form (T3).[8]

Diet

Dietary factors include synthetic and genetically engineered hormones in meat, dairy products, poultry, and eggs, which block the release of thyroid hormones. Another dietary factor is excess iodine. "Most Americans get too much iodine because it is used in baked goods as a dough conditioner, in commercial iodized salt, and in supplements such as kelp," says Dr. Lee. In excess, iodine is a powerful thyroid inhibitor.

Raw cruciferous vegetables (cabbage, broccoli, or cauliflower) contain thyroid inhibitors; lightly steaming them kills these thyroid-suppressing substances. Liver, while a nourishing food, contains thyroid inhibitors and there is some evidence that soy affects thyroid function.[9] Other dietary influences include vitamin deficiencies (particularly vitamins A and B), mineral deficiencies (zinc, copper, iron, and selenium), and excess intake of polyunsaturated fats (such as those found in soybean, safflower, and corn oils).

EDITOR'S NOTE
The position on unsaturated fats presented here is a controversial one. Many physicians advocate the dietary use and supplementation of essential fatty acids in the form of fish, primrose, borage, and flaxseed oils, among others, in the unsaturated category. There is research to support both positions.

Medications

In cases where the thyroid is already impaired, prednisone, an anti-inflammatory drug used to treat a variety of illnesses, can aggravate the condition.[10] Sulfa drugs, commonly used to treat infections, and antidiabetic agents also impair thyroid function. Birth control pills and estrogen replacement therapy (ERT) can lead to estrogen dominance (an excess of the hormone estrogen in relation to progesterone), which inhibits thyroid function. Lithium, taken for manic-depressive disorder, can produce hypothyroidism in up to 33% of long-term users. The heart drug Cordarone® and interferon-alpha (for hepatitis) can cause either an overactive or underactive thyroid.[11] Other drugs, such as methimazole and propylthiouracil (PTU), are known to cross the placental barrier in women and cause fetal hypothyroidism. These drugs, usually given to patients whose thyroid gland is releasing too much hormone, slow the body's manufacture of thyroid hormones.[12]

Stress

The action of thyroid hormones in the body is also uniquely affected by stress. The hormones released by stress, adrenaline and cortisol, interfere with the body's ability to convert the thyroid hormone T4 into the more potent T3. Dr. Lee adds that as T3 levels decrease, the body produces even more adrenaline and cortisol to try and speed up metabolism, which further inhibits the conversion. This, she adds, sets up "a vicious cycle that can only be broken by proper hormone balancing."[13] The problem of T4 to T3 conversion is referred to as "Wilson's Syndrome" (see "What is Wilson's Syndrome?" p. 211).

For more on the **weight-gaining effects of stress**, see Chapter 7: Heal Your Emotional Appetite, pp. 156-182.

Yeast Infections

Hypothyroidism is associated with the spread of *Candida albicans* (a type of yeast that is normally confined to the lower bowels, skin, and vagina) in the body. As it spreads, *Candida* takes on a toxic fungal form that affects not only the thyroid, but many other body systems. Keith Sehnert, M.D., a thyroid specialist in Minneapolis, Minnesota, has treated more than 3,000 patients with yeast-related disorders. He has noticed a significant overlap between the diagnosis and treatment of hypothyroidism and yeast infections. "In treating my patients," he says, "I see three circles intersecting: *Candida* infections, hypothyroidism, and food allergies."[17]

For more about **Candida**, see Chapter 13: Eliminate Yeast Infections, pp. 294-309. For more on **food allergies**, see Chapter 11: Break Food Allergies and Addictions, pp. 244-270.

Candida infections can cause serious damage to the intestinal lining. According to James Braly, M.D., of Fort Lauderdale, Florida, *Candida* can permeate the lining of the intestines and break down the barrier to the bloodstream. "When the fungal form of *Candida* occurs in the body, allergic substances can penetrate into the blood more easily, where they form immense complexes and perhaps even promote food allergy reactions," says Dr. Braly.[18] The damaged lining allows undigested food to pass into the bloodstream, an ailment known as "leaky gut syndrome." The immune system (SEE QUICK DEFINITION) then produces antibodies to attack these food particles as though they were allergens. This reaction of the body against itself, called an autoimmune response, can seriously damage the thyroid gland.

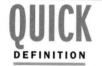

DEFINITION

The **immune system** guards the body against foreign, disease-producing substances. Its "workers" are various white blood cells including one trillion lymphocytes and 100 million trillion antibodies. Lymphocytes are found in high numbers in the lymph nodes, bone marrow, spleen, and thymus gland.

An **antibody** is a protein molecule made from amino acids in the lymph tissue and set in motion by the immune system against a specific foreign protein, or antigen. An antibody is also referred to as an immunoglobulin and binds tightly with the antigen as a preliminary for removing it from the system or destroying it.

The most severe form of this autoimmune reaction can cause Hashimoto's Autoimmune Thyroiditis (HAIT), a disease in which the body releases antibodies that attack the thyroid gland as if it were a foreign invader. Characterized by an enlarged thyroid, other symptoms of HAIT include deep fatigue, memory loss, and depression, among others. HAIT also can lead to psychological disturbances, including extreme anxiety and panic attacks. Dr. Langer explains that people with this condition often try to make themselves feel better by eating, and thus continue to gain weight, which only worsens their psychological state. HAIT predominantly strikes women between the ages of 13 and 40 (95% of HAIT sufferers are women).[19]

What is Wilson's Syndrome?

Denis Wilson, M.D., of Longwood, Florida, author of *Wilson's Syndrome: The Miracle of Feeling Well*, identified the thyroid syndrome that bears his name after many years of clinical work. The symptoms of Wilson's Syndrome include all the symptoms of hypothyroidism, according to Dr. Wilson, plus the additional symptoms of migraines, aggravated premenstrual syndrome (PMS), panic attacks, night sweats, ringing in the ears, mood swings, itchiness, allergies, and asthma.

Emotional or physical stress reduces the rate of conversion of T4 to T3, which, according to Dr. Wilson, is a natural survival mechanism that helps conserve energy. After the stressful period passes, the body should resume converting T4 to T3. However, for reasons that are still unclear, the body simply fails to do this. Dr. Wilson describes the failure as "a natural and normal starvation/stress coping mechanism gone amuck."[14]

In addition to the problem of conversion, cell membranes within the body may fail to respond to the action of the T3 hormone. Each cell has an area on its surface, a receptor site, where the T3 hormone attaches. When the chemical shape of these areas is altered, the T3 cannot attach and the metabolism of the cell consequently slows. Diets high in low-quality animal fats, particularly from red meat and chicken, will damage these receptor sites. "The thyroid hormones, especially T3, interact with the receptor in much the same way that a key turns in a lock so that it may be opened," explains Dr. Wilson.[15] When the receptors get jammed, T3 cannot get metabolism within the cell to speed up.

While stress may be a primary cause of Wilson's Syndrome, other factors also have an effect. In her book *Supernutrition for Menopause*, nutritionist Ann Louise Gittleman, M.S., says that dietary estrogens, such as those found in meat and dairy products, affect the cells' ability to take up thyroid hormones.[16] To treat Wilson's Syndrome, Dr. Wilson generally recommends T3 hormone therapy.

For information about **Wilson's Syndrome** and referrals to doctors knowledgeable in the treatment of this condition, contact: The Wilson's Syndrome Foundation, P.O. Box 916206, Longwood, FL 32791-6206; tel: 800-621-7006 or 800-533-5895.

Detecting Hypothyroidism

Despite its high incidence, hypothyroidism has remained a hidden disease that is causing many people to gain weight. The problem is that conventional tests used by most doctors to assess thyroid function are inadequate to the task. Consequently, many cases of hypothyroidism remain undetected and untreated. "Lots of people who are in fact suffering the effects of low thyroid hormone don't get classified that way when screened," says Dan Lukaczer, N.D., a naturopathic physician at Great Smokies Diagnostic Laboratory in Asheville, North Carolina.

Fortunately, there are test procedures available that can accurately assess the functioning of your thyroid. "The best way to diagnose is by using some of the newer, more sophisticated tests, which most conventional doctors don't know about or choose not to use," says Dr. Lukaczer. While most of these tests require the assistance of a health-care professional, some you can even perform yourself.

To assess thyroid function, doctors often measure blood levels of two thyroid hormones, thyroxine (T4) and tri-iodothyronine (T3), along with thyroid-stimulating hormone (TSH) secreted by the pituitary gland. These blood tests may show normal levels of all these hormones despite a weakened thyroid. Raphael Kellman, M.D., a thyroid specialist in New York City, has found that many of his patients are hypothyroid despite normal levels of T3, T4, or TSH in the blood. As a further check, Dr. Kellman correlates TSH levels with two other measurements to "triangulate" his diagnosis of thyroid function. The two other measurements are a patient's resting body temperature (called the basal temperature test—discussed below) and a thyroid sonogram, which shows if the thyroid is swollen. In some cases, he also uses a more sophisticated test, the TRH (thyrotropin-releasing hormone) stimulation test, which he calls the "gold standard" for accurately detecting an underactive thyroid.

Raphael Kellman, M.D.: Center for Progressive Medicine, 140 West 69th Street, New York, NY 10023; tel: 212-721-6633; fax: 212-721-6714.

The Thyroid Gold Standard

The TRH stimulation test is inexpensive and is performed by most laboratories. TRH is a hormone released by the hypothalamus that energizes the pituitary gland to release TSH. The physician measures the patient's TSH level (a simple blood test), gives an injection of TRH, then draws blood 25 minutes later and re-measures TSH. The TRH injection stimulates the brain's pituitary gland, which produces TSH. If the first TSH level is normal and the second TSH level is high—above ten—it indicates that the patient's thyroid is underactive, and the pituitary gland is compensating by releasing more TSH. A TSH reading of 15 is suspicious, while 20 strongly points to hypothyroidism.

"Routine testing assumes that if TSH is high, then thyroid hormone must be low, but in some cases a patient with an underactive thyroid still shows a 'normal' TSH reading," explains Dr. Kellman. Routine tests diagnose hypothyroidism by documenting its effects (such as low body temperature), while the TRH test uncovers the physiological causes behind an underfunctioning thyroid. A stressed pituitary gland, worn down by a weak thyroid, will overreact to TRH,

Success Story: Reversing a Case of Fatigue and Weight Gain

The following case from Raphael Kellman, M.D., shows how pinpointing thyroid dysfunction can lead to a successful reversal of all of the patient's symptoms:

Mona, 42, had suffered with extreme fatigue for a year, waking in the morning, after 8-10 hours of sleep, more tired than when she went to bed. During the day, she often needed a nap. While she ate relatively little, Mona was steadily gaining weight and she also experienced bloating, constipation, and abdominal pains; her skin was dry and her hair thinning; and her menstrual cycles were irregular and preceded by PMS. Mona reported that she had difficulty concentrating and was forgetful and depressed (even though she had no psychological reasons for it).

When Mona's conventional physician performed a routine thyroid hormone test (for T3 and T4 levels), the results were "normal." Although, on the basis of these results, she was advised to "rest and not worry," Mona thought otherwise and sought a different thyroid test to measure TSH levels. But this test yielded "normal" results, too. Mona's doctor, noticing her anxiety and depression, wrote her a prescription for Prozac.

"Her life seemed to be spiraling downwards," comments Dr. Kellman. "Her depression subsided a little on the Prozac, but her fatigue, weight, and other problems got worse." Dr. Kellman immediately ran the TRH thyroid test on Mona; her TSH level after stimulation was 22, indicating an underactive thyroid. He started Mona on Synthroid® (a synthetic form of T4) and Thyrostim, a natural supplement containing amino acids, vitamins, and thyroid extract to convert T4 to T3.

Mona began a nutritional program to help her body regain normal thyroid function. Dr. Kellman observes, "It's not enough to replace the low T4 with synthetics. The underlying causes of the underactive thyroid must be addressed as well." Many of these causes—nutrient deficiencies, overload of toxins and free radicals, hormonal imbalances (such as high cortisol), and mental and physical stress—benefit from improvements in diet and nutrition. By adding the nutritional program, Dr. Kellman was able to gradually lower Mona's doses of Synthroid and eventually stop the medication altogether.

"Within two weeks Mona began to feel more energy and more alive," notes Dr. Kellman. "A few weeks later, her brain fog began to lift and her attention span was significantly better. In no time, she was back to her old self and began noticing weight loss and thicker, fuller hair, and her skin was normal again. Soon her periods were more regular, her PMS became tolerable, and Mona's mood and energy level were, in her words, 'The best I can ever remember'."

while a healthy one will not. It is the best way to accurately assess thyroid function. Dr. Kellman indicates that "of the patients I've seen with three or more typical symptoms of underactive thyroid but who

"For patients who experience 'weight bounce'—losing weight only to gain it all back and more—this can be directly caused by a poorly functioning thyroid," says Raphael Kellman, M.D.

have tested 'normal' in standard tests, 35% to 40% actually have underactive thyroids based on the TRH test."

The TRH test was once widely used by American physicians, but was then replaced by the quicker, easier TSH test. "In the age of assembly line medicine, doctors jettisoned the TRH because it is cumbersome and time-consuming and opted for the easy route," comments Dr. Kellman. "But this is a grave mistake of modern medicine, causing needless suffering."

Many people with unchecked weight gain have abnormal TRH values, says Dr. Kellman. "For patients who experience 'weight bounce'—losing weight only to gain it all back and more—this can be directly caused by a poorly functioning thyroid. This means we have found the missing link in weight gain and know how to stop the weight rebound effect."[20]

Basal Temperature Test

Broda O. Barnes, M.D., Ph.D., a pioneer in thyroid research and author of *Hypothyroidism: An Unsuspected Illness*, was the first to use resting body temperature, called basal temperature, as an indicator of thyroid function. Based on more than four decades of research, Dr. Barnes found that consistently low basal temperature is a dependable indicator of problems with thyroid function. His simple test, known as the basal temperature test, involves taking underarm temperatures on consecutive mornings.

The Broda O. Barnes Research Foundation is a nonprofit information and education organization dedicated to improving endocrine function. They offer information packets, audio and video tapes, physician referrals, a 24-hour urine test to assess the health of the thyroid and other glands, and consultation services for doctors. For more information, contact: Broda O. Barnes Research Foundation, P.O. Box 98, Trumbull, CT 06611; tel: 203-261-2101

To take the basal temperature test, place a thermometer in place before getting out of bed in the morning. You can use either a traditional mercury or a digital thermometer. A digital thermometer will record your temperature in a few seconds while a mercury thermometer should be left in place for ten minutes. It is important to lie still and relax while recording the temperature. Perform the test and record your temperature for two or more consecutive days. The temperature for normal thyroid function is 97.8° F to 98.2° F. Dr. Barnes indicates that a reading below 97.8° F strongly suggests hypothyroidism.

Dr. Lee recommends taking oral temperatures instead of underarm temperatures because she feels that it is more accurate. If you elect to use oral temperatures, normal would be 98° F in the morning and between 98.6°-99° F (and not over 100° F) during the day. A reading below 98° F in the morning suggests low thyroid function.

Menstruating women should take temperatures only on the second and third days of menstruation to avoid recording the temperature fluctuations they normally experience during the menstrual cycle. Avoid all alcohol for several days before taking your temperature. In addition, do not use temperature readings taken when you are ill and do not use any heat sources in your bed, such as electric blankets, heating pads, or hot water bottles, as these may interfere with an accurate reading.

EDITOR'S NOTE
While the basal temperature and resting pulse tests are important in assessing thyroid function, they should not be used alone. Stephen Langer, M.D., warns that certain conditions other than hypothyroidism (such as chronic viral infections) can reduce a person's basal temperature. He therefore recommends, as does Dr. Kellman, that physicians correlate the basal temperature tests with hormone blood tests.[21]

Resting Pulse Test

Another way to tell if you are hypothyroid is to measure your resting pulse, according to Dr. Lee. The healthy resting pulse should be about 85 beats per minute (bpm). The national average is around 72 bpm, but if your pulse is less than 80 bpm, you may have an underactive thyroid. Infants and children have a pulse greater than 100 bpm until around the age of eight years, when the pulse slows down to around 85 bpm. "The idea of a slow pulse being healthy is folklore," Dr. Lee explains. "Studies of healthy people who have no heart disease were found to have an average pulse of 85 beats per minute. Studies on the smartest high school students showed a pulse of 85 versus a pulse of 70 in below average students." However, she cautions that "some people with low thyroid function have a high pulse of over 100 beats per minute; these are people who literally run on adrenaline."

Alternative Medicine Therapies for a Healthy Thyroid

Alternative medicine practitioners generally treat hypothyroidism by strengthening intestinal health and digestion. Dr. Spiddell emphasizes proper nutrition combined with regular exercise to help restore a weakened thyroid. "In some cases, I find that the thyroid just needs the kind of jumpstart that an exercise program, nutrients, and changes in diet can spark," he says. To help spark your thyroid back to life, here is a guide to the foods and specific nutrients that you should either include in your diet or avoid. Thyroid glandular therapy and thyroid hormone therapy are two additional options available to return the thyroid to normal functioning.

Dietary Recommendations

Goitrogens are foods that reduce the release of thyroid hormone and interfere in the conversion of T4 to T3. Examples include walnuts, sorghum, cassava, almonds, peanuts, soy flour, millet, and apples. These foods should be avoided by anyone suffering from hypothyroidism. Mustard greens, kale, cabbage, spinach, Brussels sprouts, cauliflower, broccoli, and turnips also have a mild anti-thyroid effect and should be avoided until the condition is normalized or stabilized.[22]

Thyrotrophs are foods that stimulate thyroid hormone production and increase the conversion of T4 to T3. Examples include seaweeds (bladderwrack, laminaria, kelp, and dulse), garlic, radishes, watercress, seafood, egg yolks, wheat germ, brewer's yeast, and mushrooms. Fruits and fruit juices (especially tropical varieties), watermelon, and coconut oil are also thyroid-stimulating. A two to four week diet of only raw foods, with heavy emphasis on raw greens, seaweed, nuts, seeds, sprouted beans and seeds, and freshly extracted juices, is an effective way to improve thyroid function.

Dr. Lee also makes the following general dietary recommendations to support the thyroid:

■ Adequate amounts of protein: organic beef or poultry, some kinds of fish (such as halibut and white fish), organic eggs, and organic raw milk products (such as kefir, yogurt, and cottage cheese); vegans can eat potatoes for a good protein source.

■ Fruits or fruit juices: to calm the adrenal glands and stimulate the production of thyroid hormones.

■ Avoid iodized salt: look for either organic sea salt or purified seawater with no added iodine.

■ Coconut oil: probably the most healthful type of saturated fat other than raw butter, coconut oil stimulates thyroid function.

Nutritional Supplements

A number of nutrients can play a critical role in revitalizing the thyroid:

Vitamins—A deficiency of vitamin E will reduce iodine absorption by the thyroid by 95%. This deficiency commonly occurs in women during pregnancy and menopause, which may help explain why thyroid disorders are so often triggered by these conditions. A typical recommended dosage is 800-1,200 IU of vitamin E per day.

Hypothyroid patients do not effectively convert beta carotene—the natural form of vitamin A found in yellow and green fruits and vegetables—to a biologically usable form. Vitamin A is necessary for the production of thyroxine and is required by the thyroid to absorb iodine.[23] Most vitamin A supplements are sold in the beta carotene form. As a typical recommendation, patients with impaired thyroid function should take 10,000-20,000 IU of vitamin A daily. Unless closely supervised by a physician, your intake of pure vitamin A should never exceed 20,000 IU per day.

Daily supplementation with vitamins C (3-5 g) and B complex (100-150 mg) can help strengthen the thyroid. Vitamin C deficiency will make capillaries in the thyroid bleed and normal cells in the gland will begin to multiply abnormally, a condition called hyperplasia;[24] B complex is important for keeping all cells, including those of the thyroid, in good health.

Iodine—Stephen Langer, M.D., author of *Solved: The Riddle of Weight Loss*, says that for most "first-generation hypothyroids," those whose parents did not have the disease, simply adding more iodine-containing foods to the diet is often enough to restore the functioning of the gland. "The best food supplements for iodine content are kelp and cod liver oil," he says.[25] Kelp, a type of seaweed, is best taken in tablet form. Lobster, shrimp, crab, and saltwater fish such as haddock, cod, halibut, and herring, are also good sources of iodine.

The recommended daily allowance for iodine is 100 mcg for women and 120 mcg for men. Dr. Langer advises against taking more than this amount of iodine, as too much iodine can suppress the formation of T3. He also warns patients against using too much table salt, a source of iodine that is also frequently high in sodium. Too much salt can alter the relative concentrations of sodium and potassium in the body, which, in turn, can result in serious disorders, such as heart disease, high blood pressure, and obesity.

Minerals—Zinc helps in the conversion of T4 to T3 and increases the sensitivity of cell membranes to these hormones; a typical dose is 25 mg per day along with 3 mg of copper (because zinc tends to deplete copper reserves). With medical supervision, the dosage of zinc can be increased; however, dosages should be increased with caution, as too much zinc can interfere with immune system function.

Selenium also plays an important role in the conversion of T4 to T3; the generally recommended dose is 200 mcg per day. In addition, a diet low in iron will cause anemia, which has been found to lead to low thyroid function; typical dose is 100 mcg per day.[26]

Tyrosine—The amino acid tyrosine is an important building block of both T4 and T3 hormones. Tyrosine is found in soybeans, beef, chicken, fish, carob, bean sprouts, oats, spinach, sesame seeds, and butternut squash. L-tyrosine can also be taken as a nutritional supplement; typical recommended dose is 250-750 mg per day, taken between meals.

Herbal Therapy

Gugulipid, an Ayurvedic herb that has been used in India for over 2,500 years, is helpful for supporting the thyroid. It is derived from the resin of a small myrrh tree native to Asia and is traditionally used for a number of health conditions, including rheumatoid arthritis and high cholesterol. Studies have shown that gugulipid stimulates thyroid function.[27]

Coleus forskohlii, a member of the mint family, is another Ayurvedic herb for stimulating the thyroid. Research has shown that the primary active ingredient, forskolin, increases the production of thyroid hormones and stimulates their release.[28]

Thyroid Glandular Therapy

Dr. Langer indicates that, while good nutrition is important, some patients require additional help to restore thyroid function, particularly second-generation hypothyroids—patients whose parents also had the disease. In such cases, Dr. Langer prescribes desiccated thyroid glandular extract rather than synthetic hormones. Thyroid glandular is usually derived from calves or pigs and contains both T3 and T4 hormones.

Dr. Lee also recommends the whole glandular derivatives for her clients needing additional thyroid therapy. "The whole glandular extracts are preferable rather than synthetic thyroid hormones, because they contain the protein precursors to both thyroid hormones in a natural proportion of T4 to T3," she explains. Synthroid, a synthetic thyroid medication, is a less effective form of thyroid therapy because it contains only thyroxine (T4).

Dr. Lee makes the following general recommendations for people taking thyroid glandular: typically start with ¼ grain to one grain per day, taken with food; whatever your dosage, divide it and take one portion with each meal. During thyroid therapy, be sure to monitor your metabo-

In self-administration of thyroid glandular therapy, some people increase their dosage too fast or not fast enough and they don't get well. Thyroid glandulars are not dangerous, but if not taken according to instructions they can have unpleasant side effects, such as a headache or racing pulse. Thyroid glandular therapy should be used to normalize thyroid function in cases of hypothyroidism, not as a weight-loss aid. Thyroid therapy is therefore best undertaken with the guidance of a qualified health-care practitioner.

Success Story: Glandular Therapy Stops Food Cravings

" I was almost incapacitated by fatigue and plagued by eczema, headaches, digestive problems, food and environmental allergies, and weight gain," says Karen, who was overweight—5'10" and 290 pounds—and suffered from depression. "I really examined my emotional life," she says, "but that wasn't the whole answer for me. After years of self-exploration, I was still very overweight." Karen went to see her doctor, who tested her thyroid function—the results, he told her, were normal.

Karen eventually consulted enzyme specialist Lita Lee, Ph.D., in Lowell, Oregon, who recommended that she take a thyroid glandular, a natural form of thyroid hormone, along with an enzyme supplement. An underactive thyroid interferes with enzyme production, which does not allow for proper digestion and results in poor nutrition regardless of diet. It is why some thyroid patients, including Karen, feel hungry all the time. "I had these incredible cravings for sugar," she says, "which my regular doctor had told me were all in my head. Now I know my depression was very much the result of biological imbalances and thyroid problems."

Lita Lee, Ph.D.:
P.O. Box 516, Lowell,
OR 97452;
tel: 541-937-1123;
fax: 541-937-1132.

Within a month of treatment, Karen's energy and overall health improved. "My feelings of depression were gone too," she reports. As an experiment, Karen stopped taking the thyroid treatment that Dr. Lee had prescribed, but her symptoms began to recur almost immediately; they disappeared as soon as she went back on the regimen. "Now, after one-and-a-half years of taking the thyroid treatment, my cravings have stopped," she says. "I'm not driven to overeat, my allergies are under control, headaches are gone, and I've lost 90 pounds without dieting. I feel restored in every way."

lism: take your oral temperature in the morning before arising (it should be 98° F) and repeat at around noon (98.6°-99° F); also take your resting pulse (85 bpm is normal). Slowly increase your daily dosage by ¼ grain to one grain every 7-10 days until you are feeling well and your oral temperatures and resting pulse are normal. "The reason I give a varied dosage is that some people, especially those with a toxic colon, high blood pressure, or excess adrenaline, can have side effects if they increase their dosage too rapidly," says Dr. Lee. "This is not due to thyroid hormone but to the person's toxic condition." The two major side effects of increasing your thyroid dose too fast are a transient racing pulse and headaches.

CHAPTER

10 Restore Hormonal Balance

WHEN HORMONE LEVELS in the body become imbalanced, one of the primary results for both men and women is a steady rise in body weight. Aging, stress, and an increasingly toxic environment are some of the main factors causing hormonal disruption. Alternative medicine offers a number of ways to rebalance your hormones, including natural hormone therapy, diet and nutritional support, and herbs. By restoring your hormones to their proper balance, significant weight loss can be achieved.

Success Story: Hormone and Weight Balancing

Stacey, 21, was 5'5" and weighed 273 pounds. She was a student and working to support herself. When she came to see clinical nutritionist Linda Lizotte, R.D., C.D.N., based in Trumbull, Connecticut, Stacey complained of fatigue, having difficulty getting out of bed in the morning, moodiness, and diarrhea. She was taking birth control pills but no other medications.

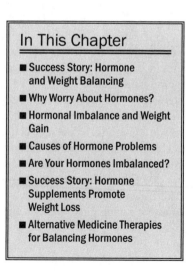

In This Chapter

- Success Story: Hormone and Weight Balancing
- Why Worry About Hormones?
- Hormonal Imbalance and Weight Gain
- Causes of Hormone Problems
- Are Your Hormones Imbalanced?
- Success Story: Hormone Supplements Promote Weight Loss
- Alternative Medicine Therapies for Balancing Hormones

When Lizotte questioned Stacey about her diet, she found that Stacey was drinking large quantities of orange juice and sodas; that is, she was taking in a lot of carbohydrates in the form of simple sugars. Lizotte also felt that the birth control pills were a factor in this case. "The pill seems to make the body sensitive to carbohydrates," says Lizotte. "Most women will tell you that they're hungrier as soon as they start the pill and they put on weight

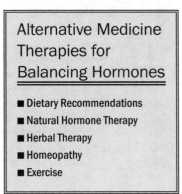

Alternative Medicine Therapies for Balancing Hormones

■ Dietary Recommendations
■ Natural Hormone Therapy
■ Herbal Therapy
■ Homeopathy
■ Exercise

faster." The hormonal changes induced by the pill cause women to crave carbohydrates, she explains, which make the body retain more water, adding to weight gain. A hormone imbalance will also cause the body to convert more carbohydrates into fat for storage.

To reduce the sugars in Stacey's diet, Lizotte limited her starch intake to two servings per day. One starch serving was allowed at breakfast (toast or cereal), but she was to avoid starch at lunch. "If people have starch at lunch, insulin [the hormone secreted by the pancreas that controls sugar levels] kicks in and causes a drop in blood sugar in the afternoon. That's when people feel a drop in energy," says Lizotte. "If they eliminate starch from lunch, the insulin doesn't kick in and they go right through the afternoon without the drop in energy."

Lizotte recommended a lunch consisting of four ounces of protein (such as chicken or hamburger), salad, and vegetables. Stacey could have another starch serving (potato, rice, or pasta) at dinner along with another four ounces of protein, plus a serving of vegetables. After one week on this program, Stacey lost 11 pounds. In addition, her diarrhea stopped when she gave up the orange juice and she no longer craved it. Both of these changes indicate that Stacey was probably allergic to orange juice, according to Lizotte.

Lizotte also took a hair sample and sent it for analysis to determine the levels of minerals in Stacey's body. Mineral levels, either too high or too low, indicate the functional status of the body's systems. The results showed that Stacey had very low levels of two minerals, sodium and potassium, which indicated that her adrenal glands were stressed out. The adrenal glands, located above the kidneys, respond to stress by producing hormones such as cortisol and adrenaline—this is the "fight-or-flight" response. In a state of constant, long-term stress, the adrenals can become exhausted. When the adrenal glands

The Endocrine System

The endocrine glands, including the pituitary, thyroid and parathyroid, adrenals, pancreas, ovaries, and testicles, are central to the regulation and normalization of all the body's complex, interconnected systems, from metabolism and heat production to sperm production and uterine preparations for pregnancy. Hormones are the chemical messengers of the endocrine system that impose order through an intricate communication system among the body's estimated 50 trillion cells. Examples of hormones include the "male" sex hormone testosterone, the "female" sex hormones estrogen and progesterone, growth hormone (pituitary), and DHEA (adrenal).

The main link between the nervous system and the endocrine system is the hypothalamus, a small gland in the lower brain that acts as a kind of hormone control center. Messages from the brain are sent to the hypothalamus, which, in turn, sends messages to the pituitary gland, located just below the hypothalamus. This bean-sized gland makes hormones that control other endocrine glands.

The pituitary produces hormones that control the menstrual cycle in women—follicle-stimulating hormone (FSH) and luteinizing hormone (LH)—and hormones that stimulate the production of male hormones, or androgens (such as testosterone). The pituitary controls the thyroid gland by releasing thyroid-stimulating hormone (TSH), activates the adrenal gland through adrenocorticotropic hormone (ACTH), and stimulates overall growth in children by releasing human growth hormone (HGH).

The thyroid gland is located just below the larynx in the throat, with interconnecting lobes on either side of the trachea. The thyroid is the body's metabolic thermostat, controlling body temperature, energy use, and, in children, the body's growth rate. The thyroid controls the rate at which organs function and the speed with which the body uses food; it affects the operation of all body processes and organs. Of the hormones the thyroid synthesizes and releases, T3 (tri-iodothyronine) represents 7% and T4 (thyroxine) accounts for almost 93%.

The adrenal glands, two small glands nestled atop the

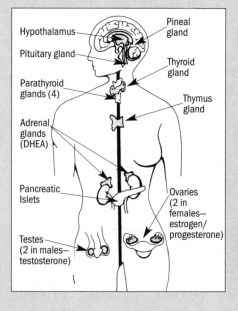

Hypothalamus

Pituitary gland

Parathyroid glands (4)

Adrenal glands (DHEA)

Pancreatic Islets

Testes (2 in males— testosterone)

Pineal gland

Thyroid gland

Thymus gland

Ovaries (2 in females— estrogen/ progesterone)

kidneys, respond to stress by producing the hormones adrenaline and noradrenaline. These hormones increase heart rate and blood sugar levels—the so-called fight-or-flight response. The adrenal glands also produce steroid (made from cholesterol) hormones, including estrogen, progesterone, DHEA, and testosterone.

For more on the **thyroid function**, see Chapter 9: Overcome a Sluggish Thyroid, pp. 202-219. For more on **insulin and its effect on weight**, see Chapter 8: Strengthen Your Sugar Controls, pp. 184-201.

organ that produces enzymes. The pancreas produces the hormone insulin, which regulates blood sugar levels and helps metabolize fats and proteins.

The gonads, or sex organs, are involved in sexual development and reproductive functions. A woman's ovaries produce the primary female sex hormones, estrogen and progesterone. A man's testes produce the male sex hormones, or androgens, the primary one being testosterone.

The pancreas, located behind the stomach, is both an endocrine gland that makes hormones and a digestive

are functioning normally, sodium and potassium levels would tend to be slightly elevated on the test. While under acute stress, when the levels of these minerals are very low (as in Stacey's case), explains Lizotte, "it means the adrenals are so weak that they're having problems just pumping out the normal hormones."

This affected Stacey's thyroid gland as well. When the adrenals are underfunctioning, the thyroid gland tries to compensate by producing more of its hormones. In a state of long-term stress, the function of the thyroid will become sluggish as well. "When these two glands are weakened together," says Lizotte, "it weakens the entire metabolic rate, that is, the person's ability to burn calories." Weight gain is one of the results.

To help Stacey's hormone function, Lizotte recommended the following supplements:

■ Adrenal Complex: contains adrenal glandulars (from desiccated animal glands), pantothenic acid, vitamin C, and B vitamins (PABA and B6), to energize and support the adrenals; three tablets daily.

■ Iron glycinate: iron is required for normal thyroid function; 18 mg daily.

■ Digestzyme: contains digestive enzymes and hydrochloric acid to support the digestive process; one capsule with every meal.

■ Thyroid L-Tyrosine Complex: contains thyroid glandulars (from animal glands) along with the amino acid L-tyrosine, to energize and nutritionally support thyroid function; three capsules daily.

For **Linda Lizotte, R.D., C.D.N.,** or information on **Adrenal Complex, Digestzyme, zinc picolinate,** and **iron glycinate,** contact: Designs for Health, 211 Pondway Lane, Trumbull, CT 06611; tel: 203-371-4383; fax: 530-618-6730. For **Thyroid L-Tyrosine Complex,** contact: Enzymatic Therapy, 825 Challenger Drive, Green Bay, WI 54311; tel: 800-783-2286 or 920-469-1313; fax: 920-469-4444.

After one month on this diet and nutritional program, Stacey had lost 19 pounds. Six months later, she had lost a total of 52 pounds. Stacey also reports that her mood is better and her energy has improved dramatically—getting out of bed is much easier now. And as far as losing weight, she's not ready to stop yet.

Why Worry About Hormones?

Stacey's weight problems were due to her hormones being out of balance. Many women will be familiar with her situation. Women going through perimenopause (SEE QUICK DEFINITION) or menopause may experience a host of symptoms, including hot flashes, fatigue, night sweats, mood swings, and weight gain. Men are not immune to these problems, either. In their fifties, men sometimes experience the "grumpy old man" syndrome or "male menopause": a condition characterized by fatigue, less muscle strength and endurance, decreased libido, short-term memory loss, and weight gain around the midriff. What is happening to produce these symptoms? The answer is in your hormones.

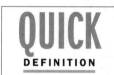

DEFINITION

Perimenopause is a condition characterized by the early onset of selected menopausal symptoms. The average American woman enters menopause around age 52; since perimenopause can begin as early as age 35, a woman may be vulnerable to the effects of menopause-related hormonal changes for as long as 17 years. Symptoms include weight gain, food cravings, moodiness, anxiety, irritability, headaches, bloating, "fuzzy" thinking, and depression. As with menopause, perimenopause (*peri* meaning "before" and *menopause* meaning "the end of the menses") is associated with a drop in progesterone relative to estrogen (two key female hormones).

These chemical messengers in the body regulate metabolism, the body's response to stress, kidney function, blood sugar balance, menstruation, and sexual function. When the hormone levels are imbalanced—from stress, medications, aging, or other causes—there can be system-wide problems. Weight gain is one of the more common results of hormonal imbalances. As Stacey found out, relief from weight problems can result from normalizing the hormone levels.

In this chapter, we look at the link between imbalances in the female and male hormones and weight problems. We outline the causes and symptoms of hormonal imbalances and how to determine if you have this problem. We then outline safe and effective alternative therapies for rebalancing hormones and shedding those extra pounds.

Hormonal Imbalance and Weight Gain

The word *hormone* comes from the Greek *hormao* meaning "to stir up." They are released by the various endocrine glands in the body in order to regulate energy production, growth, sexual development, stress responses, and many other functions (see "The Endocrine System," pp. 222-223). Because minute quantities of hormones can "stir up" so many activities in the body, when they are thrown out of balance the result can be system-wide. One of the more common symptoms of a hormone problem is weight gain or difficulty losing excess weight.

Women's Hormones and Weight Gain

For women at midlife, the natural interplay between the two primary female hormones, estrogen and progesterone (see "A Hormone Glossary," p. 228), takes on a new significance. As a woman approaches menopause, even as long as 10-15 years from menopause onset, hormone levels begin to shift. Many women don't realize that they may start having some symptoms of menopause long before what is still referred to as "The Change" is due. This early onset of symptoms is called perimenopause. These symptoms (including weight gain, night sweats, fluctuating moods, little interest in sex, and memory loss, among others) are indications that the levels of the basic female hormones are shifting out of balance. Perimenopause has been likened to "PMS from hell," an apt comparison because both are brought on by rising estrogen levels and declining progesterone levels.

When progesterone is in short supply, women become "estrogen domi-

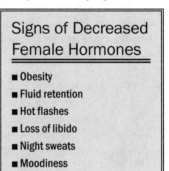

Signs of Decreased Female Hormones

- Obesity
- Fluid retention
- Hot flashes
- Loss of libido
- Night sweats
- Moodiness
- Memory loss

nant," a condition that women's health expert John R. Lee, M.D., describes as "toxic to the body."[1] Estrogen dominance can damage the pituitary gland and put stress on liver function. The liver is required to detoxify estrogen and to convert thyroid hormone to its active form. If the liver is not working properly, it will perpetuate the estrogen excess cycle by allowing estrogen to build up.

Estrogen dominance has many unpleasant results, including increased fat storage. Estrogen is manufactured and stored in body fat, which closely links this hormone with weight gain. When you have too much estrogen, you convert more food energy into fat instead of burning it as metabolic energy. Estrogen-dominant women also tend to retain fluids and salt and to crave carbohydrates, which can lead to blood sugar problems and insulin imbalances. Finally, excess estrogen

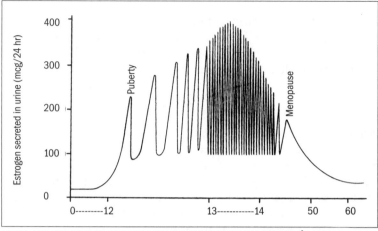

PEAKS AND TROUGHS OF ESTROGEN SECRETION THROUGHOUT A WOMAN'S LIFE.

can interfere with the function of the thyroid and the action of thyroid hormones, causing fatigue, loss of energy, and a drop in metabolism, factors which can contribute to weight gain.[2]

Men's Hormones and Weight Gain

A man's testosterone levels start to slowly decrease beginning around age 30, then more rapidly around age 60. Usually by the time a man reaches his mid-fifties (although symptoms may appear in one's forties), indications of "male menopause," also called andropause, are noticeable, according to Gary Ross, M.D., who practices in San Francisco, California. According to Dr. Ross, the andropause complex of symptoms includes fatigue, lack of energy, obesity, a loss of sexual interest and possibly some sexual dysfunction, depression or emotional malaise, panic attacks, decrease in short-term memory, and insomnia, among others.

These are signs that a man's hormones—their levels and ratios one to another—are in flux, shifting into a new configuration at midlife. "Men experience a 'lite' version of menopause, physically," says Theresa L. Crenshaw, M.D., author of *The Alchemy of Love and Lust*. "Their hormones and neuropeptides diminish, albeit less abruptly. Their bodies sag and change shape. Sexual functioning is often compromised by hormonal imbalance, disease, medications, mind, or mood. Their stamina and temperament alter as well. Yet often they are less well-equipped to deal with these extremes than women."[3]

This hormonal shift can lead to weight gain in a number of ways.

Testosterone is the hormone involved in the development of bone and lean muscle mass in men. When this hormone's levels decline, there is a loss of muscle strength and endurance during physical activities and an accompanying accumulation of body fat. Studies have shown a direct correlation between testosterone levels and abdominal fat and indicate that testosterone therapy can decrease the hip-to-waist ratio (an indicator of total body fat) and improve muscle strength in men.[4]

Testosterone is involved in blood sugar control as well. Decreased levels of the hormone are associated with increased insulin output, a risk factor for the development of diabetes and a contributing factor in obesity.[5] Decreased testosterone levels can lead to an increase in blood levels of the stress hormones adrenaline and cortisol. If this state occurs for an extended period of time, the thyroid can be affected, which may slow down metabolism and lead to an accumulation of body fat. "Testosterone has been shown to be an antagonist of the stress hormones," says Eugene Shippen, M.D., author of *The Testosterone Syndrome*. "More testosterone, less stress hormone production."[6]

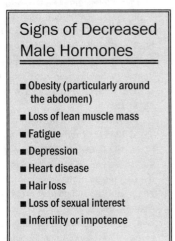

Signs of Decreased Male Hormones

- Obesity (particularly around the abdomen)
- Loss of lean muscle mass
- Fatigue
- Depression
- Heart disease
- Hair loss
- Loss of sexual interest
- Infertility or impotence

Causes of Hormone Problems

A number of factors can cause hormone imbalances in women and men. Hormone levels generally decline as a result of aging, but they can also be affected by dietary choices, mineral deficiencies, environmental toxins and synthetic chemicals, medications, smoking, and stress.

Causes of Hormone Imbalances in Women

Estrogen dominance (the excess of estrogen in relation to progesterone) can be created by numerous factors. Eating a diet high in estrogenic foods is often double exposure, because many of the foods that naturally contain estrogen are from animals that have also been pumped full of synthetic hormones to increase their weight or egg or milk production. Estrogen-mimicking chemicals, known as environmental estrogens or xenoestrogens, are found in our food, air, and water. Herbicides, pesticides, by-products of plastics manufacture, and

A Hormone Glossary

Estrogen, a female sex hormone produced mainly in the ovaries, regulates the menstrual cycle. Estrogen is important for adolescent sexual development, prepares the uterus for receiving the fertilized egg, and affects all the body's cells; its levels decline after menopause. Estrogen slows down bone loss, helps reverse the incidence of heart attacks, and acts as an antiaging factor.

Progesterone is a female sex hormone (produced in the ovaries) that prepares the uterus for a fertilized egg and then stops the cell proliferation in the uterus if pregnancy does not occur. When estrogen is high (days 7-14 of a woman's cycle), the level of progesterone is at its lowest. Its levels climb to a peak around days 14 to 24 and then drops off again just before the start of menstruation. Around age 35, a woman usually starts producing less progesterone.

Pregnenolone is the parent hormone for DHEA and other key hormones. As a brain power hormone, pregnenolone enhances memory, improves concentration, reduces mental fatigue, and generally keeps the brain functioning at peak capacity.

DHEA (dehydroepiandrosterone) is naturally produced by the human adrenal glands and gonads with optimal levels occurring around age 20 for women and age 25 for men. As an antioxidant, hormone regulator, and the building block from which estrogen and testosterone are produced, DHEA is vital to health. Low DHEA levels have been associated with diabetes, obesity, heart disease, Alzheimer's, and immune dysfunction illnesses. Test subjects using DHEA reported improved sleeping patterns, better memory, an improved ability to cope with stress, increases in lean muscle, and decreases in body fat.

Testosterone is the primary male sex hormone, important for the development of male sexual characteristics. Testosterone can help reverse male impotence, heighten virility, and increase muscle mass. After "male menopause" at midlife, testosterone levels decline.

Human growth hormone (HGH), naturally secreted by the pituitary gland in the brain, is a small, protein-like hormone similar to insulin. HGH is secreted in very brief pulses during the early hours of sleep and remains in circulation for only a few minutes. During adolescence, when growth is most rapid, production of HGH is high. After age 20, HGH production declines progressively and, by age 60, it is not uncommon to measure a growth hormone loss of 75% or more.

Cortisol is a hormone secreted by the adrenal glands, which are located atop the kidneys. Cortisol secretion occurs in daily cycles, peaking in the morning and having the lowest values at night. Cortisol promotes protein building, regulates insulin and glycogen synthesis, and helps produce prostaglandins. Under conditions of stress, high amounts of cortisol are released; chronic excess secretion is associated with obesity and suppressed thyroid function. Imbalances in cortisol secretion are linked with low energy, muscle dysfunction, and immune system depression.

many other chemicals mimic estrogen once they enter the body. The body responds as if it is real estrogen and the result is estrogen dominance and all the problems that imbalance carries with it.

Environmental estrogens are increasingly prevalent in Western societies; once in the body, they accumulate and persist for decades. There is no doubt that something is seriously interfering with normal human hormonal and endocrinal functioning, states Theo Colborn, Ph.D., a senior scientist with the World Wildlife Fund and an environmental author. Since 1945, synthetic chemicals (such as DDT, DES, PCBs, dioxin, among many others) have been released into our air, water, soil, food, and body. At least 51 of these have been conclusively shown to disrupt the human endocrine system. Each year, an estimated 1,000 new synthetic chemicals enter the world market, swelling the planetary total to well over 100,000. Evidence is accumulating that these chemicals, even at very low concentrations and exposures, can, by disrupting the endocrine system, cause "hormone havoc."[7]

Progesterone normally exerts a balancing effect on estrogen that neutralizes it, but stressful situations can disrupt the estrogen-progesterone balance. Betty Kamen, Ph.D., a psychologist and nutritionist based in Novato, California, and author of *Hormone Replacement Therapy: Yes or No?*, says that under prolonged stress, the body uses progesterone to make cortisol, one of the adrenal hormones.[8] As progesterone is used up in cortisol production, there is nothing left to balance or offset the effects of estrogen; this situation generally leads to the storage and accumulation of body fat. If a woman has chronic constipation or toxic buildup in her intestines, the excess estrogen is reabsorbed by the body instead of being eliminating, further adding to the imbalance of the hormonal ratio.

Chronic stress can exhaust the adrenal glands and lead to weight gain. The adrenal glands respond to stress by producing the hormones adrenaline and noradrenaline. Progesterone is the primary raw material the glands use for producing the adrenal hormones; the more adrenaline, the more progesterone needed. This is how chronic stress can lead to a state of progesterone deficiency (or estrogen dominance) as supplies of progesterone become depleted. When hormonal levels become imbalanced, emotional disorders can occur along with a steady rise in body weight.

Causes of Hormone Imbalances in Men

The concept that men go through major physiological changes in their fifties—the "male menopause"—of potentially equal impact as

Ten Reasons Why Women's Hormones are Imbalanced

Estrogen dominance (too much estrogen in relation to progesterone) can be created by both an excess of estrogen and a deficiency of progesterone. Here is how it happens.

Too much estrogen may be caused by:

1) foods that have hormones added to them, such as commercially produced meat, milk, eggs, and dairy products
2) herbs that have an estrogenic effect in the body, such as licorice, black cohosh, and damiana
3) birth control pills that have high levels of estrogen
4) environmental toxins that mimic the actions of estrogen (known as xeno-estrogens); the largest source of xenoestrogens is pesticides
5) exposure to radiation, which increases estrogen levels in the blood
6) chronic constipation, which interferes with the body's ability to eliminate estrogen properly; estrogen then builds up in the colon and can be reabsorbed by the body
7) synthetic estrogen supplements as part of hormone replacement therapy for menopausal symptoms

Too little progesterone may be caused by:

8) an underactive thyroid gland (hypothyroidism)
9) chronic stress
10) frequent anovulatory cycles (menstruation without ovulation)

For more on **thyroid function and weight gain**, see Chapter 9: Overcome a Sluggish Thyroid, pp. 202-219.

women's menopause is beginning to gain acceptance. But most men still remain unaware that they experience a predictable decline in hormone production at midlife, notes Julian Whitaker, M.D., a nationally recognized alternative medicine educator and editor of *Health and Healing*. As noted above, a man's testosterone levels naturally start to decrease around age 30, with a more rapid decline around age 60.

Dietary factors can influence a man's hormone levels as well. The typical Western diet with its high levels of dietary fat and low levels of fiber may have a direct influence on testosterone production, according to clinical studies.[9] Other foods that have been found detrimental to hormone balance include saturated fats (commonly found in fast foods, processed foods, and red meats), hydrogenated oils, preservatives, and products containing refined sugar.

The minerals zinc, copper, and selenium are necessary for normal hormone production in men. In one study, a group of patients was given 1.4 mg of zinc daily while a second group received 10.4 mg per day. While blood levels of zinc did not vary between groups, the low-zinc group had significantly lower levels of testosterone.[10] Selenium, in addition to being required for testosterone production, helps protect the male sex glands against free radicals and heavy metals.[11] If these minerals are lacking in the diet, hormone imbalances may occur.

Men's hormones may be thrown out of balance by environmental estrogens, foreign compounds and/or chemical toxins that mimic the effects of estrogen. Environmental estrogens, also called xenoestrogens, are present primarily in pesticides (such as DDT, PCBs, and dioxin) and industrial by-products. According to some researchers, environmental estrogens may contribute to testicular cancer, urinary tract disorders, and low sperm count. In men, a high level of estrogen slows down the production of testosterone.[12] Many prescription drugs can contribute to sexual dysfuncton in men as well. Exposure to lead, mercury, cadmium, and other heavy metals also inhibits testosterone production.[13]

Men's hormone levels can be adversely affected by certain lifestyle choices. Smoking, in particular, may be a factor in reduced production of testosterone. Animal studies have shown that nicotine and related substances in cigarettes increase the activity of enzymes that deactivate male hormones such as testosterone.[14] Excessive consumption of alcohol decreases levels of testosterone and increases estrogen levels in men. However, modest alcohol intake has not been shown to affect hormone levels.[15] In addition, physical or emotional stress can inhibit hormone production, particularly the adrenal hormone DHEA. Under conditions of chronic stress, the adrenal glands switch from producing DHEA to producing cortisol. Since DHEA is a precursor of the male hormones, less DHEA can severely limit testosterone production. A high level of cortisol also leads to blood sugar imbalances, depressed immune function, and the replacement of muscle with fat in the body.[16]

Are Your Hormones Imbalanced?

The first step in treating a hormonal imbalance is to get an accurate measurement of your hormone levels. Blood or 24-hour urine tests, which can be ordered by your physician, are the standard conventional method of determining hormone levels. However, saliva tests provide a noninvasive and simple alternative to a blood test that can also be used during the therapeutic process to determine your progress.

Aeron LifeCycles Saliva Test

If you want information about your hormone levels, you can test your saliva at home to find out where you stand. The test, called the Aeron LifeCycles Saliva Assay Report, can be ordered by both consumers and physicians and provides graphs of individual hormone levels. It can measure up to eight different hormones. Changing levels can be plotted over time on the same graph if supplementation or subsequent testing is done. Although hormones are present in saliva only in fractional amounts compared to the blood, "clinically relevant and highly accurate levels of hormones can be determined in saliva," says John Kells, president of Aeron LifeCycles in San Leandro, California. "Saliva testing provides a means to establish whether or not your hormone levels are within the expected normal range for your age."

For information on the **hormone saliva test**, contact: Aeron LifeCycles, 1933 Davis Street, Suite 310, San Leandro, CA 94577; tel: 510-729-0375 or 800-631-7900; fax: 510-729-0383. For the **Adrenal Stress Index**, contact: Diagnos-Tech, Inc., 6620 South 192nd Place, J-2204, Kent, WA 96032; tel: 800-878-3787 or 425-251-0596; fax: 425-251-0637.

The saliva assay has several advantages over traditional blood testing for hormones. It is painless and non-invasive, and tests can be performed simply at any time or place. As DHEA, cortisol, estrogen, progesterone, and testosterone levels are highest in the morning, it is far more convenient to be able to test them at home (and then immediately ship the saliva sample to Aeron's laboratory). As the test is less expensive than blood testing, you can do frequent testing to monitor changes (brought on by interventions such as diet, exercise, herbs, stress reduction, or acupuncture) and to adjust dosages of over-the-counter hormones, says Kells. In general, Kells explains that it is best to establish a baseline level of saliva hormones first, then after intervention (which can include hormone supplementation), test a second time to measure the changes.

Adrenal Stress Index

The Adrenal Stress Index (ASI) can pinpoint whether an imbalance in the adrenal glands might be contributing to hormonal imbalance and any subsequent weight gain. This test evaluates how well one's adrenal glands are functioning by tracking hormone levels over a 24-hour cycle (also known as the circadian rhythm). Four saliva samples taken at intervals throughout the day are used to reconstruct the daily adrenal rhythm in the laboratory. These samples are used to determine whether the three main stress hormones are being secreted in proper proportion to each other, and at the right times.

Success Story: Hormone Supplements Promote Weight Loss

While estrogen dominance can cause toxic effects that lead to weight gain, too little estrogen can cause similar problems. Phyllis Bronson, a Ph.D. candidate in biochemistry, and Harold Whitcomb, M.D., directors of the Aspen Clinic for Preventive and Environmental Medicine in Aspen, Colorado, relate the following case, which illustrates the powerful influence estrogen and other hormones have on mood and body weight:

Margaret, 50, weighed 189 pounds when she came to see us. At that age, she was nearing menopause and had irregular periods. She also suffered from chronic depression, for which she had been prescribed numerous antidepressants over the last ten years. Margaret had attempted unsuccessfully to lose weight numerous times; she had tried many of the popular diet programs, including Jenny Craig, Weight Watchers, and the Atkins Diet. Our blood tests revealed that Margaret was low in estrogen, progesterone, DHEA, and testosterone.

Margaret told us she was lethargic and too tired to exercise. She also experienced persistent sadness, cried frequently, continually gained weight, and retained water (a symptom associated with progesterone deficiency). Other symptoms associated with estrogen deficiency can include hot flashes, loss of sex drive, and mood swings. Her estrogen level was 54.3, whereas a woman her age should have a level between 90 and 130. Margaret's progesterone level was 0.2, but a normal reading for her was 25. Her testosterone was around 14; the acceptable reference range for women is 14 to 76, but for menopausal women we like to see it around 40 to 60. With a low level of 14, Margaret had no sex drive.

We also checked her DHEA level, which was 90. For a woman of this age to be optimally healthy, the DHEA count should be above 400 and preferably 500 to 600. Low DHEA levels such as Margaret's are often correlated with extreme exhaustion and flu-like symptoms (which she had) without apparent medical basis.

Using a procedure called electrodermal screening (SEE QUICK DEFINITION), we discovered that Margaret had many food allergies, specifically to grains such as wheat, rice, rye,

EDITOR'S NOTE

Phyllis Bronson is a nutritional biochemist and a Ph.D. candidate in biochemistry with 20 years of clinical experience in the nutrient effects of depression and anxiety. **Harold Whitcomb, M.D.**, is a board-certified internist with an emphasis in environmental and preventive medicine. They may be contacted at: Aspen Clinic for Preventive and Environmental Medicine at Internal Medicine Associates, 100 East Main Street, Aspen, CO 81611; tel: 970-920-2523 or 970-925-5440; fax: 970-920-2282.

For more on **food allergies**, see Chapter 11: Break Food Allergies and Addictions, pp. 244-270.

Electrodermal screening is a form of computerized information gathering, based on physics, not chemistry. A blunt, noninvasive electric probe is placed at specific points on the patient's hands, face, or feet, corresponding to acupuncture points at the beginning or end of energy meridians. Minute electrical discharges from these points serve as information signals about the condition of the body's organs and systems, useful for the physician in evaluation and developing a treatment plan.

Amino acids are the basic building blocks of the 40,000 different proteins in the body, including enzymes, hormones, and neurotransmitters. Eight amino acids cannot be made by the body and must be obtained through the diet; others are produced in the body but not always in sufficient amounts.

kamut, and spelt. A blood test showed that Margaret was deficient in histidine, an amino acid (SEE QUICK DEFINITION) associated with allergies; histidine deficiencies are often correlated with a hormonal imbalance. To address the food allergies and depression, we prescribed histidine (200 mg daily) and another amino acid, tyrosine (500 mg before meals), vitamin B5 (pantothenic acid; 500 mg with meals), and a supplement called Doctor's Brand 007, containing amino acids needed to produce serotonin, a key brain chemical involved in mood regulation.

We also gave Margaret a natural estrogen called E1,E2,E3 Tri-Estrogen (E123), which contains 100 mg of progesterone in cream form, and a transdermal DHEA gel. Margaret applied the E123 cream twice daily and the DHEA gel once daily, rubbing them into the skin at soft tissue sites such as the stomach and thighs; applying each in a different place and spacing the applications at least an hour apart.

A hair analysis for heavy metals revealed that Margaret had unacceptable levels of arsenic, lead, and cadmium. These created a toxic load, particularly on her nervous system, which contributed to her chronic depression. We gave her a product called OC Packs, a multinutrient package that would bind up ("chelate") the heavy metals and remove them from her system. She also started taking vitamin C buffered with calcium and magnesium (2,000 mg, four times daily). High doses of vitamin C, with calcium and magnesium, bind with toxic metals so that they can be safely excreted from the body. A hair analysis some months later confirmed that Margaret's heavy metal load was much lower.

After the first six weeks, Margaret's energy picked up, she started sleeping deeply, and woke feeling refreshed. She also had the energy

For information about **Doctor's Brand 007**, contact: Livingston Health Foods, Inc., 1324 South Sherman Street, Longmont, CO 80501; tel: 303-651-2522 or 800-672-4566; fax: 303-772-4566. For **E1,E2,E3 Tri-Estrogen** (by prescription only), contact: Women's International Pharmacy, 13925 Meeker Blvd., Suite 13, Sun City West, AZ 85375; tel: 602-214-7700 or 800-699-8143; fax: 602-214-7708. For **DHEA Transdermal Gel** (by prescription only), contact: College Pharmacy, 833 N. Tejone Street, Colorado Springs, CO, 80903; tel: 719-634-4861 or 800-888-9358; fax: 800-556-5893 or 719-634-4513. For **OC Packs**, contact: Advanced Medical Nutrition, Inc., 2247 National Avenue, P.O. Box 5012, Hayward, CA 94540; tel: 800-437-8888 or 510-783-6969; fax: 510-783-8196. For **Buffered Vitamin C**, contact: Allergy Research Group, 400 Preda Street, San Leandro, CA 94577; tel: 510-639-4572 or 800-545-9960; fax: 510-635-6730.

to start exercising. After a few weeks of treatment, Margaret's libido returned and, with it, the interest for a romantic relationship. Four months into the program, Margaret's progesterone level had climbed to 5.6. Her estrogen levels came up more slowly, which is often the case with natural estrogens. After eight months, Margaret had slimmed down to 140 pounds. After a year, her weight stabilized at 145-147 pounds.

Now, more than a year after beginning with us, Margaret's estrogen is at 95, progesterone at 8, DHEA at 350, and testosterone at 42. Margaret says she "feels great" and has plenty of energy. Her hormones have been rebalanced naturally. As you can see by Margaret's transformation, weight problems caused by a deficiency of estrogen and related amino acids can be improved dramatically by taking the proper supplements.

Alternative Medicine Therapies for Balancing Hormones

If your hormones are imbalanced, one of your priorities should be to detoxify your body systems of accumulated toxins. Both the liver and gastrointestinal system are involved in the normal processing of excess levels of hormones. When these organs are not functioning properly, your hormones may become imbalanced. Holistic practitioners generally recommend tending to these systems first in order to normalize the body's functions. Alternative medicine also offers a number of therapies to balance your hormones, including dietary and nutritional support, hormone replacement, herbal medicine, homeopathy, and exercise.

Therapies for Women
Rather than artificially manipulating your estrogen levels with synthetic hormones and ignoring the reasons behind the imbalance, it is more valuable to determine why you have the estrogen buildup or progesterone deficiency in the first place. Depending on the source of the excess estrogen, restoring hormonal balance can be more effectively achieved with dietary changes and nutritional supplements, natural progesterone cream, herbal therapy, and exercise.

For more on **cleansing the liver**, see Chapter 15: Cleanse the Liver, pp. 330-346. For more on **detoxifying the colon**, see Chapter 12: Detoxify the Colon, pp. 272-293.

Dietary Support—Eating soybeans and soybean-derived products, particularly fermented soybean foods such as tempeh and miso, can help counteract the negative effects of excess estrogen. These foods contain high levels of genistein, a substance that has a chemical structure similar to estrogen and can be used by the body as a mild estrogen surrogate. Substances like genistein are known as phytoestrogens, which are plant compounds that block estrogens from attaching to cell receptor sites, where estrogens exert their effect on the body. Phytoestrogens tend to balance estrogen in the body.[17]

Other than soy, foods that are high in phytoestrogens include flaxseeds, apples, whole grains, nuts, celery, and alfalfa.[18] Ellen Brown and Lynn Walker, Pharm.D., M.Ac., D.H.M., authors of *Menopause and Estrogen*, suggest the following foods to help balance estrogens: raw fruits, fresh fruit and vegetable juices (especially green juices), leafy green vegetables, garlic, figs, dates, cabbage, avocados, grapes, apples, beets, spirulina, chlorella, seaweed, wheat germ, and wheat germ oil.[19]

Supplementing with essential fatty acids (EFAs—SEE QUICK DEFINITION) can be an important for balancing your hormones. "Many women actually eat themselves into hormonal dysfunction," says clinical nutritionist Ann Louise Gittleman, M.S., C.N.S., of Bozeman, Montana. "They overindulge in carbohydrates, upsetting their copper/zinc ratio, and they don't get enough protein, which is also needed to support the adrenal glands.

Dietary Guidelines for Balancing Your Hormones

Women's health expert John R. Lee, M.D., of Sebastopol, California, who coined the term *estrogen dominance*, offers the following general dietary recommendations for maintaining balanced hormone levels:

■ Avoid refined sugars and processed foods; instead, eat whole organic foods, emphasizing fresh vegetables and fruit, whole grains, legumes, and nuts.

■ Consume modest amounts of meat (chicken, beef, or pork) two or three times per week at most; preferable sources of protein are eggs, yogurt, and coldwater ocean fish (4-5 servings per week).

■ Avoid hydrogenated oils (in margarine and processed foods); use primarily olive oil instead. Limit total dietary intake of fat to 20%-25%.

■ Eliminate colas and other sodas and reduce alcohol consumption; drink plenty of clean water daily.[20]

They deprive themselves of needed fats and end up lacking the building blocks of the essential sex-related hormones, which derive from fats." In the effort to cut down on fats, many women have stopped consuming the ones their bodies need.[21] Only one or two tablespoons per day of EFAs is often all it takes to restore balance to the hormones. EFAs, both omega-3s and omega-6s, can be a prime source of relief. Flaxseed oil (one tablespoon) and evening primrose oil (500 mg, twice daily) are excellent sources of EFAs.

Dr. John Lee also recommends taking the following antioxidant (SEE QUICK DEFINITION) vitamins to help cleanse the body of harmful pollutants and toxins that can lead to excessive estrogen: 1,000-2,000 mg of vitamin C daily; 400 IU of vitamin E daily; 500 mg of quercetin (a bioflavonoid) twice daily; 50 mg of B-complex vitamins daily; and 500-1,000 mg of magnesium (in the gluconate or citrate form).[22]

Natural Progesterone Therapy—To restore progesterone levels in the body, Dr. Lee recommends taking a progesterone supplement, which can help turn fat into energy and reduce water retention.[23] While progesterone supplements are available in sublingual (under-the-tongue) drops and capsules, using a progesterone skin cream or oil is best. Applying progesterone to the skin allows it to be absorbed into fat layers under the skin, where it can be taken up by the blood as needed. If taken in a capsule form, it is more difficult for the body to regulate the amount of progesterone entering the blood.

Natural progesterone can be manufactured in the laboratory from a substance called diosgenin, which is found in wild yams or soybeans. However, the body cannot manufacture progesterone from the raw diosgenin found in these foods. Dr. Lee therefore recommends using products that have been preconverted in the laboratory into progesterone, rather than try to obtain it from dietary sources. He advises consumers to check labels to make sure that a product lists the actual concentration of progesterone.

The recommended application of progesterone cream is between $1/8$ and $1/2$ teaspoon per day, or three to ten drops of the oil.

QUICK

DEFINITION

Essential fatty acids (EFAs) are unsaturated fats required in the diet. Omega-3 and omega-6 oils are the two principal types. The primary omega-3 oil is alpha-linolenic acid (ALA), found in flaxseed and canola oils, as well as pumpkins, walnuts, and soybeans. Fish oils, such as salmon, cod, and mackerel, contain the other important omega-3 oils, DHA (docosahexaenoic acid) and EPA (eicosapentaenoic acid). Linoleic acid is the main omega-6 oil and is found in most vegetable oils, including safflower, corn, peanut, and sesame. The most therapeutic form of omega-6 oil is gamma-linolenic acid (GLA), found in evening primrose, black currant, and borage oils. Once in the body, omega-3 and omega-6 are converted to prostaglandins, hormone-like substances that regulate many metabolic functions, particularly inflammatory processes.

An **antioxidant** is a natural biochemical substance that protects living cells against damage from harmful free radicals. Antioxidants work against the process of oxidation—the robbing of electrons from substances. Oxidation can lead to cellular aging, degeneration, arthritis, heart disease, cancer, and other illnesses. Antioxidants react with free radicals and neutralize them before they can damage the body. Antioxidant nutrients include vitamins A, C, and E, beta carotene, selenium, coenzyme Q10, pycnogenol (grape seed extract), L-glutathione, superoxide dismutase, and bioflavonoids. Plant antioxidants include Ginkgo biloba and garlic.

The Difference Between Progesterone and Progestins

Progestin, the primary ingredient in products such as Provera®, is the synthetic analogue of progesterone. Although progestin mimics some of the effects of natural progesterone, it does not convert into other beneficial hormones. Progestin can thus disrupt the hormonal balance essential for fat metabolism.[25] "Don't confuse natural progesterone with the synthetic variety," warns Lita Lee, Ph.D., a nutritionist from Eugene, Oregon. "They're quite different and the synthetic has severe side effects." Just a few of the many potential side effects of progestin include birth defects, epilepsy, and cardiac or kidney dysfunction.

Premenopausal women with average menstrual cycles (28 days) should apply the cream during days 12 to 26 of their cycle. Those with longer cycles should apply it from days 10 to 28. For menopausal women, Dr. Lee indicates that there can be more flexibility in applying the cream. He recommends using it over a 14-21 day period, and then discontinuing use until the following month. The cream can be applied to the palms of the hands, the face and neck, the upper chest and breasts, the insides of the arms, and behind the knees. Alternating applications among these sites will increase absorption.[24]

Various creams are available in health food stores and by mail order. When you purchase a product, there are two points to keep in mind. First, make sure it contains natural progesterone, not just wild yam (*Dioscorea villosa*). Don't be misled by claims that wild yam creams are the same as progesterone creams. As an herbal supplement, wild yam can have a mild hormone-balancing effect, but it does not provide natural progesterone. Second, make sure you use a brand of cream that contains enough natural progesterone to make a difference. Dr. Lee advises using only creams that have at least 400 mg of progesterone per ounce. Dr. Lita Lee prefers to use only creams or oils that have more than 1,000 mg of progesterone per ounce.

Herbal Therapy—Herbs that are helpful for hormone balancing include unicorn root (*Aletris farinosa*), an herb used in folk remedies for premenopausal women, and black cohosh (*Cimicifuga racemosa*). These herbs promote the normal production and conversion of the healthier forms of estrogen and contribute to the proper balance of estrogen and progesterone. Other herbs that may be helpful include *dong quai* (*Angelica sinensis*), licorice (*Glycyrrhiza glabra*), and Siberian ginseng (*Eleutherococcus senticosus*), which contribute to proper hormone regulation.[26]

Linda Ojeda, C.N.C., Ph.D., author of *Menopause Without Medicine*, generally suggests using certain herbs for their hormone-stimulating properties. Unlike synthetic hormone replacement therapy, the action of herbs is safe and gentle. Dr. Ojeda cites the following herbs as estrogen-stimulating: black cohosh, alfalfa, hops, sweetbriar, horsetail, buckwheat, sage, rose, and shepherd's purse. Among the herbs she recommends to support progesterone are: wild yam, chaste-tree berry (*Vitex agnus-castus*), sarsaparilla, and yarrow. The herbs can be taken as supplements or teas.[27]

Grape seed extract may be helpful for balancing your hormones. In one study, 165 women took a standardized extract of grape seed proanthocyanidin (a bioflavonoid or vitamin C helper) daily. After four months, they experienced a 78.8% improvement in symptoms associated with hormone imbalances—fluctuations in weight, water retention and swelling in the legs, breast pain, abdominal swelling, and pelvic pain. Researchers concluded that the bioflavonoids in grape seed block the synthesis of estrogen.[28]

Exercise—Regular exercise, in addition to having a direct bearing on weight, can alleviate the symptoms of menopause, according to recent research. In one study of postmenopausal women, 52-54 years old, those who were physically active (spending an average of 3½ hours per week exercising) had fewer and less severe hot flashes than the more sedentary women.[29] It is thought that exercise produces its beneficial effects by burning off the stores of estrogen in body fat and preventing a further buildup. Exercise is also helpful for alleviating stress, improving cardiovascular function, and increasing energy levels and mood.

Therapies for Men

Once you've determined that hormones are imbalanced, a number of alternative therapies are available to normalize them. Dietary adjustments can have a significant impact on your hormone levels, along with other therapeutic support such as nutritional supplements, hormone therapy, homeopathy, and herbs.

Dietary Recommendations—To help rebalance the hormones, the consumption of refined sugar products, saturated fats, and food preservatives must be reduced, according to Dr. Ross. He advises men to eat more fresh fruit and vegetables with a high nutrient content. Increase your intake of legumes (especially soy), dark-green leafy vegetables (for their protective antioxidant content), essential fatty

Boost Your DHEA

One of the key hormones supportive of a healthy body weight and vulnerable to stress is DHEA (dehydroepiandrosterone). DHEA, generally the most abundant hormone in the bloodstream, has been called the "mother of all hormones," because it is used as a building block for many other essential hormones. When the adrenal glands are chronically stressed, your production of DHEA can be greatly reduced.

A recent study at Temple University Medical School showed that DHEA effectively reduces the production of fat tissue and aids in the conversion of fat to muscle. Dr. Arthur Schwartz, one of the researchers, found that participants who were given DHEA showed a 31% decrease in body fat balanced by a gain of lean muscle mass.[30] DHEA can also have beneficial effects on libido. In men who have decreased testosterone production resulting in lowered libido, DHEA can boost libido almost as well as testosterone.

Since 1994, DHEA has been classified as a dietary supplement and requires no prescription. Nevertheless, it is best to consult a health professional when taking DHEA. C. Norman Shealy, M.D., Ph.D., of Springfield, Missouri, recommends blood testing to determine your exact DHEA dosage. A typical dosage is 25 mg daily, but since DHEA levels fluctuate significantly, it is important to accurately identify your optimum dose.

Some experts argue that, rather than taking DHEA directly, it's better to take the substance your body uses to make DHEA, namely pregnenolone. "I'm against taking DHEA for weight loss," says Lita Lee, Ph.D. "Supplied with the proper materials, the body can manufacture it's own supply of this hormone from pregnenolone." A typical dose is 50 mg of pregnenolone daily, taken in the morning.

Should You Take DHEA? A Saliva Test Will Tell You—

Depending upon a person's genetic makeup, a certain amount of DHEA from a supplement may be converted into the hormones testosterone and estradiol (a type of estrogen). You may experience unwanted side effects with supplementation as a result of the increased amounts of these hormones, including fatigue, insomnia, irritability, acne, oily skin, deepening of the voice, and an increase in body hair.

Using a saliva sample, the DHEA Challenge Test determines whether DHEA supplements will improve or worsen your health. The test works by measuring levels of the two hormones (testosterone and estradiol) in the saliva both before and after a five- to seven-day treatment with DHEA (15 mg daily for women, 25 mg for men). If your levels are too high following the "challenge," continuing to take DHEA supplements is probably not advisable.

For more information on the **DHEA Challenge Test**, contact: Diagnos-Tech, Inc., 6620 South 192nd Place, J-2204, Kent, WA 96032; tel: 800-878-3787 or 425-251-0596; fax: 425-251-0637.

CAUTION

Since DHEA can convert to estrogen and testosterone, it is best to proceed with caution. DHEA supplements are contraindicated in people with diabetes, especially women. DHEA can produce unwanted side effects, including acne, facial hair in women, breast enlargement in men, rapid heart rate, irritability and anxiety, headaches, and difficulty sleeping.

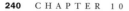

acids (flaxseed, evening primrose, and borage oils), and nuts and seeds (a good source of zinc).

During male menopause, low levels of testosterone may lead to a relative excess in estrogen; this female hormone can reduce the effects of testosterone in the body. Dr. Shippen emphasizes eating more soy, which contains phyto-estrogens that can block the action of estrogen in the body. He recommends eating plenty of cruciferous vegetables, such as cauliflower and broccoli, as these vegetables help rid the body of excess estrogen.[31] Maintaining an adequate level of dietary fiber is also important for clearing estrogen from the body.

Since environmental estrogens and other toxins are a factor in male hormonal imbalances, you should reduce or eliminate your exposure to these substances. One way is to select meats produced without the use of hormones or antibiotics, eat free-range chicken, and choose organic sources for your dairy products, fruits, and vegetables.

Testosterone Replacement Therapy—

According to Dr. Whitaker, easing male menopause requires its own hormone therapy, testosterone replacement. Studies have shown that testosterone replacement can heighten sex drive, increase bone density, and improve mood, among other effects. If you are considering testosterone replacement, the first step is a blood or saliva test to assess your levels of

Supplements for Male Hormone Support

Sandra Cabot, M.D., author of *Smart Medicine for Menopause*, offers a nutritional strategy that men can apply to start improving the functioning of their endocrine system. Here are Dr. Cabot's daily male menopause recommendations:

- Vitamin E: 500 IU
- Magnesium: 500 mg
- Zinc: 50 mg
- Selenium: 50 mcg
- Manganese: 5 mg
- Ginseng: 2,000-4,000 mg
- Royal Jelly: 2,000-4,000 mg
- Vitamin B complex: 1 tablet
- Evening primrose oil: 3,000 mg

These supplements, taken daily, are designed to help the male body cope with the natural decline of testosterone. Ginseng, for example, acts as a glandular tonic, helping to improve the function of the testes. Royal Jelly, rich in choline, indirectly helps improve sexual performance and response. Evening primrose oil supplies fatty acids that aid the production and release of hormones. Zinc can boost male virility and reduce prostate problems such as swelling. Vitamin E and magnesium strengthen the heart and circulation, including blood supply to the pelvic region.[32]

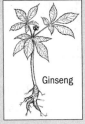

Ginseng

Michael Borkin, D.C., N.M.D.: 310 26th Street, Santa Monica, CA 90402; tel: 310-451-8599; fax: 818-248-5434. For **Libidex Creme** (available to health-care practioners only), contact: Market Resource International, 310 26th Street, Santa Monica, CA 90402; tel: 888-674-9556. For **ginseng supplements**, contact: Prince of Peace Enterprises, Inc., 3450 Third Street #3G, San Francisco, CA 94124; tel: 800-PEACE2U or 510-887-1899. Nature's Herbs, 600 East Quality Drive, American Fork, UT 84003; tel: 800-437-2257 or 801-763-0700. Futurebiotics, 145 Ricefield Lane, Hauppauge, NY 11788; tel: 800-FOR-LIFE or 516-273-6300.

the hormone, says Dr. Whitaker. If your levels are low or even average for your age, testosterone therapy can help alleviate andropause symptoms and improve overall health, he explains.

The goal of supplementation is to restore blood testosterone levels to those of a healthy 25- to 30-year-old man. For this, Dr. Whitaker recommends weekly injections of testosterone cypionate (100 mg) or biweekly injections of testosterone enanthate (200 mg). These long-acting versions of the hormone are considered the safest and most effective preparations for use in testosterone replacement, says Dr. Whitaker. As injection guarantees consistent absorption, he considers this to be the preferred method of testosterone supplementation. Skin patches and oral lozenges can also be effective, he reports. However, Dr. Whitaker advises against testosterone in pill form. "With oral testosterone, there is a potential for liver dysfunction and a decrease in protective HDL [high-density lipoprotein] or 'good' cholesterol levels," he cautions. In addition to the benefits of testosterone replacement cited above, according to Dr. Whitaker, positive effects include increased lean muscle mass and protection for the heart, as certain forms of testosterone can improve the ratio between "good" and "bad" cholesterol and lower cholesterol levels overall.[33]

Another option is a gel called Libidex Creme, which can be applied to the skin to stimulate testosterone production and support the endocrine system. Developed by Michael Borkin, D.C., N.M.D., of Santa Monica, California, Libidex contains DHEA, androstenedione (a testosterone precursor), alpha-lipoic acid, oat extract (*Avena sativa*), saw palmetto, colloidal silver, vitamins A, B12, and E, plus homeopathic support and ten flower remedies. The typical daily dosage is ⅛ to ½ teaspoon, depending on age, applied to areas of soft skin, preferably upon rising in the morning.

Herbal Medicine—As an accompaniment to andropause treatment, Dr. Whitaker generally suggests taking the herb saw palmetto (120-360 mg daily). This medicinal plant has been shown to reduce the conversion of testosterone into dihydrotestosterone, a stronger version of the hormone. Too much testosterone has been linked to various health problems, including prostate cancer.

The herb ginseng has an ancient history and has accumulated much folklore about its actions and uses. One variety, Oriental ginseng (*Panax ginseng*), has received a great deal of attention as a potential aid to virility and animal studies have shown that *Panax ginseng* does increase testosterone levels.[34] Ginseng should not be abused, however, as serious side effects can occur, including headaches, skin problems, and other reactions. For this reason, the proper dosage for the individual should be determined and respected.

Studies indicate that Chinese wolfberry (*Lycium chinense*) may be able to boost testosterone levels.[35] Oats (*Avena sativa*) have traditionally been used as an energy and nerve tonic and may be useful for stimulating male hormone levels. In Ayurveda, the traditional medicine practiced in India for thousands of years, the herb ashwagandha (*Withania somnifera*) is indicated for the treatment of impotence and infertility.

Gary S. Ross, M.D.: 500 Sutter Street #300, San Francisco, CA 94102; tel: 415-398-0555. For information on **complex homeopathic remedies**, contact: Heel/BHI, 11600 Cochiti Road SE, Albuquerque, NM 87123; tel: 800-621-7644; website: www.heelbhi.com.

Homeopathy—An important step in andropause treatment is to balance and correct any hormone deficiencies, says Dr. Ross. Here he finds certain complex homeopathic (SEE QUICK DEFINITION) remedies helpful, either alone or in conjunction with prescribed hormones. Among these are *Testis compositum*® (stimulates male sexual, brain, and adrenal function and reduces fatigue); *Coenzyme compositum*® (a multiple vitamin in homeopathic form, containing vitamin C and several B vitamins needed for metabolism); *Cerebrum compositum*® (enhances brain and nervous system function and memory, reduces anxiety and depression); and Galium-Heel® (for body detoxification and inflammation reduction). "Depending upon each individual's case, any or all of these homeopathic preparations can be used in the treatment plan," says Dr. Ross. Response time can vary from quickly to several months, he adds.[36]

DEFINITION

Homeopathy was founded in the early 1800s by German physician Samuel Hahnemann. Today, an estimated 500 million people worldwide receive homeopathic treatment; in Britain, homeopathy enjoys royal patronage. Homeopathy is now practiced according to two differing concepts. In classical homeopathy, only one single-component remedy is prescribed at a time, in a potency specifically adjusted to the patient; the physician waits to see the results before prescribing anything further. In complex homeopathy, typified by *Hepar compositum*, a prescription involves multiple substances given at the same time, usually in low potencies.

11

Break Food Allergies and Addictions

DO YOU FIND certain foods irresistible? Are you often a victim of uncontrollable bingeing? If so, you may be suffering from a food allergy. Although largely ignored by mainstream medical practitioners, food allergies and addictions affect millions of Americans, causing a variety of symptoms including weight gain. Alternative medicine offers testing procedures that can determine if you suffer from such an allergy and help you to finally break your addiction. For many, pinpointing hidden food allergies has been the key to finally realizing permanent weight loss and a healthier life.

Success Story: Rescued From Food Allergy Hell

For Claudia, 39, a simple meal always meant bloating, cramps, and intestinal misery shortly after eating. This had been her digestive reality for many years. So, too, were weight problems, chronic sinus and ear problems, muscle and joint pain, mood swings, and hyperactivity. One day, however, her condition dramatically worsened.

Claudia took some conventional cold medicine with orange juice and, soon after, she began to bleed from her rectum—a sign that the bleeding originated in her bowel. She rushed to her family doctor and came home with a prescription that only worsened the problem, known as ulcerative colitis. Claudia started having esophageal reflux, in which stomach acids leak upwards into the esophagus producing an intense sensation of heartburn. In addition to physical symptoms, she reported emotional disturbance, describing herself as irritable, argumentative, and overbearing, adding that, most of the time, she "didn't feel good inside."

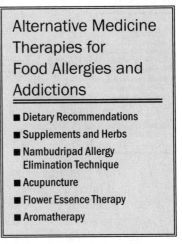

Alternative Medicine Therapies for Food Allergies and Addictions

- Dietary Recommendations
- Supplements and Herbs
- Nambudripad Allergy Elimination Technique
- Acupuncture
- Flower Essence Therapy
- Aromatherapy

Bouncing around among specialists, Claudia discovered that none was able to improve her condition or even ferret out its causes. She decided to conduct her own research into her problem and she learned that food allergies were probably involved. However, she was unable to accurately correlate allergic reactions with specific foods she ate, especially since her's were delayed food allergies. Claudia experimented with eliminating suspected allergic foods from her diet, but that hit-or-miss approach proved to be unsuccessful. Then she made a lifestyle choice which for many other people would have resulted in better health, but for Claudia was the last step in a disastrous food allergy cascade—she became a vegetarian. After three months on this new supposedly health-promoting diet, which was also dairy-free, Claudia had gained 12 pounds and was excessively bloated all the time; none of her other symptoms improved.

Wondering why the vegetarian diet proved such a disaster, Claudia consulted James Braly, M.D., of Fort Lauderdale, Florida, author of *Dr. Braly's Food Allergy and Nutrition Revolution.* "It's because, typically, such a diet is high in grains, such as wheat, rye, oats, and barley, that contain gluten, a highly allergenic protein now linked with at least 100 medical conditions," explains Dr. Braly. "Eggs, also commonly included in a vegetarian regimen, are ranked among the top five allergens found in the American diet." (The other top allergenic offenders are dairy milk, corn, citrus fruit, and chocolate.)

The only way to get to the core of Claudia's food allergy distress was to employ a precise laboratory test to pinpoint the foods that were producing the allergic symptoms. Dr. Braly used the Immuno 1

Bloodprint, a test for delayed food allergies based on monitoring levels of IgG antibodies (immune system proteins arrayed against food antigens) for any of 102 suspected allergenic foods. The presence of IgG antibodies means that the immune system is reacting to food proteins it judges as hostile. Dr. Braly ran the test on Claudia and found she had significant allergies to 17 foods. Claudia's allergenic foods included bananas, green, kidney, and yellow wax beans, chili peppers, clams, eggs, oysters, green peppers, pineapples, scallops, spinach, sugar cane, wheat, and yeast (baker's and brewer's).

To reach **James Braly, M.D.**, or for **Information on the Immuno 1 Bloodprint**, contact: Immuno Laboratories, 1620 West Oakland Blvd., Fort Lauderdale, FL 33311; tel: 800-231-9197 or 954-486-4500; fax: 954-739-6563.

Claudia also had an infestation of *Candida albicans*, a yeast-like fungus that often overgrows in the intestines as a result of a faulty diet, such as one high in sugar and yeasted foods. "*Candida* establishes a vexing biological loop," says Dr. Braly. "The yeast robs the person of simple sugars and carbohydrates, which it uses as food, and secretes toxins that poison the individual. These factors lead the person to crave more of the allergenic foods that support *Candida* growth."

Dr. Braly recommended that Claudia not eat any of her allergenic foods and that she avoid all foods and beverages containing yeasts, including buttermilk, cereals, cheeses, mushrooms, olives, wine, soy sauce, and pickles. He advised Claudia to rotate the foods that produced no allergies and to not consume the same foods or drinks two days in a row. "To prevent the development of new allergies and get over your current food allergies, rotate what you can eat and avoid what you cannot," he explains.

Claudia had excellent results from these dietary changes. Over the next few months, she lost 22 pounds without any restriction of calories, her bowel stopped bleeding, and her remaining symptoms cleared up. Not only did Claudia's physical symptoms resolve, but her state of mind improved as well—she no longer felt tense, hyperactive, and argumentative.

The Allergy Connection

Like Claudia, you may not suspect that weight problems or other health conditions could be related to food allergies. We tend to think of allergies in terms of pollens, dust, and animal hair—the things that make us sneeze or give us a rash. However, the truth is that we can be allergic to many different types of substances, including foods, and suffer a wide variety of symptoms. "The majority of Americans suffer from allergies," says Dr. Braly. "This is particularly true of food allergy, which, along with undernutrition, is the most commonly undiagnosed condition in the United States today." Dr. Braly believes that food allergies are the reason why so many Americans are overweight and why they fail to lose weight using methods that focus only on cutting calories. "Until you get rid of your food allergies," he says, "you will find it all but impossible to lose the weight you want to lose, and even harder to keep it off."

An allergy is the immune system's abnormal reaction to a substance that is harmless to most people. The immune system usually responds to only dangerous invaders, such as bacteria or viruses, and ignores "normal" substances such as foods. People develop allergies when the immune system has become weakened or compromised and can no longer distinguish between harmful and harmless substances. In response to these otherwise normal substances, the immune system releases chemicals, such as histamines, resulting in many of the symptoms associated with allergies (see "A Primer on Allergies," pp. 250-251). Allergies are a contributing factor in a number of health problems, including depression, hyperactivity and learning disabilities, gastrointestinal problems, diabetes, arthritis, and obesity.

Dr. Braly has identified 88 possible food allergy symptoms—in addition to weight gain, they include stomach pains, joint pain, insomnia, mood swings, and apathy. A food allergy specifically leads to weight gain in a number of ways. It can slow down your metabolism, the rate at which the body burns calories, or cause the body to produce too much insulin, the hormone that manages how the body processes sugar in the blood. Allergies may also cause food addictions and the related problems of food bingeing behavior, bloating, and cravings, all significant in weight gain.

Metabolism Slows

Metabolism is the biological process by which energy is extracted from food, or, put another way, how fast or slowly the body burns calories. Basal (or base) metabolism refers to the number of calories used by the body at complete rest to maintain basic functions such as breathing and circulation. Basal metabolism is controlled by the thyroid gland (SEE QUICK DEFINITION) and keeps the body at a normal temperature of 98.6° F. When the thyroid is dysfunctional or underactive—a condition called hypothyroidism—it sends out fewer hormones, causing basal metabolism to slow down and fewer calories to be burned off. Food allergies are one of the causes of hypothyroidism, as the overactivated immune system can damage the thyroid. Hypothyroidism causes a

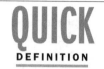

QUICK
DEFINITION

For more about **Insulin and hypoglycemia**, see Chapter 8: Strengthen Your Sugar Controls, pp. 184-201.

number of problems, including general feelings of sluggishness and increases in body weight.

Insulin Imbalance

High levels of the hormone insulin can lead to a condition called hypoglycemia (SEE QUICK DEFINITION), an illness that can cause significant weight gain. Insulin is the body's chief sugar (glucose) regulator and also controls appetite, affecting your choice of when and how much you eat. The physiological mechanism that regulates insulin can be thrown off balance by food allergies, as the immune system becomes stressed and overburdened by the constant response to allergenic foods. This causes too much insulin to enter the blood, precipitating a condition called insulin resistance, in which the body's cells no longer respond to insulin. As a result, insulin, unable to get glucose into the cells, converts more and more sugar into fat. High insulin levels lead to salt and water retention (making you feel bloated and adding pounds) and can also increase your appetite. Studies have shown a clear connection between chronic obesity and high insulin levels.

Food Addictions

Although overweight individuals are often accused of laziness or having no willpower, the truth is that, for some, the failure to control eating habits is due to a food addiction brought on by an allergy. Dr. Braly says that a food addiction is no small challenge to overcome. "The dieter is often asked to perform the Herculean feat of having every day just a little bit of the foods to which he is physiologically and psychologically addicted—the equivalent of insisting that the alcoholic take one small drink every day," says Dr. Braly.[1] Moreover, like alcoholics, most food addicts are not likely to recognize that they even have a problem.

With food allergies, the person often becomes addicted to a food that produces an allergic response. When the person stops eating an allergy-producing food to which their body is addicted, such as coffee or chocolate, they experience unpleasant withdrawal symptoms. Eating more of this addictive substance can alleviate the situation by suppressing these withdrawal symptoms. Similar to the withdrawal from other substance addictions, withdrawal from a food addiction only occurs when the person stops eating the food. Such reactions to food were first noted by Theron Randolph, M.D., a Chicago allergist and pioneer in environmental medicine. Dr. Randolph observed that the symptoms that a person normally experiences when eliminating a craved-for food from the diet can improve or be suppressed if the individual eats more of the food. Dr. Randolph called this phenomenon "masking," which is clearly illustrated in coffee addictions. Coffee addicts experience severe fatigue if they fail to have a cup of coffee every few hours. They therefore reach for a cup as soon as they begin to feel fatigued, thus remaining forever trapped in their addiction.

This becomes an unhealthy cycle of addiction, craving, and fulfillment that eventually leads to serious health problems, like obesity. "Persons addicted to certain foods are usually not aware of their dependency on them. If they even give the subject a thought, they usually attribute their preference to a natural food craving," says Stephen Langer, M.D., of Berkeley, California, author of *Solved: The Riddle of Weight Loss*.[2] At best, addicts may confess to liking or, as Dr. Langer indicates, craving a certain food, and some may even tell themselves they can give up any food at will. This is called the "food addict's fallacy."

Causes of Food Allergies and Addictions

While we inherit some allergies from our ancestors, our food choices, stress, and lack of exercise exert a larger influence on our susceptibility to allergies. Indeed, as the pace of our lives has increased and the quality of our food has declined, allergies have become increasingly commonplace. It is why Dr. Braly calls them "a side effect of modern life." Allergies are usually rooted in underlying problems and their onset is linked to a weakened immune system, leaky gut syndrome, and a repetitive diet.

Weakened Immune System—The immune system is the body's first line of defense against harmful substances. However, a weakened immune system has difficulty distinguishing the good from the bad, and thus reacts to some foods as if they were harmful invaders. Fuller Royal, M.D., of Las Vegas, Nevada, explains the failure of the immune function this way: "The immune system is no longer able to tell friend from foe. When that happens, it starts reacting to all sorts of things which are not foes, and these substances then become treated as aller-

A Primer on Allergies

An allergy is an adverse immune system reaction—sometimes mild, sometimes severe—to a substance that other people find harmless. Quite often, an allergen (a substance provoking an allergy symptom) is a protein that the body judges to be foreign and dangerous. The adverse reaction that follows is called an allergic response. Common manifestations of this allergic response include fatigue, headaches, sneezing, watery eyes, and stuffy sinuses following exposure to an allergen. Allergies fall into two categories, those caused by environmental factors and those caused by food. The most common source of environmental allergies is the pollen of plants, particularly trees, weeds, and grasses. The most common culprits in food allergies are yeast, wheat, corn, milk and other dairy products, egg whites, tomatoes, soy, shellfish, peanuts, chocolate, and food dyes and additives.

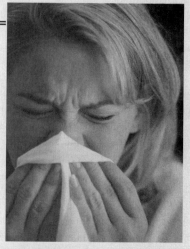

Common Symptoms of a Typical Allergic Reaction—Breathing congestion, inflamed, bloodshot, or scratchy eyes, watery eyes, tears, sneezing, coughing, itching, nosebleeds, puffy face, flushing of the cheeks, dark circles under the eyes, runny nose, swelling, hives, vomiting, stomachache, intestinal irritation or swelling.

The Cycle of Food Allergies—With food allergies, there is a strange paradox: often a person becomes addicted to a food that produces an allergic response. When a person stops eating an allergy-producing food to which their body is "addicted," such as coffee or chocolate, there is a three-day period in which they experience unpleasant withdrawal symptoms, such as fatigue; eating more of this addictive substance can suppress these withdrawal symptoms. Allergy experts call this suppression of symptoms "masking," because it masks or disguises the true allergic symptoms. This becomes an unhealthy cycle of addiction, food craving, and masking that eventually leads to serious health problems.

What Happens in an Allergic Response—The typical allergic reactions people have to foods, dust, pollen, and other substances are the body's way of fending off the intrusion of toxins that disrupt the body's equilibrium. Allergens enter the body through breathing, absorption through the skin, by eating or drinking foods, or by injection, such as insect bites or vaccinations. Because the body judges the substances to be dangerous to its health, the immune system identifies them as antigens. Antigens trigger an allergic inflammatory response. The mobilized immune system then releases specific forms of protein called antibodies to deactivate the allergenic antigens, setting in motion a complex series of events involving many biochemicals. These chemicals then produce the inflammation or other typical symptoms of an allergy response. The antibody most commonly involved in the allergic response to pollens and environmentals is IgE, one of five immunoglobulins, or specially designed antibody proteins, involved in the immune system's defense response to foreign substances. The main types of immunoglobulins, grouped according to their concentration in the blood, are: IgG (80%), IgA (10%-15%), IgM (5%-10%), IgD (less than 0.1%), and IgE (less than 0.01%). Mast cells, which produce the allergic response, next come into play; they tend to be concentrated in the skin, nose, and lung linings, gastrointestinal tract, and reproductive organs. When the IgE antibody senses an allergen, it triggers the mast cells to release histamine and other chemicals and the allergic response flares into action. The IgE molecules also attach themselves, like a key fitting a lock, to the allergens.

Immediate vs. Delayed Allergic Reactions—The most common allergic reactions occur immediately after exposure to a certain substance (peanuts, pollen, bee stings, or cats). These reactions are typically caused by IgE immunoglobulins, resulting in a runny nose, watery eyes, itching, and skin rashes; more severe reactions include constriction of the bronchial tubes and difficulty breathing. Delayed allergies are another type of allergic reaction, which can manifest symptoms up to 72 hours after exposure to a triggering substance. These can commonly appear as seemingly unrelated illnesses such as lethargy, attention deficit disorder, fatigue, hyperactivity, acne, itchy skin, mood swings, insomnia, and inflammation. Many of these reactions are caused by IgG immunoglobulins. Up to 100 different medical conditions—from arthritis, asthma, and autism to insomnia, psoriasis, and diabetes—have been clinically associated with IgG food allergy reactions. Many patients display little or no immediate sensitivity reactions (produced by IgE), but instead show moderate to severe delayed reactions (produced by IgG).

gens."[3] Allergies can precipitate the body into a downward spiral of illness, because histamine, a substance produced by the immune system during an allergic reaction, is an immune suppressant, which only worsens the situation.

Heredity may be a factor in immune system dysfunction. Charles Gableman, M.D., a practitioner of environmental medicine in Encinitas, California, explains that allergies also occur "when the immune system becomes stressed due to an overload of toxins." Among the toxic factors are environmental pollution, repeated vaccinations and immunizations, and the destruction of "friendly bacteria" in the intestines due to frequent use of antibiotics or steroids.

Leaky Gut Syndrome—Related to the problem of a weak immune system is a condition known as leaky gut syndrome. As its name indicates, this illness occurs in the intestines, where most of the digestion and absorption of nutrients occurs. In leaky gut, the lining of the intestines breaks down, creating tiny fissures that allow partially digested food particles to seep out of the intestines and into the bloodstream. Dr. Braly explains that the immune system reacts to the particles of partially digested foodstuffs that leak through the gut as if they were foreign material.

Nutritionist Inez d'Arcy-Francis, Ph.D., who practices in Kentfield, California, says that a food addiction is actually a process founded on malabsorption of nutrients. As she sees it, there are three phases to this addictive process. The initial factor precipitating the addiction is the trauma to the body of undigested food particles. It's a trauma, says Dr. d'Arcy-Francis, because the body does not know what to do with these food particles once they have inappropriately entered the bloodstream.

The second stage in the addictive process is adaptation. This is the strange situation in which the body actually craves foods that it cannot digest; these foods—typically, dairy, wheat, eggs, chocolate, sugar, alcohol—must be consumed in increasing amounts so the body can avoid the pain of withdrawal. The third stage is degeneration, in which a serious illness emerges, such as diabetes, alcoholism, obesity, or Crohn's disease, among others.

One of the leading causes of a leaky gut syndrome is a harmful overgrowth of the yeast-like fungus *Candida albicans*, a microbe found in the intestines and other parts of the body. According to Dr. Braly, *Candida* microbes cause leaky gut by burrowing beneath the intestinal lining, literally eating away at the walls of the intestine. In addition to *Candida* overgrowth, other causes of leaky gut syndrome include alcohol consumption; vitamin, mineral, amino acid and/or essential fatty acid deficiencies; excessive stress; premature birth; and radiation.

For more on *Candida*, see Chapter 13: Eliminate Yeast Infections, pp. 294-309.

Repetitive Diet—Food allergies are also caused by a repetitive and monotonous diet. Dr. Randolph has observed that the diets of allergy patients normally consist of 30 foods or less, which they eat repeatedly. These 30 foods all have the potential of causing an allergy. "If someone eats bread every day, he could easily develop a wheat allergy due to the immune system's continuous exposure to it," says Marshall Mandell, M.D., medical director of the New England Foundation for Allergies and Environmental Diseases. "The likelihood of having an allergic reaction to any given food is directly proportional to how often a person eats it," Dr. Gableman explains. "This is not true in all cases, but as a rule the foods that we eat the most as a culture tend to be the ones we are most allergic to."

Success Story: Overcoming a Carbohydrate Addiction

William, 42, was 5'11" and weighed 253 pounds. He was constantly hungry even though he was overeating. Unable to control his appetite, he sought advice from clinical nutritionist Linda Lizotte, R.D., C.D.N., based in Trumbull, Connecticut. William also complained that he was tired all the time, had intermittent chest pains, and suffered from indigestion and high blood pressure.

How can someone be eating all the time and still be hungry? The problem, says Lizotte, was that William was a carbohydrate addict. "When we eat carbohydrates, we should produce serotonin [a neurotransmitter], which makes us feel satisfied," explains Lizotte. "But some people, in response to carbohydrates, do not make enough serotonin and, on top of this, their insulin production is higher than normal, which compounds into not feeling satisfied and feeling very hungry soon after eating." This chemical imbalance sets up a carbohydrate addiction: the more carbohydrates they eat, the more they crave them. Lizotte estimates that about 10% of overweight people are carbohydrate addicts. William, who had been eating high amounts of carbohydrates for years, was putting on about 20 pounds per year because of his addiction.

To control William's cravings, Lizotte recommended that he eat only proteins, vegetables, and a little fat (healthy fats like flaxseed or olive oils)

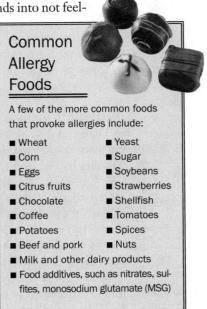

Common Allergy Foods

A few of the more common foods that provoke allergies include:

- Wheat
- Corn
- Eggs
- Citrus fruits
- Chocolate
- Coffee
- Potatoes
- Beef and pork
- Yeast
- Sugar
- Soybeans
- Strawberries
- Shellfish
- Tomatoes
- Spices
- Nuts
- Milk and other dairy products
- Food additives, such as nitrates, sulfites, monosodium glutamate (MSG)

for breakfast and lunch, and avoid carbohydrates, such as bread and rice, until dinner. Breakfast could include proteins like eggs, chicken, or ham. For lunch, William could eat vegetables like green beans or broccoli, salad with chicken or shrimp, or a hamburger without the bun. For dinner, William could eat just about anything. "By dinner, he was really missing his carbohydrates. Plus he's Italian and wanted his pasta," said Lizotte. "So, if he wanted pasta with tomato sauce and meatballs for dinner followed by a piece of fruit for dessert, that was fine." Any of the carbohydrates that couldn't be eaten during the day—potatoes, rice, pasta—could be included in dinner.

There are two reasons for limiting carbohydrates to only the evening meal. First, it keeps insulin production down to once per day, which reduces food cravings. Second, it can lead to a greater loss of excess fat. "When insulin is in the system, it tells the body not to use stored fat as a fuel source, but rather to burn the sugar that just came in through the meal," says Lizotte. "If insulin is not being produced during the day, the body will burn stored fat as fuel, leading to much greater fat loss."

She also suggested a supplement program for William as nutritional support and to help burn fat. Amino Acid Stabilizers is a combination formula of all 22 amino acids (protein building blocks) used by the body. This formula provides extra protein and decreases appetite by preventing blood sugar levels from dropping between meals; recommended dose was three capsules at mid-morning and at mid-afternoon. Lizotte also recommended Mitroplex, an energy-boosting and fat-burning supplement containing carnitine, coenzyme Q10, and lipoic acid (two capsules daily).

After one week, William lost eight pounds. Lizotte then recommended that William take zinc (zinc picolinate, 50 mg daily). "Zinc helps insulin work more effectively and efficiently," says Lizotte. "Studies have shown that zinc deficiency can decrease the body's response to insulin." William's doctor had determined that his chest pains were due to heartburn, so Lizotte recommended Pancreatin, a pancreatic enzyme formula to help his digestion. After two months, William had lost 21 pounds, his heartburn had disappeared, and his blood pressure was almost normal. William was amazed at how much his energy levels had increased. Also, he could easily make it from meal to meal without being hungry. He had won the appetite battle.

To reach **Linda Lizotte, R.D., C.D.N.**, and for information on **Amino Acid Stabilizers, Mitroplex, zinc picolinate**, and **Pancreatin**, contact: Designs for Health, 211 Pondway Lane, Trumbull, CT 06611; tel: 203-371-4383; fax: 530-618-6730.

Diagnosing a Food Allergy

"Accurate diagnosis of food allergies has always been the bane of allergy treatment," says Dr. Braly. The problem with diagnosing a food allergy is that reactions are often varied, inconsistent, and may take several days to develop after eating an allergy-causing food. How much or how often you eat an allergenic food or how it is cooked may be factors in whether or not you have a reaction. Or the allergy may be caused by an additive or ingredient rather than the food itself.[4] In addition, more than one food is frequently involved in causing the reaction, and, as explained earlier, symptoms are often "masked" by regular consumption of the foods.

Despite the complexity surrounding the detection of a food allergy, mainstream medical practitioners generally take a highly simplified approach to the problem. Most rely on a procedure called the scratch or prick-puncture test, a procedure which is only about 20% accurate in detecting food allergies.[5] In truth, this test is only useful for identifying allergens that cause immediate reactions, such as those caused by pollen or dust, and is not effective in pinpointing food reactions. Another common test procedure is the RAST (Radio Allergo Sorbent Test). This blood test is useful for diagnosing allergies to pollens, dust, molds, bee venom, and other allergens. Again, this test is not very accurate in testing food allergies and can be very expensive. Most alternative medicine practitioners rarely use these tests. Instead, they recommend self-testing and laboratory procedures, such as the elimination diet, pulse test, and ELISA test, designed specifically to assess food allergies.

Do You Suffer From Food Allergies?

The following questionnaire, developed by naturopath Leon Chaitow, N.D., D.O., of London, England, can help you determine if you have a food allergy. If your answer is "no" or "never" to any question, give yourself a score of zero for that particular question; the other scores are provided with each question.

■ Do you suffer from unnatural fatigue? (Score 1 if occasionally, 2 if regularly—three times a week or more.)

■ Do you sometimes experience weight fluctuations of four or more pounds in a single day, accompanied by puffiness of the face, ankles, or fingers? (Score 1 if infrequently, 2 if frequently—more than once a month.)

■ Do you have hot flashes (apart from menopause) or find yourself sweating for no obvious reason? (Score 1 if infrequently, 2 if several times a week or more.)

A Food Allergy Timetable

Michael Lessner, M.D. of Berkeley, California, has created a timetable that can be used to determine the foods or liquids you may be allergic to.[6] When experiencing the symptoms below, notice if they began within the given time after eating a particular food. If so, they may be due to food allergies.

Symptom	Elapsed Time
Indigestion or heartburn	30 minutes
Headache	Within 1 hour
Asthma, runny nose	Within 1 hour
Stomach bloat/diarrhea	3 to 4 hours
Rashes or hives	6 to 12 hours
Weight gain by fluid retention	12 to 15 hours
Fits, convulsions, mental disturbance	12 to 24 hours
Mouth ulcers, joint/muscle pain, backache	48 to 96 hours

■ Does your pulse race or your heart pound strongly for no obvious reason? (Score 1 if infrequently, 2 if several times a week or more.)

■ Do you have a history of food intolerance, causing any symptoms at all? (Score 2 if your answer is yes.)

■ Do you crave bread, sugary foods, milk, chocolate, coffee, or tea? (Score 2 if your answer is yes.)

■ Do you suffer from migraine or severe headaches, irritable bowel syndrome, eczema, depression, asthma, or muscle aches? (Score 2 if your answer is yes.)

The most anyone could score on this test would be 14, explains Dr. Chaitow. "If your score is five or higher, there is a strong likelihood that allergies are part of your symptom picture."

The Elimination Diet

Despite the name, this is not really a diet in the conventional sense, but a test procedure to help you identify your allergy foods. It involves three steps: 1) eliminating the potential allergic foods from your diet for ten to 14 days; 2) carefully observing any changes in your symptoms; and 3) testing the eliminated foods by bringing them back into your diet, one by one, and noting any return of symptoms.

The foods you choose to eliminate should be from those that you eat every day or nearly every day, ones that you crave, or foods that make you feel weak. It is important to eliminate all of the suspected foods on your list, as multiple allergies are quite common and, if all are not eliminated, it could skew your testing results. Also, read the ingredients on any packaged foods very carefully to ensure you do not inadvertently consume whatever it is you are trying to eliminate (sugar, for example, or perhaps a flavor enhancer such as monosodium glutamate). Remember that delayed food allergies can take as long as 72 hours to exhibit symptoms. If you experience symptoms such as irritability, fatigue, headaches, and intense cravings during the elimination period, you may be going through withdrawal, which is a sure sign that you have been suffering from an allergy.

The Pulse Test

This is a relatively simple test developed by Arthur Coca, M.D., a pioneer in the field of environmental medicine. Dr. Coca based his test on many years of clinical observations of patients, during which he noticed that a common symptom of many food allergies is increased heart rate. Although the pulse test can help identify food allergies, you should not conclude you are allergy-free if the foods you test do not affect your pulse rate. The problem is that not all food allergens will increase heart rate. "The weakness of this particular approach lies in the frank possibility that not every allergic reaction will necessarily produce the biochemical responses that result in a faster heartbeat," says Ralph Golan, M.D., a holistic physician from Seattle,

How to Take the Pulse Test

The pulse test is easy to self-administer and involves simply recording your pulse rate before and after meals. Dr. Langer observes that "certain of my patients who use the pulse test have seen their heartbeat rise from 72 to as high as 180 after they have eaten an allergenic food."[7] To take the test, follow these simple instructions:

- Find the pulse point on your wrist by placing the second finger of the opposite hand on the inside of your wrist.
- Count the beats (pulses) for six seconds and multiply the number by ten; this is your resting pulse.
- Record your resting pulse first thing in the morning before getting out of bed.
- Record your pulse 30 minutes before each meal, then 30 minutes and 60 minutes after each meal.

If the difference between the morning pulse and either of the two after-meal rates is more than 12 to 16 beats, chances are you have a food allergy. Once you have identified a meal that triggers a rise in your pulse rate, you can begin testing individual foods eaten during that meal. However, in some cases, you may find that your resting pulse is higher than your after-meal pulse or that your before-meal pulse is higher than your after-meal pulse. If you observe such a pattern, it is possible that dust or some other airborne allergen is interfering with your test.[8]

For **ELISA tests**, contact: Immuno Laboratories, 1620 West Oakland Blvd., Fort Lauderdale, FL 33311; tel: 800-231-9197 or 954-486-4500; fax: 954-739-6563. Meridian Valley Clinical Laboratory, 24030 132nd Avenue, S.E., Kent, WA 98042; tel: 800-234-6825 or 206-631-8922. MetaMetrix Clinical Laboratory, 5000 Peachtree Industrial Blvd., Suite #110, Norcross, GA 30071; tel: 800-221-4640 or 770-446-5483; fax: 770-441-2237.

Washington, and author of *Optimal Wellness*.[9] If you have no success in identifying a food allergen using the pulse test, but still suspect that you are suffering from such an allergy, you should try one of the other tests.

The ELISA Test

The ELISA (or enzyme-linked immunoserological assay) test is a blood test considered by many alternative medicine practitioners to be among the most sensitive and useful in detecting food allergies. Unlike other allergy blood tests, it is able to pinpoint delayed allergic reactions. It also tests for a wide variety of substances, subjecting a patient's blood sample to 102 different food extracts. Blood samples can be sent by mail to any one of several specialized laboratories that perform this test. You can have your doctor arrange to submit a sample of your blood to the lab.

Success Story: Losing 71 Pounds by Treating Food Addictions

Zoë, 53, was 5'4" and weighed 310 pounds when she first consulted Dr. d'Arcy-Francis. She had a dangerous condition called "morbid obesity" and had suffered from alcohol addiction for years. "This woman was a walking time bomb on account of her weight," comments Dr. d'Arcy-Francis. "As a result of her body's inability to break down foods, her fat cells had become 'storage bins' for unutilized nutrients and she was suffering malnourishment as a result."

In the course of her medical history, Zoë had had her gallbladder removed, suffered physical disabilities as a result of excess weight, endured chronic depression, and currently had irregular and painful menstruation, tender breasts, hot flashes, and alternating constipation and diarrhea. Many of these conditions are directly traceable to inefficient digestion, says Dr. d'Arcy-Francis. Zoë was also a compulsive overeater, subject to strong food cravings. "I was always hungry," Zoë says. "The amount of fear I ate away with chocolate cake is overwhelming. The eating was killing me."

"The goal is for clients to master the keys to their own optimal biochemical and physiological balance," says Dr. d'Arcy-Francis. "I try to find the key to nourishing the body so that if there is still any physiological memory of healthy function, the body kicks in again." One way to rekindle the body's memory of correct functioning is precise nutritional supplementation.

The nutritional program for Zoë began with unsweetened fruit juice diluted with water as a carbohydrate source (up to 24 oz daily) with Designer Protein (predigested whey protein; 4 tbsp). She also took Vegetable Glycerin, a liquid nonsugar sweetener that provides the energy of fat at only 80 calories per tablespoon (4 tsp daily). In addition, Zoë took two teaspoons daily of dolomite powder for easily absorbed calcium and magnesium (for her muscle aches and painful periods), and 1-2 teaspoons (4-8 g) of vitamin C ascorbate, buffered to reduce intestinal upset. For thyroid support, Zoë took ten drops daily of dulce, a sea vegetable high in iodine, a nutrient essential to thyroid function.

Zoë started taking Mega III, a full-spectrum multivitamin/mineral (initially one tablet daily, building to three). She took vitamin B6 (250 mg daily) to support protein digestion and Vitex (three capsules daily), which contains plant-based hormones and cofactors required for hormone secretion, to help stabilize her menstrual cycle. She took the essential fatty acid gamma-linolenic acid (GLA; 180 mg, three times daily) as a nutritional aid. GLA helps to stabilize menstruation and moods and nourish the skeletal system, explains Dr. d'Arcy-Francis.

Hydrochloric acid capsules (one with each meal) were prescribed to facilitate better breakdown of nutrients in the stomach, where the first stage of digestion occurs. When this stage fails, the addictive process begins, says Dr. d'Arcy-Francis. If the stomach's acid level is not sufficient, then proteins are not properly broken down in the stomach and ferment. These fermentation products act as "food" for unwanted bacteria, yeasts, and other parasites in the small intestine. From here, large particles of undigested food are able to get through the intestinal wall, which should act as a barrier against them, and enter the bloodstream. "Undigested food molecules are toxins once they're in the blood and cause chaos in the body," explains Dr. d'Arcy-Francis. The liver gets overwhelmed, the immune system becomes overactive and confused, and chronic allergic reactions are set in motion.

Dr. d'Arcy-Francis gave Zoë Super-Enzyme Digestive Caps (containing the essential digestive enzymes; two capsules with each meal) to support the digestive process at the intestinal stage and the amino acid L-glutamine (1,000 mg, five times daily) to help regulate her blood sugar and reduce her food cravings. It was largely these

"Undigested food molecules are toxins once they're in the blood and cause chaos in the body," explains Dr. Inez d'Arcy-Francis. The liver gets overwhelmed, the immune system becomes overactive and confused, and chronic allergic reactions are set in motion.

blood sugar irregularities that led to her food cravings, explains Dr. d'Arcy-Francis. When the body is unable to digest a substance, such as wheat or dairy, this causes trauma to the body. "The trauma itself causes the blood sugar to drop and produce a food craving. This is a physiological reaction by the body trying to protect itself from this toxic substance."

Finally, Zoë radically simplified her diet, eliminating sugar, grains, caffeine, dairy products, processed foods, breads, and flours. Instead, she ate at least 24 ounces of cooked root vegetables every day (especially yams, parsnips, and turnips) and the same amount of other cooked vegetables (raw foods are harder to digest), plus three pieces of fruit, 6-8 ounces of protein, and herbal teas.

The results of this nutritional strategy, after ten months, were impressive. Zoë lost 71 pounds; she was no longer depressed and her food cravings were gone; her periods had become regular, her hot flashes stopped, and her breasts were no longer tender; her constipation and diarrhea disappeared; and she no longer had pains throughout her body. Alcohol and other drugs had no appeal whatsoever. "She is amazed," says Dr. d'Arcy-Francis, "that chocolate, coffee, and cigarettes no longer interest her at all."

Alternative Medicine Therapies for Food Allergies

The first step in treating a food allergy is to remove problem foods from your diet. In addition, a number of nutrients and herbs are helpful for treating allergies and supporting the digestive system. Finally, a unique alternative medicine therapy based on acupressure, called the

Inez d'Arcy-Francis, Ph.D.: P.O. Box 386, Kentfield, CA 94914; tel: 415-924-2079; fax: 415-927-1873. For more about **Designer Protein Powder**, contact: Next Nutrition, P.O. Box 2469, Carlsbad, CA 92018; tel: 619-431-8152 or 800-468-6398; fax: 619-431-9969. For **Vegetable Glycerin**, contact: Now, 550 Mitchell Road, Glendale Heights, IL 60139; tel: 630-894-2553 or 800-469-5552; fax: 630-894-0206. For **Dolomite Powder**, contact: KAL Supplements, 6415 De Soto Avenue, Woodland Hills, CA 91365; tel: 800-755-4525 or 801-626-4900; fax: 800-767-8514. For **Mega-III** and **Super-Enzyme Digestive Caps**, contact: Twin Labs, 2120 Smithtown Avenue, Ron Kon Kuma, NY 11779; tel: 800-645-5626 or 516-467-3140; fax: 516-467-3080.

Nambudripad Allergy Elimination Technique, can help reprogram your allergic reactivity.

Dietary Changes

Once you have identified the foods you are allergic to, the next step is to eliminate them from your diet. Initially, you should completely refrain from eating all allergenic foods for 60 to 90 days. After this period, you can begin to slowly reintroduce them into your diet. You should also vary the foods that you eat on a daily basis to avoid developing new allergies. You are likely to find that as you reintroduce the foods to which you were once sensitive, your old symptoms will not reappear. This is because most food allergies are temporary and can be cured through abstinence. Dr. Braly estimates that only about 5% of delayed food allergies are permanent.

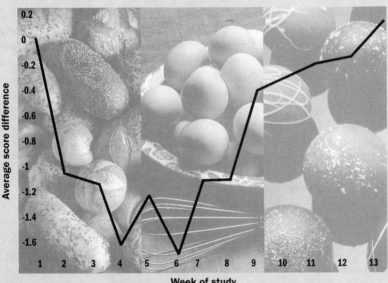

Week of study

HOW TO STOP YOUR FOOD ALLERGIES FAST—The graph shows the rapid decline in reactions to suspected allergenic foods when patients completely avoided them for about two months, in a study sponsored by Immuno Laboratories. Maximum freedom from food allergy–related symptoms was achieved between the third and sixth weeks. Among foods most commonly identified as allergenic are wheat, eggs, and chocolate (pictured above), as well as milk and corn.

Remember that eliminating an allergenic food can cause withdrawal reactions. "The majority of people who give up foods they're allergic to go through a mild to moderate withdrawal phase, lasting one to five days, while the body detoxifies itself," says Dr. Braly. Allergic symptoms may get worse during this period and cravings can be intense. If the allergy foods were also your comfort foods, you may experience emotional feelings of loss and distress. Dr. Braly explains that "once the withdrawal phase has passed, the cravings also abate, and the allergy sufferer is free of dependence on that food, free of both the physiological and psychological desire to consume it so frequently, and in such great quantities."[10]

Many individuals have discovered that identifying and treating their food allergies was the key to solving their weight problems. However, it is important to understand that the desire to lose weight is rarely the source of the kind of driving desire needed to beat a food addiction and break a food allergy. To overcome an allergy, people often need to completely overhaul their eating patterns. "I don't think that just wanting to be thin will give anyone the motivation they need to completely change how they shop, cook, and eat," says Dr. Braly. "Depending on how many foods a person is sensitive to, the process can be a very demanding, very daunting task. It often means saying no to popular foods, party foods, or the foods we grew up eating. It takes discipline and effort." Because the task is so difficult and yet so important for health, Dr. Braly suggests that food allergy sufferers focus on embracing health rather than just losing weight. In effect, what is necessary is a total commitment to healthy living. This commitment, combined with the know-how for making the changes needed to bring the body back into balance, is the way to get in the right shape.

Supplements and Herbs

A combination of quercetin and bromelain is one of the most effective supplements available to combat a food allergy. Quercetin is a bioflavonoid derived from plants, such as blueberries, cranberries, cherries, onions, or tomatoes. It enhances the body's ability to use vitamin C, increasing its absorption by the liver, kidneys, and adrenal glands. Bromelain, a digestive enzyme derived from pineapple, enhances the absorption of quercetin. Taken together, quercetin and bromelain strengthen the membranes of the body's cells so that they are less likely to be damaged in the presence of an allergen. This, in turn, lessens the effect and reduces the symptoms of an allergy. "Patients using quercetin/bromelain find that, within a period of one to two months, their allergy problems significantly diminish," says Dr. Braly. "Formerly allergic foods can often be reintroduced without the usual symptoms." The typical recommended dosage is 250 mg of quercetin and 125 mg of bromelain, taken three times daily, 20 minutes before each meal.

Herbs can also help to counteract the effects of an allergy. Curcumin, an extract from the spice plant turmeric, decreases the symptoms of an allergic reaction; typically take one capsule, three times daily. Another allergy-relieving herb is cayenne (*Capsicum annuum*) or red pepper. This herb is a systemic stimulant, meaning it invigorates the function of the whole body, and is especially helpful for digestive function.

You can reduce the reaction of the digestive system to offending foods by using the appropriate plant enzyme supplements: protease digests protein, lipase digests fats, amylase digests carbohydrates, lactase digests dairy products, and disaccharidases digest sugars. Supplementing with betaine hydrochloric acid, the dietary form of the primary acid in the stomach, may also help digestive function. As digestion improves, the allergic reactions should be minimized or eliminated. Other nutrients useful for supporting overall digestion include the amino acid glutamine, vitamin E, chlorophyll, and aloe vera. Herbs for digestive support include slippery elm, marshmallow root, comfrey, and pau d'arco.

Since imbalances of intestinal flora are common among allergy sufferers, Dr. Chaitow stresses the need to restore bowel flora balance with a daily program of probiotics, the beneficial bacteria that inhabit the intestines under healthy conditions. *Lactobacillus acidophilus*, *L. bulgaricus*, and *Bifidobacteria* are the key players in this process, according to Dr. Chaitow. Probiotic supplements are available at most health food stores.

For **quercetin/bromelain supplements**, contact: Doctor's Best, 1120 Calle Cordiller, San Clemente, CA 92673; tel: 800-333-6977 or 714-498-3628; fax: 714-498-3952. For **curcumin** (available only to health-care professionals), contact: Metagenics, Inc., 971 Calle Negocio, San Clemente, CA 92673; tel: 800-692-9400; fax: 714-366-0818. For **cayenne**, contact: Arise & Shine, P.O. Box 1439, Mount Shasta, CA 96067; tel: 800-688-2444 or 530-926-0891.

For more on **supplements**, see Chapter 3: Supplements for Weight Loss, pp. 76-97.

Nambudripad Allergy Elimination Technique

The Nambudripad Allergy Elimination Technique (NAET) is a unique alternative therapy that relies on altering energy flow through the body to treat allergic symptoms. The technique's creator, Devi S. Nambudripad, D.C., O.M.D., Ph.D., uses the energy pathways, also called acupuncture meridians (SEE QUICK DEFINITION), to diagnose an allergy and reprogram how the body reacts to different substances. According to Dr. Nambudripad, when our bodies interpret a particular substance as potentially harmful, energy pathways freeze in defense

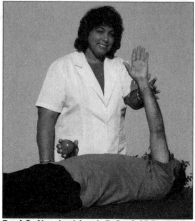

Devi S. Nambudripad, D.C., O.M.D., Ph.D.

against the substance. "Allergens cause a reaction in the central nervous system," she explains, "and messages travel from the brain, through the spinal column, to every cell in the body." These blocked energy channels are what produces the allergy.

Dr. Nambudripad uses acupressure and acupuncture to diagnose and restore the energy flow in an allergic body. She applies these techniques while patients hold the allergic substance (in a vial) in their hand. The effect is to reorganize the body's way of reacting to a substance. As the energy pathways are reopened, the body does not defensively recoil but rather perceives the allergen as a harmless, acceptable substance. "This produces a totally new and irreversible response to the allergen," Dr. Nambudripad says. "The new message is that this substance is safe. Then, you are no longer allergic." She adds that you only have to stay away from the substance for 24 hours as your energy meridians "reset" themselves.

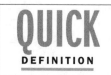

DEFINITION

Acupuncture meridians are specific pathways in the human body for the flow of life force or subtle energy, known as *qi* (pronounced CHEE). In most cases, these energy pathways run up and down both sides of the body, and correspond to individual organs or organ systems.

Success Story: Treating Allergies With NAET—Catherine had just received a diagnosis of hepatitis C. She was also severely overweight—194 pounds on a five-foot frame—and had struggled with her weight for the past ten years. Catherine complained of fatigue, constipation, and almost continual respiratory infections. "She came to see me to get healthy," says Helen Thomas, D.C., a chiropractor practicing in Santa Rosa, California. "She knew that under the present circumstances, with the hepatitis C diagnosis, she needed to have a healthy body."

Dr. Thomas is an Ayurvedic physician and employs this traditional medicine of India in her diagnosis. She took Catherine's pulses—pulse diagnosis reads patterns in the pulse as indications of the health of the body's systems. Catherine's pulse was very fast and light, indicating an imbalance in her nervous system (a *vata* imbalance). She also looked at Catherine's tongue to assess her health. Her tongue had a thick, white coating, indicating that her system was toxic. "When the body is overloaded with toxins, this indicates a clogged-up liver," Dr. Thomas explains.

Ayurveda also uses body typing as part of diagnosis. There are three metabolic, constitutional, and body types (*doshas*), in association with the basic elements of Nature: *vata* (air and ether, rooted in intestines), *pitta* (fire and water/stomach), and *kapha* (water and earth/lungs). Ayurvedic physicians use these categories to prescribe individualized formulas of herbs, diet, massage, breathing, meditation, exercise, and detoxification techniques.

By observing Catherine's facial expressions, height and weight, complexion, skin tone, and speech patterns, Dr. Thomas determined that Catherine was a *vata* type, which is basically a thin body type. Growing up, Catherine was short, thin, and wiry, so her current weight problem confirmed how much she was out of balance. "She ran into lots of emotional imbalance and experimented with drugs early on in her life," says Dr. Thomas. "Then she became overweight and just stayed there." Catherine's metabolism, the biological process by which energy is extracted from food, was stuck, explains Dr. Thomas, so that no matter what diet she tried, she just couldn't lose weight. The toxins in her system set up a system-wide allergic response which upset Catherine's normal metabolic rate.

To get Catherine 'un-stuck', Dr. Thomas used a special allergy desensitization approach called NAET (Nambudripad Allergy Elimination Technique). First, she muscle-tested Catherine for allergic sensitivity to ten basic nutrients: vitamins A, B complex, and C, calcium, chloride, egg, protein, iron, salt, and sugar. Catherine showed weakness in her muscle responses in six of the ten substances. According to NAET, these underlying allergies block the flow of energy, causing a "shortage" in the body's meridian system. "With NAET, what you're doing is testing the meridian or subtle-energy body," explains Dr. Thomas. "If there's a 'shortage' or disruption in those ten substances, then the body is not working properly."

She then used acupressure to apply gentle pressure of the fingers on the meridian points to clear these energy pathways and stimulate the organs. "An allergy, as far as NAET is concerned, means 'altered reactivity'," says Dr. Thomas. "Once the body is full of little landmines of altered reactivity, it gets stuck in the patterns. NAET breaks the patterns and allows the body's innate intelligence to restore itself." By normalizing the energy flow

Helen Thomas, D.C.: 2200 County Center Drive #B, Santa Rosa, CA 95431; tel: 707-527-7313. **Devi Nambudripad, D.C., O.M.D., Ph.D.:** Pain Clinic, 6714 Beach Blvd., Buena Park, CA 90621; tel: 714-523-0800.

Helpful Hints for Breaking a Food Addiction

Breaking a food addiction is never easy. Nevertheless, there are a few basic measures to follow that can help you make it through the cravings and withdrawal:

- Have plenty of non-allergy foods on hand at all times, including when you're away from home.

- Drink at least six to eight glasses of pure water every day, as adequate water intake is essential for good health; use spring, distilled, or filtered tap water.

- Don't go it alone—you may need extra help to break an addiction, so consider the support of a trained counselor.

- Maintain good nutrition because malnourishment only increases cravings; try working with a nutritional expert to determine your unique nutritional needs.

- Engage in light exercise on a regular basis—a brisk walk twice a day is all it takes to obtain some health benefit.

through the acupuncture meridians, NAET is able to turn off allergic reactions and prevent them from recurring.

She also put Catherine on a diet based on her Ayurvedic body type. Catherine was a *vata* type, but her body had become toxic and plugged up, so Dr. Thomas recommended a *kapha*-pacifying diet. "I wanted to give her food that would heat her up, that would increase her digestive fire," explains Dr. Thomas. "The *kapha*-pacifying diet helps the metabolism stimulate itself." The diet includes foods that are hot and pungent (to add heat), bitter (to purify), and astringent (to pull fluids out of the body). She recommended using peppers and any spices (except salt) in cooking; vegetables included leafy greens, beets, carrots, and cauliflower; all beans except tofu; fruits included apples, pomegranates, cranberries, and pears. Soymilk and rice milk were suggested instead of dairy products and uncooked honey was the only sweetener allowed. Since Catherine was not a vegetarian, Dr. Thomas recommended chicken and turkey only. She also encouraged Catherine to drink plenty of distilled water.

Catherine started an exercise program as well, walking five days per week, ten minutes per day to start, then gradually increasing to 30 minutes daily. She also meditated for 10-15 minutes a day to help relieve her stress. On this therapy program, Catherine lost 45 pounds in nine weeks. Her cholesterol levels normalized, her energy increased, and she was no longer troubled with constipation. She continued to test positive for hepatitis C on blood tests, but Catherine's biopsies showed a healthy liver.

Help Control Your Food Addictions

Overcoming a food addiction can be a formidable challenge, despite a carefully planned menu and nutritional supplements. Acupuncture, flower essence therapy, and aromatherapy, three alternative medicine therapies used to help treat addictive behaviors, can give you the extra support you need to curb your desire for sugar or other addictive foods.

Acupuncture

Acupuncture, a branch of traditional Chinese medicine, is a proven means of combating cravings and controlling weight. "Acupuncture points, especially on the ears, can be used to help a person control carbohydrate cravings and regulate appetite so they feel full from eating less food," says Richard Shwery, O.M.D., L.Ac., director of the Acupuncture Center of Cary in Cary, North Carolina. The "points" Dr. Shwery refers to are also used by acupuncturists in controlling other addictions, such as alcoholism.

Success Story: Reprogramming Hunger With Acupuncture—Guy, 34, stood 5'7" tall and weighed 249 pounds. He worked long days as a traveling sales representative and, due to the stress of his job, he tended to eat erratically, relying on fast foods and late-night snacks. His food choices were high in calories, fats, and salt, all of which contribute to weight gain. While he had tried different diets, herbs, and weight-loss drugs, nothing had yielded permanent weight loss. His body mass index (BMI) was 37 (his normal range was 20 to 25). Guy was still fat and unhappy about it when he made contact with Tim Tanaka, Ph.D., D.Ac., of the Pacific Wellness Institute in Toronto, Canada.

Dr. Tanaka knew that through acupuncture he could help Guy permanently shed pounds, but he cautioned him that "we never try for quick weight reduction. We prefer to see a slow reduction which generally brings a consistent and perma-

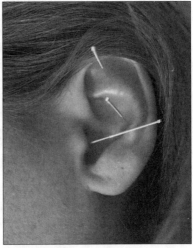

EAR ACUPUNCTURE.

Needles are placed mainly on points on the ear to influence two parts of the brain located in the hypothalamus: the feeding center, which is responsible for the feeling of hunger, and the satiety center, which tells you when you've eaten enough.

Tim Tanaka, Ph.D., D.Ac., C.S.T., R.M.T.: Pacific Wellness Institute, 80 Bloor Street West, Suite 1100, Toronto, Ontario M5S 2V1, Canada; tel: 416-929-6958; fax: 416-929-6365; website: www.toronto.com/pwi.

nent change." He adds that many strictly dietary approaches to weight loss tend to fail over time because they are too restrictive and leave people feeling deprived, with no joy in their life regarding food.

Dr. Tanaka uses acupuncture to reduce the appetite, activate metabolism (energy conversion from food), and enhance digestion, so more nutrients are extracted and absorbed from what is eaten. The placement of acupuncture needles can activate the parasympathetic nervous system, which controls appetite, metabolism, and digestion, he explains. The goal is to "decrease nervous tension that frequently triggers the desire to consume sugar."

The needles are placed mainly on points on the ear (plus some points along the spine and abdomen) to influence two parts of the brain located in the hypothalamus: the feeding center, which is responsible for the feeling of hunger, and the satiety center, which tells you when you've eaten enough. "These systems may sometimes become oversensitive or inactive, which can lead to weight problems," says Dr. Tanaka. Acupuncture can reset the operation of these two centers, so you feel less hunger and feel more satisfied after eating less food.

Dr. Tanaka also employed a technique he calls SES, a systemic acupuncture treatment in which the needles are placed very shallowly. While the patient sits upright, exceedingly tiny acupuncture needles are placed just below the skin surface at treatment points as the patient exhales. This procedure, performed before the ear acupuncture, takes about two minutes and is repeated at the end of the treatment session. The purpose is to "correct imbalances in the autonomic nervous system and to create favorable conditions for altering metabolic activity," Dr. Tanaka explains. "This type of needling elicits a parasympathetic response."

At the same time that Dr. Tanaka was energetically reducing Guy's food cravings with acupuncture, he asked him to voluntarily eat 10%-30% less at each meal. He also placed a kind of acupuncture "earring" (a tiny silver pellet) in Guy's ear so that merely by pressing on it, Guy could activate the treatment point to reduce his food cravings whenever he felt the need.

Dr. Tanaka referred Guy to the Center's expert in healthy cooking, Cathy Wong, B.Sc., who showed Guy new ways of cooking that would not lead to weight gain. "Changing acquired eating habits and food preferences is not easy," says Wong. "Guy learned how to create low-fat meals that do not taste 'light' even though, calorically, they are. This minimized the feelings of deprivation and eased his transition to a healthier diet." For example, Wong substituted baked Atlantic salmon with shiitake mushroom pesto for Guy's unhealthy penchant for fried foods. Guy was used to eating apple pie with ice cream as a late night snack, but Wong showed him that chilled almond pudding with fresh berry sauce could appealingly be substituted. "Combined with low-fat cooking techniques, this approach provides optimum levels of both nutrients and taste."

It took only three months of acupuncture and dietary substitutions for Guy to lose 37 pounds and for his BMI to drop to 31.5. His weight continues to gradually decrease. What pleased Guy the most is that he achieved the ongoing weight reduction without the "feeling of sacrifice" so typical of other weight reduction programs.

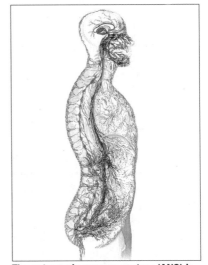

The autonomic nervous system (ANS) is like your body's automatic pilot. It keeps you alive through breathing, heart rate, and digestion, without your being aware of it or participating in its activities. The ANS has two divisions: the sympathetic, which expends body energy (prepares us physically when we perceive a threat or challenge by increasing heart rate, blood pressure, and muscle tension), and the parasympathetic, which conserves body energy (slows heart rate and increases intestinal and gland activity).

Flower Essence Therapy

Flower essence therapy helps control addictive behaviors by treating underlying emotional, psychological, and spiritual issues. The approach was pioneered by British physician Edward Bach in the 1930s, when he introduced the Bach Flower Remedies, based on English plants. Flower essences are made by floating blossoms in spring water, then letting them sit in the sun for a few hours. The blossoms are removed, leaving the essence of the flower, which is then diluted to a dosage level. Drops of the essences are either placed under the tongue, ingested in a tonic, or diluted in a bath. Although you can administer a flower essence treatment yourself, a trained practitioner can help tailor a treatment program specific to your psychological needs.

Aromatherapy

Another way to control appetite is through aromatherapy. Rather than water-based flower essences, aromatherapy relies on oils extracted from the leaves, flowers, or roots of plants. The size of the molecules in these oils allows them to penetrate bodily tissues via the skin or the olfactory nerves, affecting central nervous system activity.[11] Aromatherapy can be performed at home, using either a diffuser, which spreads microparticles of the oils into the air, or floral waters, which can be sprayed. Roberta Wilson, author of *Aromatherapy for Vibrant Health and Beauty*, recommends an aromatherapy appetite suppressant formula made from 15 drops of bergamot oil and ten drops of fennel oil.[12]

Inhalants are essential oils that you can breathe directly from the bottle. As the soothing aromas travel through your respiratory system, they trigger a positive reaction in the brain. You might feel the difference—elevated mood, lower stress level, or reduced appetite—in as little as a few seconds. To make an inhalant, just place your choice of essential oils in a small glass bottle with an airtight cover. Then blend the oils by gently turning the container upside down or rolling it between your hands (but not by shaking, as this upsets the chemical balance between the oils). After a few minutes, the oils are well blended and your inhalant is ready for use. If you would like to use your inhalant throughout the day, try placing a few drops of the blend on a tissue or handkerchief, then carry the scented item with you to enjoy an aromatherapy break anytime.

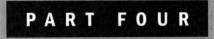

PART FOUR

Detoxify
the Body

12 Detoxify the Colon

A HEALTHY COLON teems with beneficial microorganisms that contribute to the healthy digestion and absorption of food. However, years of poor diet, reliance on medications, stress, and other factors can throw our intestinal ecology severely out of balance, causing a variety of illnesses as well as weight gain. Alternative medicine offers natural, gentle, and effective methods that can restore the intestinal environment and simultaneously facilitate weight loss.

Nutritionist Lindsey Duncan, C.N., director of the Home Nutrition Clinic in Santa Monica, California, says, "I've consulted with 8,000 clients, who come to me with a variety of health problems ranging from fatigue, depression, impaired immune function, and obesity to chronic constipation, gas, acne, and lower back pain. The vast majority of these complaints and symptoms are alleviated by cleansing, healing, and supporting the intestinal system."

Indeed, many illnesses arise from problems in the intestines. Most of the digestion and absorption of nutrients that happens in the body occurs along the 25-foot-long passageway that comprises the small and large intestines. Keeping this passageway clean and alive with healthy digestive microbes is vital to maintaining a healthy body weight. In her 26 years of practice, Carol Port, D.C., M.A., a chiropractor and holistic practitioner based in Los Angeles, California, found that many conditions were associated with an unhealthy colon, including food cravings, fatigue, insomnia, irritability, anxiety, depression, headaches, and allergies. These conditions, along with a general malaise, are what contribute to the self-destructive eating habits that translate into weight gain. "Detoxification and permanent weight loss go hand-in-hand," she says, "because it addresses the cause, not the symptom."

Similarly, Daniel Reid, a Chinese medicine expert who practices in

> ## Alternative Medicine Detoxification Therapies
>
> ■ Dietary Recommendations
> ■ Colon Cleansing
> ■ Enemas and Colonic Irrigations
> ■ Chiropractic, Massage, and Reflexology

Taiwan and author of *The Tao of Health, Sex, and Longevity*, explains that a colon cleanse is necessary to undo the harm done by years of eating an unhealthy diet and to help the body better absorb needed nutrients. "There's no point in changing your diet or taking any sort of supplements if the body can't handle what's coming in," says Reid. "In Chinese medicine, obesity is viewed as a problem of stagnation. The first step in a truly successful weight-loss program must be to cleanse the internal body."

In this chapter, we'll look at the link between a toxic colon and weight gain as well as the dietary and lifestyle factors that may be harming your intestinal function. We review the tests available for assessing the state of your colon and digestive system. And, finally, we outline the alternative medicine therapies, including colon cleansing programs and dietary recommendations, which can help you restore your colon to health.

Success Story: Colon Cleansing Reduces Excess Weight

"My weight crept up on me so slowly that I hardly noticed what was happening," says Nancy, 30, who was 5'1" and weighed 140 pounds. Nancy tried diet drinks, such as Slim Fast™, to reduce her weight and succeeded in losing a few pounds; however, she soon gained it all back and more. She also began to feel increasingly run down and, when she tried to have a baby, suffered a miscarriage.

Nancy went to see a holistic nutritionist, whose exam revealed that her problems were related to a buildup of fecal material in her colon (the end portion of the large intestine). The nutritionist recommended that she undergo a colon cleanse. "At first, the idea seemed a little

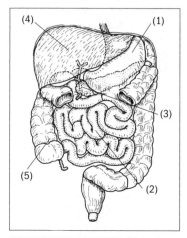

THE DIGESTIVE SYSTEM. Digestion begins in the mouth, then food travels to the stomach (1), where it is further broken down by gastric juices. Next, the partially digested food goes to the small intestine (2) where enzymes from the pancreas (3) and bile produced by the liver (4) act upon the food to extract nutrients for absorption into blood and lymph cells. The unusable food materials are sent to the large intestine (5) for evacuation from the body.

weird to me and I was scared," Nancy remarks. She didn't think she had a problem with her colon, as she was neither constipated nor had diarrhea. Nevertheless, she decided to give the cleanse a try.

"I went on a brief, supervised juice-and-water fast and took herbal cleansing formulas in the morning and before bed," she said. Nancy was also given enemas and a series of colonic irrigations, a treatment which involves flushing out the entire colon with warm, filtered water. Soon after the treatment, Nancy began to see results. "Thick black and dark brown matter literally poured out of my body," she reports. "I couldn't believe all that stuff was inside me or how much better I felt once it was gone."

After the fast and colonic irrigations, the therapist also flushed out Nancy's liver and gallbladder, using herbs and a cleansing diet. The treatment restored her vitality and brought her down to a healthy weight. "I don't worry about dieting now," she says. "My body has more muscle and less fat. I weigh around 100 pounds and I've stayed at that weight for the past four years."

How a Toxic Colon Leads to Weight Gain

At birth, the inner lining of our intestines is pink, clean, and supple. Over time, however, the combination of poor diet, stress, and exposure to environmental toxins causes the intestines to become caked with debris, swollen, and stagnant. Nutritionist Robert Gray, of San Francisco, author of *The Colon Health Handbook*, explains that while the small intestine and even the stomach become impacted with food debris, the colon is where the most severe buildup occurs.[1] The accumulated material can often contribute several pounds to the weight of the colon.

"At the simplest level, weight loss can be a natural outcome of cleaning the colon because accumulated waste is solid, it has weight," explains Jack Larmer, N.D., a naturopath and homeopath in Nashua, New Hampshire. "Most people are walking around with at least seven pounds of fecal matter in their large intestine, and I have seen patients lose that much weight, and their tummy bulge, immediately following colon treatment."

False Linings

Intestinal mucus makes the stools gummy, causing them to stick to the intestine walls. Mucus also leaves a residue as it passes, which builds up and eventually hardens into plaque. Mucoid plaque can be up to one-inch thick with a texture from stiff and hard to soft and gooey, and is often blackish-green in color, somewhat resembling rubber or leather. This "false lining" in the intestine reduces the diameter of the intestinal passageway, leaving only a narrow opening through which waste can travel. As the condition of the lining worsens, it becomes increasingly difficult to regularly empty the bowel.

As the false lining builds up, it also blocks absorption of essential nutrients into the bloodstream and offers a hiding place for bacteria, fungi, yeast, and parasites that are harmful to human health. When these abnormal life forms start growing too freely, they kill off the "friendly" bacteria, such as *Lactobacillus acidophilus*, that inhabit the intestines, leading to an imbalance in the intestinal microflora (see "Friendly and Unfriendly Bacteria," p. 276). When this happens, the contents of the intestines putrefy and harmful chemicals are generated,

Transit Time

About 100 years ago, most people in the United States had a short intestinal "transit time," meaning it took only about 15-20 hours from the time food entered the mouth until it was excreted as feces. Today, many have a seriously delayed transit time of 50-70 hours. One reason transit times have increased is that our diets now include less fiber from fresh fruits and vegetables. As fiber is indigestible, it helps give stools bulk, while also making them soft and flexible. Another reason is that our modern lifestyle, high in stress, excessive antibiotics, and certain acid-forming foods (such as sugar, eggs, and meat), causes the intestinal tract to accumulate a slimy, sticky substance called mucus.

This means there is more time for the stool to putrefy, for harmful microorganisms to flourish, and for toxins to develop and poison the body. Optimal transit time is about 18-20 hours; an acceptable transit time is 24-48 hours. Ideally, everyone should have comfortable, unforced bowel movements about 20 minutes after every meal, just like a baby. A healthy colon produces an easy-to-eliminate stool that is soft but formed, consisting of about 70% water but having enough bulk so that it readily responds to the muscular contractions of the bowel.

Friendly and Unfriendly Bacteria

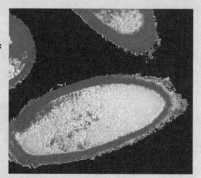

The estimated 100 trillion bacteria that live in the human intestines do so in a delicate balance. Certain bacteria, such as *Lactobacillus acidophilus* and *Bifidobacterium bifidum*, are "friendly" bacteria that support numerous vital physiological processes. They help ensure that bowel movements are regular and frequent and they also oppose the overgrowth of yeasts and parasites. Other bacteria, such as *Staphylococcus* and *Clostridrium*, are also present, but are considered "unfriendly" because they produce a variety of toxic substances. A healthy proportion of microorganisms in the colon is 85% friendly bacteria to no more than 15% unfriendly bacteria. Unfortunately, in most people, the proportions are the exact opposite.[2] A number of factors can throw off the balance of intestinal flora, including stress, the use of antibiotics and other drugs, and processed foods.

leading to condition called bowel toxemia (characterized by inflammation and swelling in the bowel), which can lead to numerous health problems, including weight gain.

Serafina Corsello, M.D., director of the Corsello Centers for Nutritional Complementary Medicine in New York City and Huntington, New York, states that the large and small intestines are the active front of the immune system, trapping and eliminating pathogens and harmful debris. "The intestines constitute the largest immunological system of the body," Dr. Corsello observes. "The digestive system is one of the first screening systems against the daily load of bacteria, viruses, and parasites that, if left unchecked, would constitute a grave threat to our entire immune system."

Toxins that build up in the colon pass through the intestinal wall and accumulate in the lymphatic system—a network of vessels and nodes that clean and drain the body of toxic substances. When the flow of toxins from the colon becomes too heavy, the lymph can become blocked and cause toxins to back up throughout the body. The result can be swelling of the torso and legs, damage to the liver and other detoxification organs, and blood toxicity, eventually compromising the entire immune system.[3] "When the colon is impacted with mucoid layers, the lymphatic system gets blocked and backup develops—this is one of the main reasons for obesity," explains naturopath Richard Anderson, N.D., N.M.D., of Mt. Shasta, California.[4]

Toxins Tack On the Pounds

Unhealthy or compromised intestinal function can have a major impact on your weight. Many people with a toxic colon simply may not be able to absorb the nutrients from the foods they're eating and may overeat as a result. "When the bowel fails, the whole body goes into a nutritional crisis. Metabolic shock waves flow to every cell and tissue," says nutritionist and chiropractor Bernard Jensen, D.C., Ph.D., of Escondido, California, who has treated thousands of colon patients during his 60 years of practice.[5]

"The intestines constitute the largest immunological system of the body," Dr. Serafina Corsello observes. "The digestive system is one of the first screening systems against the load of bacteria, viruses, and parasites that, if unchecked, would constitute a grave threat."

Nutritionist Lindsey Duncan agrees that a clean colon aids in digestion and the ability to metabolize food. "Over 90% of the people I see are metabolizing less than 55% of what they are eating," he says. "They think it's normal to have a bowel movement once every few days. I often startle my clients with the question, 'If we eat three meals daily but only eliminate once a day, or once every other day, where do you think all the rest of that food is hiding?'"

However, it is not just the weight of the accumulated fecal matter itself that contributes to excess body weight. Toxic by-products from the colon can drain the body of energy, lower metabolism (SEE QUICK DEFINITION), and over-burden other detoxifying organs, such as the liver and kidneys. "The real importance of removing toxic waste from the bowel is to stop damaging by-products from recycling back into other parts of the body," explains Dr. Larmer. "Once the colon is clean, the metabolism is more likely to work as it should, and when that happens, a major obstacle to weight loss is eliminated."

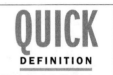

QUICK
DEFINITION

Metabolism is the biological process by which energy is extracted from the foods consumed, producing carbon dioxide and water as by-products for elimination. There are two kinds of metabolism constantly underway in the cells: anabolic and catabolic. The anabolic function produces substances for cell growth and repair, while the catabolic function controls digestion, disassembling food into forms the body can use for energy.

Factors That Harm the Colon

These factors can contribute to the formation of mucoid plaque, throw off the balance of the intestinal microflora, and cause a toxic bowel.

Acid Diet–Acid-forming foods, such as sugars, processed grains, eggs, and meat, contribute to the formation of intestinal plaque. They deplete the body of electrolytes, substances which prevent the bile (the intestinal fluid that helps digestion) from becoming too acidic. Bile that is acidic cannot digest food normally, causing mucoid plaque to develop. Other ways of causing too much acid in the intestines is by overeating during a meal.

Processed Foods–Foods made from bleached white flour, such as white bread, pastries, and cakes, contribute to the buildup of intestinal plaque. These foods are almost totally devoid of fiber. Because most of the nutrients have also been bleached out, they tend to deprive the body of enzymes and other wholesome nutrients. Enzymes are specialized living proteins that break down food and change it into a form the body can absorb. Without adequate enzymes, food tends to putrefy in the intestines rather than being digested and absorbed.

Stress–Stress can cause excess acid in the intestine, contributing to the formation of intestinal plaque. Tension also causes the walls of the bowel and sphincter muscles to constrict, hindering the passage of fecal material. Dr. Corsello has observed a direct relationship between stressful events and exponential growth of harmful organisms in the intestine.

Allergies–The intestines may produce mucus in response to a food allergy. Ralph Golan, M.D., of Seattle, Washington, says that "any food can be an allergen and cause constipation, cramps, bloating, diarrhea, and other bowel symptoms."[6] He warns that many individuals are allergic to whole wheat and wheat bran, two foods commonly ingested to increase fiber intake. Although these foods are often eaten to relieve constipation, if an allergy exists, they may only increase the problem.

Parasites and Yeast–Parasite and yeast infestations in the colon can also cause digestive problems. Parasites commonly enter the body through contaminated food or water supplies (both domestic and from foreign travel). Intestinal parasites can induce a wide variety of reactions, including swelling of joints, asthma, and weight gain. Dr. Corsello is concerned that many physicians refuse to acknowledge that parasite infestation is a major factor in systemic illness. She notes that physicians at her clinic have observed a strong correlation in their patients between having intestinal parasites and a range of chronic conditions such as arthritis, respiratory problems, heightened allergies, menstrual disorders, and prolonged bowel disorders.

For information about **enzymes**, see Chapter 4: Enzymes and Weight Loss, pp. 98-120. For more on **food allergies**, see Chapter 11: Break Food Allergies and Addictions, pp. 244-270. For more about **parasites**, see Chapter 14: Eradicate Parasites, pp. 310-328. For more about **yeast infections**, see Chapter 13: Eliminate Yeast Infections, pp. 294-309.

Antibiotics—Antibiotics are prescribed by physicians to kill the harmful bacteria causing an infection. Unfortunately, these drugs do not distinguish between the unfriendly and friendly microbes that live in our bodies—they cause a massive die-off of friendly bacteria (steroids and birth control pills can have a similar effect). When friendly bacteria are not replaced through diet or supplements, unfriendly bacteria quickly lay claim to the intestines, causing a buildup of toxic materials.

Carbohydrate Intolerance—Elaine Gottschall, M.S., nutritional scientist from Ontario, Canada, and author of *Breaking the Vicious Cycle: Intestinal Health Through Diet*, says that, in some individuals, starches (also called carbohydrates) can cause intestinal problems that lead to a toxic bowel. The problems arise when carbohydrates in the small intestine are not completely digested, which attracts bacteria from the colon. "The presence of undigested and unabsorbed carbohydrates in the small intestine can encourage microbes from the colon to take up residence in the small intestine and multiply," explains Gottschall.

Bacteria from the large intestine destroy enzymes in the small intestine, which further reduces the body's ability to digest and absorb carbohydrates, resulting in what Gottschall describes as a "vicious cycle." Moreover, both the small intestine and colon respond to the bacterial bloom by secreting mucus. "Excess mucus may be triggered as a self-defense mechanism whereby the intestinal tract attempts to 'lubricate' itself against the injury caused by the microbial toxins, acids, and the presence of incompletely digested and unabsorbed carbohydrates." Although the mucus may protect the intestinal lining from damage, it also slows transit time and hampers digestion.[7]

Success Story: Reversing Obesity Through Detoxification

Florrie, 49, had a host of debilitating symptoms, including obesity, severe gastrointestinal dysfunction (chronic diarrhea and diverticulitis, an inflammation of the intestinal lining), gum disease, possible food allergies, and recurring depression. Florrie, who weighed 220 pounds, had almost never exercised in her life and her weight gain had become such a problem that "I can't even see my knees anymore."

She consulted clinical nutritionist Monika Klein, B.H.Ec., C.N., in Malibu, California. Florrie explained that for the last 14 years she had consumed an average of 16-18 diet colas every day. She had started this habit during her student years when she needed the quick caffeine boost the sodas provide. As a self-described "sodaholic," Florrie kept two cases of sodas in her car, just in case she needed a boost while on the road.

She had tried numerous popular diet plans, such as Weight Watchers, Jenny Craig, and Slim Fast, but had gained no benefit. Her life wasn't working and she knew it. "Every morning I woke up feeling bad," she reflects. "I was in a lot of pain from my diverticulitis. I never cooked. I primarily ate out, and when I did eat vegetables (which was seldom), they were the microwaved, frozen variety."

For someone in this state of ill health and gastrointestinal dysfunction, you cannot rush into a detoxification program, explains Klein. In patients who are chronically ill and whose systems are deeply imbalanced, the body lacks the energy and proper organ function to run the complex processes of detoxifying itself. "You must prepare for detoxification carefully and in stages. The body (and mind) of such a person is deeply entrenched in a ruinous lifestyle but which to them seems like an ordinary way of living," says Klein. As evidence of this habituation to harmful dietary habits, Florrie had to wean herself off diet sodas for five months before she was ready or able to drop the "addiction."

To prepare Florrie for detoxification, Klein started her slowly on supplements that would help her immune and digestive systems. Specifically, vitamin C, garlic, and a supplement to build up her immune vitality, while pancreatic enzymes, hydrochloric acid (the stomach's primary digestive "juice"), and flaxseed oil would assist her digestion. Klein also encouraged Florrie to start eating more fresh vegetables and fish. After five months of preparation, Florrie was still unable to handle detoxification. Klein decided to focus on repairing Florrie's gastrointestinal tract using a product called UltraClear Sustain®. This is a "medical food" that provides vegetarian-based nutritional support for patients with chronic gastrointestinal problems.

A lifetime of poor eating habits and 15 years of steady diet soda intake had seriously imbalanced the intestinal bacteria that Florrie needed for good digestion. Klein added the probiotics UltraDophilus and UltraBifidus, along with Probioplex, a formula that supplies concentrated whey protein to promote the growth of beneficial microflora. Aloe vera juice was added to improve her intestinal health.

After about five months, as she realized her weight was dropping, Florrie finally gave up the daily sodas. Her decision to abstain completely from these soft drinks was a psychological victory for her. Her bowel movements were much improved, which indicated healthier function returning to both the lining of her intestines and its ability to eliminate more materials through peristalsis.

Florrie now seemed ready to begin the full detoxification regimen. This consisted of a two-week "intensive" phase in which she ate primarily foods that produced no allergic reactions or excessive mucus, avoiding foods such as dairy products, white flour, wheat, corn, and sugar. The core of this two-week phase was another medical food called UltraClear®, billed as a "metabolic detoxification program for food-based clearing." This product contains high-protein white rice concentrate, rice carbohydrates, safflower oil, and other beneficial essential fatty acids and can be combined with foods as part of a meal.

UltraClear helps the liver, the body's chief organ of detoxification, begin its processes of ridding the body of toxins and accumulated waste matter. Toxins are also cleared from the kidneys, bladder, intestines, skin, lungs, lymph, and even the mind. "In a curious but physiologically rational way, the state of our intestines has a lot to do with the state of our mind and the tenor of our emotions," says Klein. As toxins are flushed out, many people report feeling uplifted in their

Monika Klein, B.H.Ec., C.N.: Healing Arts West, 1411 5th St., Suite 405, Santa Monica, CA 90401; tel: 310-458-0400; fax: 310 458-7551. She may also be contacted at: Malibu Health & Rehabilitation, Pacific Coast Highway, Suite 220, Malibu, CA 90265; tel: 310-456-7721; fax: 310-456-9482. For information about **UltraClear Sustain, UltraClear, UltraDophilus, Inflavanoid, UltraBifidus, ProAntho C, Bio-zyme, Oxygenics,** and **Cal Apatite** contact: Metagenics, Inc., 971 Calle Negocio, San Clemente, CA 92673; tel: 800-692-9400; fax: 714-366-0818. For **Zymex, Multizyme,** and **Immuplex,** contact: Standard Process, 1200 W. Royal Lee Dr., Palmyra, WI 53156; tel: 414-495-2122; fax: 800-438-3799. For **Garlicin,** contact: Emerson Ecologics, 18 Lomar Park, Pepperell, MA 01463; tel: 800-654-4432; fax: 800-718-7236. For **Aloe Herbal Juice,** contact: Pacific Resources, P.O. Box 4043, Malibu, CA 90264; tel: 310-457-3164; fax: 310-457-3396. For **Similase** and **Metazyme,** contact: Tyler Encapsulations, 2204-8 NW Birdsale, Gresham, OR 97030; tel: 800-869-9705. To order **Essential Balance** and **Udo's Choice,** contact: Health from the Sun, P.O. Box 360, Georges Mills, NH 03751; tel: 800-339-5999.

Florrie's Weight Loss Detoxification Plan

Initial Preparatory Protocol—

- Zymex: two capsules, three times daily with food
- Multizyme (enzymes): two capsules, three times daily with food
- Immuplex: one capsule, three times daily with food
- Flaxseed oil: one to two tablets daily
- Garlicin: one capsule, three times daily with food

Follow-up Preparatory Plan—

- UltraClear Sustain: ½ scoop daily for the first week, increasing ½ scoop per week up to two scoops daily
- Probioplex: one teaspoon daily, taken with UltraClear Sustain
- UltraDophilus® (a special strain of *Lactobacillus acidophilus*): ½ tsp daily taken with UltraClear Sustain
- UltraBifidus® (*Bifidobacteria adolescentis*): ½ tsp daily taken with UltraClear Sustain
- Aloe Herbal Juice: two ounces daily, on an empty stomach

Two-Week Intensive Protocol—

- UltraClear: two scoops per drink; day 1, two drinks; day 2, three drinks; day 3, four drinks; days 4-8, five drinks; day 9, four drinks; day 10, three drinks; days 11-12, two drinks; days 13-14, two drinks
- Esterol: 6-10 capsules daily for three days
- Oxygenics: twice daily on an empty stomach

Maintenance Program—

- UltraClear Sustain: 1-2 drinks daily (four scoops total)
- Multigenics (a multiple mineral/vitamin): four times daily with food
- Cal Apatite: twice daily with food
- Metazyme or Similase: one capsule, three times daily with food
- Esterol: one capsule, three times daily with food
- Essential Balance or Udo's Choice: 1-2 tablets daily
- Garlicin: twice daily
- Cat's claw: one capsule, three times daily, on an empty stomach
- Aloe vera: one ounce daily, on an empty stomach

thoughts and a lightening of their mood. On the other hand, in the process of clearing toxins there may be moments of mental agitation, irritation, and sudden mood shifts, and there may also be headaches and muscle pains, but these negative reactions are temporary (usually one or two days at most).

If a person complains of headaches or other detoxification symptoms within the first few days, Klein suggests nutritional supplements.

In Florrie's case, Klein gave her antioxidants to help flush out toxins and free radicals from her cells: Oxygenics™, a free radical quencher and antioxidant, containing herbs, vitamins, fatty acids, and minerals; and ProAntho-C, containing vitamin C with proanthocyanidin, a vitamin C helper from grape seeds.

Florrie had no significant problems during the two-week detoxification program, because her system was now strong enough to handle it. In the middle of the intensive phase, Florrie remarked, "This is a process. It doesn't happen overnight. It is a gradual change in lifestyle." When it was over, she said: "I felt as if somebody had taken a vacuum cleaner through my insides and cleaned it all out. My taste buds suddenly felt alive again, for the first time in years. I started 'craving' foods that were good for me, such as broccoli and okra."

That was two years ago. Since that time, Florrie has gone through four more detoxification programs, spaced about six months apart. She has clearly developed a committment to her health. She feels better than ever, has dropped 60 pounds and two dress sizes, and grown leaner in terms of body fat. Florrie continues with several of the program's key supplements, such as vitamin C, UltraClear Sustain, digestive enzymes, and Cal Apatite (a mineral supplement including calcium, phosphorus, vitamin D3, magnesium, zinc, copper, and manganese). Her food choices are primarily fresh vegetables, some fruits, fish, chicken, eggs, and a limited amount of grains. Reversing a lifetime of indolence, Florrie also began a regular exercise program in the form of lunchtime walks. In fact, this year Florrie walked the 26-mile Los Angeles marathon, and next year she intends to run it.

Do You Have a Toxic Colon?

One way to get an idea of the condition of your colon is by paying attention to your symptoms. An obvious sign of trouble is painful, difficult bowel movements. "Few people have any inkling as to how much old, hardened feces are chronically present within their bodies," says nutritional counselor Robert Gray.[8] Also, transit time can be used as a measure of bowel health (as stated above, optimal transit time is about 18-20 hours). Other symptoms of a toxic bowel include headaches, bloating and gas, weight gain, fatigue and depression, lower back pain, sallow complexion or dark circles under the eyes, tender abdomen, abnormal body odor, and bad breath.

In addition to observing your symptoms, you may also want to consider undergoing a test that can give you more detailed information about the condition of your colon. Some of these tests are also helpful in determining the exact treatment remedy you need.

■ Testing Your Transit Time—Dr. Golan recommends a simple procedure you can follow to test your food transit time. Begin by eating a "test food" (test foods include corn on the cob, sesame or sunflower seeds, beets, or any other material likely to be visible in the stool). You should note the time that you ingest the test food. Then, watch for the material to appear in your stools—specifically, whole undigested kernels or seeds or a marked red color from the beets. The time between eating the test food and the appearance in your stool is the transit time.[9]

■ Bacterial Breath Test—This test helps determine whether bacteria have invaded your small intestine. The test measures the levels of methane and hydrogen in your breath after you are given a specially formulated drink containing non-digestible sugar (lactulose). If you have bacteria in your small intestine, the levels of the two substances in your breath will increase.

■ Urinary Indican (Obermeyer Test)—This test measures the amount of indican (a bacterial waste product) in your urine. High levels of indican may reflect a colon loaded with putrefactive bacteria. This test is available through your health-care practitioner.

■ Iridology—A useful alternative medicine technique for assessing the state of the colon is iridology, a diagnostic tool that studies the iris (the colored portion) of the eye. Iridologists have mapped the entire body on the iris, and look for small markings such as black spots, speckles, tiny yellow clumps, or white circles on its surface to detect disease in various organs and systems. Toronto naturopath James D'Adamo, N.D., indicates that when the colon is toxic a ringed formation will appear on the iris.[10]

For information about the **Bacterial Breath Test** and the **Comprehensive Digestive Stool Analysis**, contact: Great Smokies Diagnostic Laboratory, 63 Zillicoa Street, Asheville, NC 28801; tel: 800-522-4762 or 704-253-0621. Lab staff will also make referrals to physicians around the country using these tests.

■ Tongue Analysis—In traditional Chinese medicine, the tongue is used to diagnose a host of internal conditions. To do a tongue analysis, do not eat any food after 5 P.M. on the day before you will do the diagnosis; also do not include any meat in your last meal. Upon arising the next morning, immediately look at your tongue. A coating on the tongue may indicate a clogged colon—the thicker the coating, the more severe the problem.

■ Comprehensive Digestive Stool Analysis—An excellent "window" into seeing how digestive inadequacies can contribute to a variety of illnesses is a stool analysis, which consists of a group of nearly two dozen tests performed on a stool sample and can be ordered by your physician. The tests reveal how well you are digesting your food and absorbing nutrients, the proportions of friendly versus unfriendly bacteria in your intestine, and whether or not your diet contains adequate fiber (see "What a Stool Analysis Can Tell You," pp. 286-287). The test provides a great deal of information about digestion of various foods, whether or not fats are being absorbed, and the status of digestive enzymes. It also tells you whether yeasts such as *Candida* are present. All of these factors may be contributing to your symptoms.

Alternative Medicine Detoxification Therapies

Colon cleansing is commonly recommended by natural health practitioners as an effective method of detoxification. There are a number of colon cleansing programs available to help you scrub and remove hardened fecal matter and other toxic materials from the intestines. Enemas and colonic irrigations, in which water or some other fluid is used to flush out the lower portion of the colon, can also help restore intestinal health. In addition, physical therapies such as chiropractic and reflexology are useful in stimulating and normalizing digestive function.

Before the Cleanse
The foundation of any colon cleansing program must begin with a healthy diet, adequate intake of fiber and water, and measures that help restore friendly bacteria to the colon.

Diet—Your diet during a colon cleanse should be very high in fiber and fresh raw vegetables and fruits, and low in acid-forming foods that stimulate the intestines to secrete mucus. During the cleansing period, it is preferable to stop eating all milk products and refined white flour products, such as pastas, breads, and baked goods, and eliminate all sugar. You should also reduce your intake of eggs, meat, chicken, most fish, nuts, seeds, and unsprouted beans and grains.

Fiber—"A diet deficient in fiber is an important causative factor in the development of obesity," says Michael Murray, N.D., a naturopath based in Seattle, Washington, and author of *Natural Alternatives for Weight Loss*.[11] Fiber acts like a sponge, absorbing water as it goes through the stomach and the small intestine, and arrives in the colon

What a Stool Analysis Can Tell You

The following is a glossary of terms used in stool analysis along with an explanation of each of the values:

Colonic Environment—

■ Dysbiosis index: Intestinal dysbiosis refers to an imbalance of intestinal flora. Specifically, these flora include friendly, beneficial bacteria (for example, *Lactobacillus acidophilus*) and unfriendly or harmful bacteria (for example, *Pseudomonas aeruginosa*). In dysbiosis, the unfriendly bacteria predominate; they begin fermentation, producing toxic by-products that interfere with normal elimination.

■ *Lactobacillus* and *Bifidobacteria*: These bacteria are involved in vitamin synthesis and detoxification of cancer-causing substances, and they support the immune system. Deficiencies have been linked with a higher risk for chronic diseases.

■ *gamma Streptococcus*: This is a bacteria normal to the intestines; its presence is not necessarily an indication of digestive imbalance.

■ *Pseudomonas aeruginosa*: Associated with wound and urinary tract infections, this bacterium causes infections in the context of a weakened immune system. *P. aeruginosa* can contribute to diarrhea and inflammation.

■ Macroscopic (appearance): Yellow to green stools may indicate diarrhea and a bowel sterilized by antibiotics; black or red may reflect bleeding in the gastrointestinal tract; tan or gray can indicate a blockage of the common bile duct; and mucus or pus can point to irritable bowel syndrome, polyps, diverticulitis, or intestinal wall inflammation.

■ pH: pH is a reflection of the acid/alkaline balance in the colon. The preferred range is 6.0 (mildly acidic) to 7.2 (mildly alkaline).

■ N-butyrate: This is a form of butyric acid, a primary energy source for the colon; it must be present in adequate amounts for healthy metabolism. Butyric acid is needed to digest short-chain fatty acids (SCFAs).

■ Total SCFA: Short-chain fatty acids are produced when the colon ferments soluble fibers. SCFAs provide 70% of the energy needed by the cells lining the colon.

■ SCFA distribution: Elevated levels of any of the four SCFAs can indicate poor nutrient absorption or bacterial overgrowth, while decreased levels suggest lack of dietary fiber, unbalanced metabolism, or dysbiosis.

■ Beta-glucuronidase: This is an enzyme produced by various bacteria in the colon. Elevated levels may result from bacterial overgrowth, an abnormal pH, too much dietary fat, or low levels of beneficial bacteria.

■ Fecal sIgA: Fecal secretory IgA is a specialized immunoglobulin, one of a class of five antibody proteins involved in the immune system's response to foreign substances. Fecal sIgA serves as the first line of defense against invading pathogens, toxins, and food allergens. Low levels mean an increased susceptibility to infection and food allergies.

Measures of Digestive Dysfunction—

■ Triglycerides: Most dietary fats are triglycerides; during digestion, lipase (a pancreatic enzyme) breaks down triglycerides into glycerol and fatty acids. Elevated fecal triglyceride levels indicate incomplete fat metabolism and possible problems in the pancreas.

Colonic Environment

Microbiology

Beneficial Bacteria

Lactobacillus	0+
Bifidobacter	4+
E Coli	4+

Additional Bacteria

gamma Strep	3+
Pseudomonas aeruginosa	1+

Mycology

presumptive C. albicans	3+

Microscopic yeast from parasite exam: N/A

▮ normal flora   ▯ imbalanced flora   ▮ possible pathogen

Metabolic Markers

n-Butyrate (μmoles/gm)	6	0 10 30 ... 100
ß-Glucuronidase (IU/gm)	685	70 ... 1000 ... 2000
pH	7.3	5 6.0 7.2 9

SCFA distribution:

Acetate (54 - 67%)	65	
Propionate (16 - 24%)	21	
Butyrate (14 - 23%)	14	0 25 50 75 100

Immunology

Fecal sIgA (μg/gm)	63	0 22 ... 140 ... 200

Macroscopic

	Optimal	Abnormal	Ref.
Color	Brown		Brown
Mucus	None		None
Occult blood	None		None

Histograms represent idealized data based upon large populations

---

Digestion

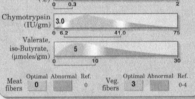

	Optimal	Abnormal	Ref.			Optimal	Abnormal	Ref.
Triglycerides (%)	0.1			0 0.3 ... 2				
Chymotrypsin (IU/gm)	3.0			0 6.2 ... 41.0 ... 75				
Valerate, iso-Butyrate, (μmoles/gm)	5			0 ... 10 ... 30				
Meat fibers	0		0		Veg. fibers	3		0-4

Absorption

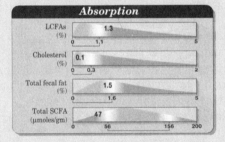

LCFAs (%)	1.3	0 1.1 ... 5
Cholesterol (%)	0.1	0 0.3 ... 2
Total fecal fat (%)	1.5	0 1.6 ... 5
Total SCFA (μmoles/gm)	47	0 56 ... 156 ... 200

■ Chymotrypsin: Levels of this digestive enzyme can indicate the patient's enzyme status. Decreased levels mean the pancreas is not releasing enough enzymes and/or that the stomach is low on digestive acids (needed to activate chymotrypsin). Elevated levels suggest a rapid transit time.

■ Valerate and iso-butyrate: Valerate and iso-butyrate are SCFAs produced

---

Dysbiosis Index

12		
0 OPTIMAL SLIGHT MODERATE 10 SEVERE >10		

when intestinal bacteria ferment protein. Elevated levels indicate that the protein was not digested properly.

■ Meat and vegetable fibers: These are crude markers for digestive function. Elevated levels indicate inadequate chewing, stomach acid, or digestive enzymes.

Measures of Absorption—

■ LCFAs: Long-chain fatty acids are normally absorbed directly by the intestine. Elevated levels reflect malabsorption of fats, a result of maldigestion or inflammation of the lining of the small intestine.

■ Cholesterol: Cholesterol in the feces comes from either dietary fats or the breakdown of the cells lining the intestines. Generally, fecal cholesterol levels remain stable, despite dietary intake; elevated levels suggest malabsorption or irritation.

■ Total fecal fat: This represents the sum of all fats, except for SCFAs, and can indicate either maldigestion or malabsorption.

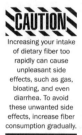

full of moisture. Diets low in fiber cause fecal material to become dry and hard to expel, whereas a diet high in fiber will greatly reduce transit time. Fiber consists of the cell walls of plants and certain indigestible food residues. There are two basic types of fiber: soluble and insoluble. The insoluble fibers are found in wheat and corn bran, whole grains, nuts, legumes, and some vegetables; they increase fecal size and weight and promote regular bowel movements. However, insoluble fibers can also irritate the bowel, especially if it is already inflamed. Soluble fibers are not irritating to the bowel. They are found in fruits and vegetables, oat bran, barley, beans, and peas. Ingesting foods containing these fibers stimulates bowel movements, decreases appetite, and leads to weight loss. Good forms of fiber are powdered psyllium husk, flax seed, guar gum, and apple pectin.

Water—Soluble fiber requires copious amounts of water to carry it to the colon. Without sufficient water, the colon tries to extract every possible drop from the food we eat, which contributes to fecal matter becoming extremely dry and compacted. Adults need at least 8-10 cups of water daily, but few people drink that much. Other liquids, such as milk, coffee, tea, juice, and soda, are not substitutes for pure water. Even if you drink plenty of these other liquids, you need to consume 60-80 ounces of purified water daily.

Probiotics—Whenever you undergo any form of intestinal cleansing, all of the bacteria, both friendly and unfriendly, are washed out. It is therefore important that you repopulate your intestines with friendly bacteria, particularly *Lactobacillus acidophilus* and *Bifidobacterium bifidum*. Cabbage is one of the best food sources of friendly bacteria; eat it raw or juice it daily. Other foods that can help revitalize the colon and encourage the growth of normal bacteria include rice protein, chicory, onions, garlic, asparagus, and bananas. Friendly bacteria are also found in yogurt and kefir (a fermented milk drink). Another way to repopulate the intestines with beneficial bacteria is to take a probiotic supplement.

Colon Cleansing Programs

Increased interest in colon health has led to a surge in the development of colon cleansing programs. Most of these programs utilize a cleansing supplement in addition to recommending a basic dietary program. The supplements generally contain a combination of herbs, nutrients, enzymes, and toxin-absorbers designed to help remove the false lining in the colon and enhance digestion and absorption of food. Many of these supplements include ingredients that also cleanse the liver, gallbladder, and lymph.

A.M./P.M. Ultimate Cleanse™

A.M./P.M. Ultimate Cleanse is a cleansing program designed by Lindsey Duncan, C.N., of Santa Monica, California. The program includes two herbal and fiber formulas called Multi-Herb™ and Multi-Fiber™. The formulas are made from 29 cleansing herbs, amino acids, antioxidants, digestive enzymes, vitamins, and minerals, and five kinds of fiber. Both the Multi-Herb and Multi-Fiber formulas are taken in the morning and evening, in gradually increasing dosages for several weeks. The key to the effectiveness of the formula, Duncan explains, is that of timing: the morning formula stimulates while the evening formula relaxes. Duncan's formulas target not only the bowel, but the liver, lungs, skin, and lymph. "The goal is to stimulate, feed, and detoxify the complete internal body, not just the bowel," states Duncan. At the end of the program, a person should be having two to three bowel movements every day.

Nature's Pure Body Program™

Nature's Pure Body Program is made by the Pure Body Institute of Beverly Hills, California. The program relies on an herbal supplement that is a blend of 27 herbs specifically chosen for their ability to flush toxins out of the organs and old fecal matter from the intestines. The program consists of two sets of pills: colon and whole-body blends. Users start with one colon pill and three whole-body pills taken twice daily with water, 30 minutes before breakfast and 30 minutes before dinner. The colon pills can be increased to three pills twice daily (or more) until the bowels move twice daily. The whole-body pills are increased from three up to 4-7, taken two times daily. Users also need to increase their intake of pure water (at least 64 ounces daily), take one day off from the pills every week, and take a daily multivitamin. The program is designed to last about 30 days. First-time users may find that three courses of the program are required for complete inner cleansing and detoxification.

Cleansing supplements should not be confused with laxatives. The latter are not considered to be a healthy alternative. According to colon hydrotherapist Joyce Koleno, of Cleveland, Ohio, laxatives only stimulate the muscular movement of the colon. But they can also cause dehydration and do nothing to loosen and remove the colon's false lining. Laxatives may also weaken the colon by irritating and over-stimulating it.

For **A.M./P.M. Ultimate Cleanse™**, contact: Nature's Secret, 4 Health Inc., 5485 Conestoga Court, Boulder, CO 80301; tel: 303-546-6306; fax: 303-546-6416. For **Nature's Pure Body Program™**, contact: Pure Body Institute of Beverly Hills, 423 East Ojai Avenue #107, Ojai, CA 93023; tel: 800-952-7873 or 805-653-5448; fax: 805-653-0373.

For more about the **liver and weight gain**, see Chapter 15: Cleanse the Liver, pp. 330-346. For more about the **lymph and weight gain**, see Chapter 16: Get the Lymph Flowing, pp. 348-363.

Cleanse Thyself™: The Arise & Shine Program–Naturopath Richard Anderson, N.D., N.M.D., of Mt. Shasta, California, introduced the Cleanse Thyself self-care colon cleansing program in 1986. This four-phased program enables users to "clean your entire alimentary canal from your tongue to your stomach, to your organs, all the way down to your colon," says Dr. Anderson. Dr. Anderson recommends that the prospective user first test both saliva and urine for pH balance, using pH test papers included in the kit. pH is the degree of acidity and alkalinity of a solution, measured on a scale of 1 (acidic) to 14 (alkaline).

Psyllium Reduces Obesity

Recent research conducted at the University of London has demonstrated that psyllium husks, a type of bulk fiber, causes a reduction in calorie consumption and increased feelings of fullness. A group of female subjects were given 20 grams of psyllium seed granules with 200 ml of water three hours before meal times and again immediately before the meal. Those taking the psyllium consumed an average of 15 grams less fat per day than the group that didn't receive the extra fiber.[12]

The results of the pH test determine what level of the Cleanse Thyself program should be used, from the Mildest Phase to the Master Phase. The Mildest Phase of the Cleanse Thyself program is designed for those whose bodies are weaker, chronically or severely ill, or elderly enough that they need a gentle approach to cleansing, Dr. Anderson explains. "Persons who use the Mildest Phase generally show a severely over-acid condition (which can also appear as over-alkalinity) prior to preparing for cleansing. For such a person, the first step before beginning to cleanse must be to alkalinize so that the body has enough resources to handle cleansing."

Those on the Mildest Phase start with a breakfast of fresh fruit, while their lunch and dinner should emphasize alkaline-forming foods, such as salad greens, raw vegetables, potatoes, and more fresh fruits. The user on this phase also consumes two Cleanse Thyself Shakes, consisting of liquid bentonite (a purifying clay), psyllium husk powder, and pure water. The Master Phase involves fasting from solid foods while taking the supplements along with fresh juices. "The Master Phase should only be attempted by persons whose bodies have already attained an adequate reservoir of electrolytes and strength to handle this level of cleansing," says Dr. Anderson.

To soften and break up toxic waste material while detoxifying, the program provides two customized elements called Chomper and Herbal Nutrition. Chomper is an herbal laxative containing plan-tain, *Cascara sagrada*, barberry, peppermint, sheep sorrel, fennel seed, ginger root, myrrh gum, red raspberry, rhubarb root, golden seal, and lobelia. Herbal Nutrition is a vitamin supplement (containing alfalfa, dandelion, shavegrass, chickweed, marshmallow root, yellow dock, rosehips, hawthorne, licorice root, Irish moss, kelp, amylase, and cellulase) that helps strengthen and nourish the body during detoxification.

Each successive stage in the Cleanse Thyself program involves stricter dietary controls and a higher intake of program supplements and a correspondingly deeper cleansing. Typically, the overall cleansing program takes four weeks, in which three are devoted to the Pre-Cleanse, and one week for the Power or Master Phase. "What took months, years, or a lifetime to create cannot be cleaned up in a week's time," says Dr. Anderson.

Enemas and Colonic Irrigations

Some health-care practitioners recommend using either an enema or colonic irrigation to augment a colon cleansing program. Colon hydrotherapist Joyce Koleno of Cleveland, Ohio, says that colonics should be used at the very beginning of any weight loss or colon cleansing program. An enema involves injecting water into the colon via a small plastic tube inserted into the rectum. The tube is attached to a compressible sack called an enema bag and generally about one cup to one quart of warm water is used. The water flushes out the lower portion of the colon.

A colonic irrigation, also called a colonic or a "high enema," follows a similar procedure; however, it goes further and accomplishes more. A colonic irrigation moves water slowly through the entire length of the colon, so that the waste matter lining the walls of the intestine will soften and detach. To administer a colonic, therapists generally have their patients lie on a treatment table and a specially designed funnel, called a speculum, is inserted into the rectum. Several gallons of water flow in and out of the colon during the irrigation. The therapist monitors the temperature and pressure of the water and also massages the abdomen. A single treatment can take anywhere from 20 to 45 minutes.

You can administer your own colonic irrigation, using a home colonic unit called a Colema Board. The principle and procedure is basically the same as that employed in a clinic, but the device is less

For information about the **Cleanse Thyself**™ program, contact: Arise & Shine, 401 Berry Street, P.O. Box 1439, Mt. Shasta, CA 96067; tel: 916-926-0891 or 800-688-2444; fax: 916-926-8866.

It is common to have physical reactions to the colon cleansing process. These reactions may include headaches, vomiting, diarrhea, fatigue or dizziness. For all the discomfort, this is actually a sign that the process is working and that you are eliminating toxins from your body. If these symptoms occur, you may need to temporarily cut back on your cleansing procedure.

Dietary Guidelines for a Clean Colon

As your colon becomes clean, you will begin to shed pounds. One way to maintain your intestinal health—and keep your weight down—is to follow these simple dietary guidelines:

- Eliminate or significantly reduce your consumption of white sugar, white flour, white rice, and fried foods
- Make 50% of each meal fresh, raw, unprocessed foods
- Chew each mouthful of food 10-20 times
- Do not eat when emotionally upset
- Every day, eat one serving of protein, at least ½ pound each of two different fruits, six different vegetables (including two ounces of raw fresh sprouts), and at least one serving of whole grain
- Vary foods from meal to meal and from day to day
- Eat your largest meal of the day at noon; do not go to sleep on a full stomach
- Drink a minimum of ½ ounce of water per pound of your body weight daily; for example, a 128-pound person needs 64 ounces of water; unsweetened fruit and vegetable juices or herb teas are acceptable
- Drink liquids before and after meals, not with them, to avoid diluting your digestive fluids
- Eliminate or cut back on stimulants like coffee, black teas, colas, chocolate, and alcohol, as well as aspirin and nicotine

high-tech, using a gravity-feed system to supply water rather than a mechanical pump; the unit is designed to fit over a standard toilet. To ensure that your irrigations are proceeding safely, it's always best to obtain guidance from a trained health-care professional.

The number and frequency of irrigation or enema treatments needed will vary, depending on the condition of the colon and the nature of the overall cleansing program. It's not unusual for some people to require 6-18 treatments, which can be given daily or weekly. Your colon therapist should be a trained, licensed professional, though they need not be a doctor.

After the Cleanse

Nutritionist Lindsey Duncan tells his clients that, while a periodic colon cleanse will help improve your digestion and shed unwanted pounds, it's what you do every day that counts. This means eating the right foods, drinking plenty of water, exercising, and managing stressful situations.

While intestinal health depends on the daily consumption of fiber, it is important that you do not use a fiber supplement, or any other aspect of a treatment program, to compensate for a colon-clogging diet. "There is no substitute for a healthy diet," says Dr. Murray. "It is clear from the scientific literature that whole foods provide the best source of dietary fiber."[13]

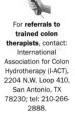

For **referrals to trained colon therapists**, contact: International Association for Colon Hydrotherapy (I-ACT), 2204 N.W. Loop 410, San Antonio, TX 78230; tel: 210-266-2888.

If you have spent most of your life eating foods or engaging in behaviors harmful to the colon, making the necessary changes may be difficult. However, it is important to understand that the lifestyle changes you make may not only end your battle with weight, it may also give you an entirely new outlook. "It may sound odd, but cleansing the bowel can be an inspirational experience," says Dr. Larmer. "Many people have told me that after a cleansing they feel motivated to make a new start in their lives. They have a strong desire to be healthy and stay clean and that outlook provides just the impetus and attitude that's needed for permanent weight control."

Physical Therapies

Chiropractic adjustments can prompt bowel movements. "The waves that move material through the colon occur as a result of nerve excitement which originates at the spinal nerves," explains Dr. Port. Chiropractic adjustments can help normalize the action of the ileocecal valve, the valve that separates the large from the small intestine. If this valve goes into spasms and shuts too tightly, material remains in the small intestine longer than it should, extending transit time.

Massage can help relax the abdominal muscles and encourage normal peristalsis (the wave-like contractions that push food through the intestines), thus helping to prevent the build-up of fecal material. As stress is also a factor in colon problems, massage acts as a "natural tranquilizer" to restore calm and soothe the digestive tract.[14] Another treatment modality often used by alternative medicine practitioners to treat the colon is reflexology (SEE QUICK DEFINITION). Reflexology therapy stimulates organs of the body through gentle pressure applied to the foot. Inge Dougans, a Danish reflexologist, explains that the foot has a reflex influence throughout the body. "Stimulating the areas of the feet has an effect on the internal organs via simple reflex action," she says.[15] The reflex areas for the colon are found on the soles of both feet.

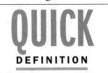

DEFINITION

Reflexology is based on the idea that there are reflex areas in the hands and feet that correspond to every part of the body, including the organs and glands. By applying gentle but precise pressure to these reflex points, reflexologists can release blockages that inhibit energy flow and cause pain and disease.

13 Eliminate Yeast Infections

CANDIDA ALBICANS is a yeast-like fungus normally present in the body. An unhealthy overgrowth of these microbes, however, can result in a variety of conditions and symptoms, including fatigue, migraines, depression, out-of-control food cravings, and weight gain. Because it produces such a wide array of symptoms, yeast overgrowth often goes undetected for years. For many individuals, correctly diagnosing and treating the problem is the key to health and a healthy weight.

Success Story: Eliminating the Yeast for Weight Loss

Darlene, 56, had dealt with a variety of health and weight problems most of her life. She often caught colds, had recurring vaginal yeast

infections, and hypoglycemia (a blood-sugar disorder). Although Darlene had managed to maintain her weight between 120 pounds and 140 pounds through her thirties, she began gaining weight rapidly when she turned 44, reaching 200 pounds within a year—a considerable weight for her 5'2" frame. She also became very weak and tired, had muscle pain throughout her body, experienced regular bouts of nausea, and had to use a wheelchair to get around.

"I saw more doctors than I can count, was tested at two major medical centers, and took eleven experimental drugs," she said. "Nothing helped." At the recommendation of a friend, Darlene went to William G. Crook, M.D., based in Jackson, Tennessee, author of *The Yeast Connection and the Woman.* Upon hearing her symptoms, Dr. Crook told Darlene that she had a type of yeast growing in her intestine called *Candida albicans.* He immediately put her on a special diet and gave her medication (nystatin) to kill the yeast.

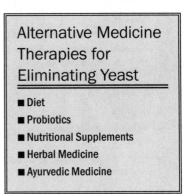

Alternative Medicine Therapies for Eliminating Yeast

■ Diet
■ Probiotics
■ Nutritional Supplements
■ Herbal Medicine
■ Ayurvedic Medicine

"Within a couple of weeks, all my nausea was gone," Darlene reports. "A year after my treatment began, I'd lost 70 pounds." Darlene's weight stabilized at 119 pounds, which is how much she still weighs today, more than ten years after beginning her treatment. "I feel good, almost never catch a cold, and my blood sugar is under control," she said. "If you could have seen me then and see me now, you'd never know I was the same person."

What's Yeast Got to Do With It?

Had it not been for Dr. Crook's diagnosis and treatment, Darlene's condition would have continued to deteriorate. She might have ended up like many other thousands of people, forever struggling with a weight problem and suffering from symptoms that their doctors failed to understand or effectively treat. Destroying the yeast that had bloomed in her intestines was the key to restoring Darlene's health. Doctors regularly treat women for localized yeast infections in the vaginal tract, but many do not consider that these same yeasts are able to cause illnesses in other parts of the body.

"Yeast overgrowth in the gastrointestinal tract is not understood or accepted by most members of my profession," says Robert Waters, M.D., of the Waters Preventive Medical Center in Dells, Wisconsin. "This is primarily because we don't learn anything about it in medical school and are slow to adopt new ideas." Nevertheless, an increasing number of doctors are discovering that weight problems can be the result of a *Candida* infection (a condition called candidiasis).

Recognizing Candidiasis

Candidiasis can cause a wide array of symptoms, including the following:

- Chronic fatigue
- Weight gain
- Depression, anxiety, and irritability
- Hyperactivity, confusion, and loss of memory
- Gastrointestinal problems, such as bloating, gas, intestinal cramps, chronic diarrhea, constipation, or heartburn
- Allergies (to both food and airborne allergens)
- Severe premenstrual syndrome (PMS)
- Sexual dysfunction and loss of sexual interest
- Memory loss, severe mood swings, and feeling mentally "disturbed"
- Recurrent fungal infections (such as "jock itch," athlete's foot, or ringworm) or vaginal/urinary infections
- A feeling of being lightheaded or drunk after minimal wine, beer, or certain foods
- Rashes, hives, acne, and scaly skin
- Respiratory problems, including asthma and nasal or lung congestion
- Sinus pressure, hay fever–like attacks, and coughing
- Eye or ear irritation
- Migraines and headaches
- Sleep disturbances
- Heart palpitations

Dr. Crook says that *Candida* treatments offer hope for a large number of overweight individuals. And, unlike mainstream weight-loss treatments, the results are often permanent. "Many of my overweight patients have found that a comprehensive *Candida* treatment program has enabled them to lose weight and keep it off," he says. In this chapter, we explain the symptoms and causes of yeast infections and their direct connection to weight problems. We review the diagnostic tests that determine if you have a yeast problem, and offer effective treatment options to rid yourself of *Candida* and restore your body—and weight—to a proper balance.

The Yeast Connection

A yeast is a type of single-celled organism found throughout nature—in the soil, on vegetables and fruits, and in the human body. *Candida albicans* is a very common variety of yeast, frequently present in small quantities in the intestines and in a woman's vagina. It is not harmful under normal conditions (that is, when its numbers are few), but it can cause considerable damage when its colonies grow and multiply. *Candida* then becomes pathogenic, transforming from a simple yeast into an aggressive fungus.

This potential for mutating from a benign organism to a pathogenic one is why Dr. Crook describes

Candida as a kind of microbiological "Dr. Jekyll and Mr. Hyde." Candidiasis causes a lengthy and diverse list of allergic reactions, which makes it particularly difficult to diagnose. The symptoms can range from skin rashes, fatigue, and digestive difficulties to joint pains, food cravings, and emotional problems (see "Recognizing Candidiasis," p. 296).[1]

According to Stephen Langer, M.D., author of *Solved: The Riddle of Weight Loss*, one classic symptom of candidiasis, particularly in women, is excess body weight.[2] He indicates that the weight gain from candidiasis can range between 15 pounds and 50 pounds. A *Candida* infection may cause you to gain weight in several ways: it lowers metabolism, creates food allergies and sugar cravings, interferes with the digestion of sugars, and increases fatigue.

For more about the thyroid and body weight, see Chapter 9: Overcome a Sluggish Thyroid, pp. 202-219. For more about food allergies and addictions, see Chapter 11: Break Food Allergies and Addictions, pp. 244-270.

Metabolism—*Candida* can affect the thyroid gland, the endocrine gland that is primarily responsible for controlling metabolism, the rate at which the body uses energy. A yeast infection interferes with the body's ability to use thyroid hormones and may even block the hormones from entering cells. This leads to many of the symptoms associated with hypothyroidism (low thyroid function), including feelings of sluggishness, cold extremities and low body temperature, and depression. The thyroid hormones regulate how the body burns calories from food—when their effectiveness is impaired, the excess calories are stored as fat, resulting in weight gain.[3]

Food Allergies—*Candida* can also cause a person to develop food allergies, according to James Braly, M.D., medical director of Immuno Laboratories in Fort Lauderdale, Florida, by burrowing into and damaging the intestinal lining.[4] This may cause breaches in the lining, allowing food particles to seep out of the intestines and into the bloodstream (a condition known as leaky gut syndrome). Dr. Braly says that the immune system responds to these particles of partially digested food as if they were foreign material (such as a virus) and produces antibodies to fight off the invaders.

Food allergies can lead to weight gain by slowing the body's metabolic rate. They can also trigger the overproduction of insulin, the hormone that controls blood sugar levels; a blood sugar imbalance (hypoglycemia) can potentially result in significant weight gain. Allergies may also cause food-bingeing behavior, bloating (fluid retention), cravings (particularly carbohydrates and sugars), and food addictions, all significant in terms of weight gain.

For more information about **blood sugar** problems and how they contribute to **weight gain**, see Chapter 8: Strengthen Your Sugar Controls, pp. 184-201.

Sugar Balance—*Candida* is also known to interfere with the body's ability to use sugar as an energy source. Toxins excreted by *Candida* organisms block the ability of sugar to be absorbed by the cells of the body. When these sugars cannot get into the cells, the body converts and stores them as fat. At the same time, the body starts to develop intense sugar cravings and the person may then binge on carbohydrates. The excess insulin released to deal with the elevated levels of sugar in the blood interferes with your body's ability to break down and burn fat, another factor in weight gain.[5]

Fatigue—One of the common symptoms of candidiasis is fatigue, often resulting in reduced exercise levels among its sufferers. This may be due to the fact that *Candida* interferes with the body's ability to extract energy from fats and sugars or to reduced thyroid function. *Candida* may also interfere with the body's ability to get oxygen into and waste materials out of muscle cells during exercise, leading to muscle aches and stiffness. Whatever the exact cause, those with candidiasis generally do not get enough exercise—lack of exercise is a contributing factor in obesity.

What Causes *Candida* Infections?

Candida infections were rare as recently as a generation ago, but now the illness is relatively commonplace, affecting the health of one in three individuals. That's why Jack Tips, N.D., Ph.D., a naturopath, nutritionist, and educator based in Austin, Texas, calls *Candida* "the plague of the late 20th century."[6] Why the increase in *Candida* infections? According to Dr. Langer, the widespread use of antibiotics, frequent high doses of cortisone (a steroid used to treat arthritis and other conditions), and increased levels of refined starches and sugars in the diet have all contributed to the proliferation of candidiasis. Several other factors may also be responsible, including the more common occurence of diabetes, use of the birth-control pill, chemotherapy and radiation, stress, and overeating.[7]

Antiobiotics—Antibiotics are considered to be the prime cause. In a healthy individual, *Candida* competes with and is held in check by the presence of beneficial bacteria (*Lactobacillus acidophilus*, *Bifidobacterium bifidum*, and others) that live in the intestinal tract. However, these healthy bacteria are destroyed by antibiotics. When this occurs, the *Candida* yeast may quickly take advantage of the situation, multiplying and filling the void left by the beneficial bacteria.

Dr. Waters says that physicians are often too quick to dispense antibiotics to their patients. He remarks that he only learned about the harmful effects of antibiotics after observing how it affected his patients. "I saw that the antibiotics often made things worse, clearing up one problem while creating new ones," he says. "I was not taught in medical school about the dangers of antibiotic therapy and the need to repopulate the intestinal tract with healthy bacteria." Dr. Waters recognizes that antibiotics play an important role in controlling infections and saving lives, but he cautions that they must be used judiciously and consideration must always be given to restoring the healthy intestinal ecology that they disrupt.

In addition to medications, we are also exposed to antibiotics and other drugs in the meats and other animal products we consume. Antibiotics and steroids are fed to livestock in large quantities to prevent infection and stimulate growth. "If you eat a lot of meat that contains even traces of antibiotics, you may develop a bacteria-yeast imbalance in your intestines," according to Dennis Remington, M.D., and Barbara Higa Swasey, R.D., authors of *Back To Health*.[9]

It's Not Just in Your Head

Individuals who suffer from a *Candida* infection sometimes have a sense that they are not themselves, that something is seriously wrong. Unfortunately, their doctors often cannot find a physical cause and send them home without an adequate diagnosis. Because these patients suffer from depression, anxiety, and moodiness—all symptoms of candidiasis—they are often told that their ailments are psychological in origin. Many doctors will prescribe antidepressant medications and recommend a psychiatrist or therapist.

C. Orian Truss, M.D., of Birmingham, Alabama, a *Candida* expert and author of *The Missing Diagnosis*, says that chronic candidiasis is almost always labeled psychosomatic and treated as a nervous disorder. "Yeast may lead to such a variety of symptoms that the condition is easily confused with illnesses that are psychological in nature," he says. "This has resulted in the heavily disproportionate application of psychiatric methods of treatment in patients whose only psychological problems are those that have been brought on by the failure of the medical profession to correct their long-standing, frustrating illnesses."[8]

Dietary Factors—Milk and dairy products also carry traces of antibiotics, but milk should be avoided for another reason: it contains lactose, a type of sugar that promotes *Candida* growth. Other foods that promote candidiasis are those that contain molds or yeasts, such as

Candida and Gender

Approximately 75% of *Candida* sufferers are women, or about eight women for every man who has *Candida*. Hormonal fluctuations during pregnancy and a woman's monthly cycle (menstruation) are considered to be responsible for the higher *Candida* incidence. Although exactly how these fluctuations aggravate *Candida* is not known, most alternative medicine practitioners agree that the problem is linked to imbalances between progesterone and estrogen, two hormones produced in a woman's ovaries.[13]

Birth control pills and hormone therapy for menopause also make women's bodies more vulnerable to *Candida* infestations, according to Ralph Golan, M.D., author of *Optimal Wellness*.[14] Another less obvious con-

For more information about **hormonal imbalances and weight gain**, see Chapter 10: Restore Hormonal Balance, pp. 220-243.

tributor to *Candida* in women may be how often women see their doctors. Women visit their doctors far more often than men for routine checkups, Pap smears, pregnancy, and other reasons, and consequently are more likely to receive medications, particularly antibiotics. These medications can contribute to *Candida* overgrowth.[15]

Despite the greater prevalence in women, men should not think themselves immune to *Candida*. It is important to note that the statistics showing *Candida* to be more prevalent in women are based on numbers of reported cases—because men generally visit their doctors less often than women, male *Candida* may be a seriously under-diagnosed and under-reported disease.

---

alcoholic beverages, breads and pastries, cheeses, dried fruits, and peanuts. However, not all the experts agree that it is necessary to eliminate yeasted foods. They maintain that some foods with yeast—commercially prepared breads and rolls, pastries, and doughnuts—also contain sugar and/or white, processed flour. White flour and sugar are converted into simple sugars (monosaccharides) in the body, the food of choice for yeast. These substances, and not yeast, may be responsible for the *Candida* overgrowth.

Many of your food choices may be contributing to yeast problems. The standard American diet now contains higher amounts of refined carbohydrates and sugar than ever before—in breads, pasta, pastries, potato chips, desserts, candy, sodas, and junk foods. High-carbohydrate diets provide plenty of sugars in the body, which support the growth of *Candida*.[10]

Other Factors—Environmental factors can also contribute to candidiasis. Damp environments, like musty or moldy basements, may encourage yeast growth. Also, regions with rainy climates tend to have a higher incidence of *Candida*, according to Ann Louise Gittleman, M.S., of Bozeman, Montana, author of *Supernutrition for Women*.[11] Exposure to environmental pollutants, such as pesticide residues, car exhaust, industrial chemicals, and heavy metals (particularly from mercury amalgam fillings), may foster the growth of *Candida* as well.[12]

Diagnosing Candidiasis

Candidiasis causes systemic illnesses that produce a wide variety of symptoms. This makes candidiasis difficult to accurately diagnose, since it shares symptoms with so many other conditions. Leon Chaitow, N.D., D.O., of London, England, notes that when symptoms are chronic rather than acute or sudden, he generally suspects a yeast infection. Another clue is if specific symptoms have been previously treated without success, then the diagnosis usually suggests candidiasis.

Some physicians rely on laboratory test results to diagnose the condition. However, while these tests are helpful, it is important not to depend on them exclusively. For example, blood tests can be used to pinpoint *Candida* antibodies. But since most people normally have *Candida* organisms in their systems, the tests may show antibodies even if the patient is not suffering from candidiasis. The truth is there is no single diagnostic test. Dr. Langer indicates that "the clincher to any diagnosis is not so much what is happening in the laboratory as what is happening in the patient." The combination of an individual's complete medical history and examination, the patient's response to treatment, and information culled from laboratory tests is the key to a correct diagnosis.[16]

Are You a Candidate for Candidiasis?

Dr. Chaitow describes the likely candidate for *Candida* overgrowth as someone whose medical history includes steroid hormone medications (cortisone or corticosteroids, often prescribed for skin conditions such as rashes, eczema, or psoriasis), prolonged or repeated use of antibiotics, medications for treating ulcers, or oral contraceptives. Certain illnesses, such as diabetes, cancer, and AIDS, can also increase susceptibility to *Candida* overgrowth.

"All too often more than one influence is operating," says Dr. Chaitow. "Over a few years, a patient may have had antibiotics for a variety of conditions, while using steroids as well, perhaps in the form of the contraceptive pill. If the patient also happens to be living on a diet rich in sugars, then the *Candida* is very likely to have spread beyond its usual borders into new territory."[17]

A qualified practitioner should take a complete medical history to determine if you have a *Candida* infection, but here are a few questions to ask yourself to see if you are at risk (the more questions that you answer affirmatively, the greater your risk):

■ Have you taken repeated courses of antibiotics or steroids (e.g., cortisone)?

■ Have you used birth-control pills?

■ Have you had repeated fungal infections ("jock itch," athlete's foot, ringworm)?

■ Do you regularly have any of these symptoms—bloating, headaches, depression, fatigue, memory problems, impotence or lack of interest in sex, muscle aches with no apparent cause, brain fogginess?

■ Do you experience symptoms of PMS (pre-menstrual syndrome)?

■ Do you have cravings for sweets, products containing white flour, or alcoholic beverages?

■ Do you repeatedly experience any of these health difficulties—inappropriate drowsiness, mood swings, rashes, bad breath, dry mouth, post-nasal drip or nasal congestion, heartburn, urinary frequency or urgency?[18]

Blood Tests

Blood tests can look for *Candida* antibodies (SEE QUICK DEFINITION) in the body. When *Candida* assumes its fungal form, the immune system responds by producing special antibodies to fight off the infection. Consequently, if a large concentration of these antibodies are found in the blood, you may be experiencing a *Candida* outbreak. Dr. Langer notes that "if the yeast antibodies are elevated and the test is positive, the yeast infection is active and threatening."[19] However, as noted earlier, the antibody test may be misleading, because most individuals normally have *Candida* in their bodies. The Anti-Candida Antibodies Panel, from Great Smokies Diagnostic Laboratory, in Asheville, North Carolina, is a blood test that measures the levels of antibodies (specifically, the immunoglobulins IgG and IgM) against *Candida*. The IgG levels indicate both past and ongoing infection, while the IgM level may be a truer reflection of present infection.

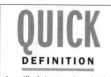

QUICK

DEFINITION

An **antibody** is a protein molecule made by white blood cells in the lymph tissue and activated by the immune system against specific foreign proteins (antigens). An antibody, also referred to as an immunoglobulin, binds to the antigen as a preliminary for destroying it.

The blood can also be examined visually using a darkfield microscope to detect the presence of the *Candida* fungus. Darkfield microscopy is a way of studying living whole blood cells under a specially adapted microscope that projects the image (magnified 1,400 times) onto a video screen. The skilled physician can detect early signs of illness in the form of microorganisms in the blood known to produce disease. Specifically, darkfield microscopy reveals distortions of red blood cells (which indicates nutritional status), possible undesirable bacterial or fungal life forms (like *Candida*), and other blood ecology patterns indicative of health or illness.[20]

Stool Analysis

Another test used to diagnose candidiasis is a stool analysis, which can help assess digestive function through laboratory examination of a stool sample. The Great Smokies Comprehensive Digestive Stool Analysis (CDSA) can measure how much yeast is actually present in the intestines. If the stool contains abnormally large amounts of *Candida*, this may indicate candidiasis. The CDSA can also look at levels of beneficial bacteria in the intestines as well as other digestive markers for determining *Candida* levels. Another stool analysis test, the Yeast Screen-Candascan, from Diagnos-Techs, Inc., measures levels of all types of yeast, including *Candida*.

For more about the **Comprehensive Digestive Stool Analysis**, see Chapter 12: Detoxify the Colon, pp. 272-293.

Electrodermal Screening

Electrodermal screening (EDS) is a form of computerized information gathering that can be used to identify the presence of *Candida*. EDS works by placing a blunt, noninvasive electric probe at specific points on the patient's hands, face, or feet, corresponding to acupuncture points at the beginning or end of energy meridians. Minute electrical discharges from these points serve as information signals about the condition of the body's organs and systems, useful for the physician in evaluation and developing a treatment plan. Using EDS, the trained practitioner conducts an "interview" with the patient's organs and tissues, gathering information about the basic functional status of those systems.

For the **Anti-Candida Antibodies Panel** and **Comprehensive Digestive Stool Analysis**, contact: Great Smokies Diagnostic Laboratory, 63 Zillicoa Street, Asheville, NC 28801; tel: 800-522-4762 or 704-253-0621; fax: 704-252-9303. For the **Yeast Screen-Candascan**, contact: Diagnos-Techs, Inc., 6620 South 192nd Place, J-104, Kent, WA 98032; tel: 800-878-3787 or 425-251-0596; fax: 425-251-0637. For **electrodermal screening**, contact: Occidental Institute Research Foundation, P.O. Box 100, Penticton, B.C., Canada V2A 6J9; tel: 604-497-6020; fax: 604-497-6030.

Alternative Medicine Therapies for Eliminating Yeast

One way that conventional doctors treat their patients for candidiasis is to simply prescribe anti-fungal drugs such as nystatin, ketoconazol, and Diflucan®. However, these drugs should be used as a last resort rather than a first line of defense. Naturopath Michael Murray, N.D., of Bellevue, Washington, author of *A Textbook of Natural Medicine*, says that "a comprehensive approach is more effective in treating chronic candidiasis than simply trying to kill the *Candida* with a drug or natural anti-*Candida* agent."[21] The problem with just using drugs is that they fail to address the underlying factors that promote *Candida* overgrowth. Alternative medicine physicians employ a comprehensive approach for treating candidiasis, which includes diet, probiotics, nutritional supplements, herbal medicine, and Ayurvedic medicine.

Diet

Avoidance of certain foods is important for both treating and preventing *Candida* overgrowth. While an anti-yeast diet can keep *Candida* at bay and help people feel better, it is not a cure. Nevertheless, proper diet does contribute to repairing the damage *Candida* has likely caused and helps minimize the chance of flare-ups. It is best to always combine dietary prescriptions with the other elements of an anti-fungal treatment program.

Yeast thrives on sugar, so to overcome candidiasis, sugar must be avoided in all its various forms. These include sucrose, dextrose, fructose, fruit juices, honey, maple syrup, molasses, milk products (which contain lactose), most fruit (except berries), and potatoes (their starch converts into sugar). Candidiasis patients should also stay away from all alcohol, since it is composed of fermented and refined sugar. "In treating candidiasis, my basic dietary taboos are sweets, alcohol, and refined carbohydrates," reports Leyardia Black, N.D., of Lopez Island, Washington.

Meat, dairy, and poultry consumption can also foster *Candida* growth because of the large amount of antibiotics used on the animals. Traces of antibiotics given to dairy cows can later show up in milk. Organic (hormone- and antibiotic-free) meat and poultry should be consumed as a substitute. For those with candidiasis, seafood (free of mercury toxins) and vegetable protein are preferable, since they are not only antibiotic-free, but lower in fat.

Many candidiasis sufferers have allergies or sensitivities to various foods. Although *Candida albicans* yeast is not synonymous with the yeasts found in certain foods, such as breads, a cross-reaction between food yeast and *Candida* frequently occurs. As a result, foods containing or promoting yeast (such as baked goods, alcohol, and vinegar) should be avoided until possible sensitivities are clearly diagnosed.

Molds are another aspect of *Candida* sensitivity, according to Murray Susser, M.D. These include food molds (found in cheeses, grapes, mushrooms, and fermented foods) and environmental molds (found in wet climates, in damp basements, in plants, and outdoors). Mold and yeast can exchange forms; therefore, avoid the ingestible molds of cheeses and fermented foods. Avoiding food yeast and mold does not treat the *Candida* yeast itself, but it can ease stress on the immune system caused by allergenic substances.[22] Even so, food yeast and mold avoidance should be considered on an individual basis. As Dr. Susser says, "My personal opinion is that most anti-*Candida* diets are too strict. It is unnecessary to take *Candida* patients off vinegar and mushrooms unless they are allergic to these things."

Dr. Susser advises patients to avoid yogurt because of its high sugar content, despite its concentration of *Lactobacilli*, which suppress unhealthy bacteria in the intestines and keep other organisms (like *Candida*) under control. He finds that freeze-dried *L. acidophilus* supplements in capsule form are more effective in promoting healthy bacteria than even unsweetened raw yogurt.

Probiotics

Every anti-fungal treatment for candidiasis will reduce the numbers of "friendly" bacteria that inhabit the intestines. In the long run, a healthy growth of these bacteria—particularly *L. acidophilus* and *B. bifidum*—is the best defense against yeast infections. Cabbage is one of the best food sources of friendly bacteria; eat it raw or juice it daily. Other foods that can help revitalize the colon and encourage the growth of normal bacteria include rice protein, chicory, onions, garlic, asparagus, and bananas. *B. bifidum* is also found in yogurt and kefir (a fermented milk drink). Another way to repopulate the intestines with friendly bacteria is to take a probiotic supplement, particularly one containing *L. acidophilus* and *B. bifidum*.

Another useful supplement is FOS (fructo-oligosaccharide), a sugar that specifically encourages friendly bacteria to multiply. FOS acts like an intestinal "fertilizer," selectively feeding the healthy microflora in the large intestine so that their numbers can usefully increase. FOS is found

A Diet to Rid Yourself of *Candida*

Acupuncturist and psychologist Jacqueline Young makes the following dietary recommendations to eliminate *Candida*:

Eliminate for at least one month:

- All foods containing yeast, including bread, biscuits, and cakes
- All fermented foods, such as vinegar, soy sauce, and pickled foods
- All forms of sugar and products containing sugar, including sweets, chocolate, honey, maple syrup, sweetened drinks, and sweetened yogurt
- Milk and dairy products
- All refined white flour products
- Alcohol, tea, and coffee
- Foods with artificial sweeteners, colorings, preservatives, and additives

Include these foods:

- Fresh vegetables and salads
- Whole grains—unlike processed white flour, whole grains (such as rye or millet) do not produce much sugar in the intestinal tract; as these grains are digested, they are converted into polysaccharides (long-chain sugar molecules), which do not stimulate the growth of yeast organisms
- Garlic—crushed or finely sliced on salads or vegetables
- Olive oil—extra virgin, cold-pressed olive oil should be the only oil used
- Fresh fruits—only moderate amounts of fruit should be eaten; eliminate them completely from the diet for the first week due to high sugar content, then limit to two fruits per day; avoid sweet varieties and all citrus fruits.[23]

in small amounts in garlic, honey, Jerusalem artichokes, soybeans, burdock, chicory root, asparagus, banana, rye, barley, tomato, onions, and triticale. NutraFlora®, a FOS supplement found in most health food stores, contains 95% pure FOS to be used as a dietary supplement.

Nutritional Supplements

As routine supplementation for treatment of candidiasis, Dr. Braly offers the following regimen:

- Vitamin C (8-10 g daily)
- Vitamin E (400 IU daily)
- Evening primrose oil (6-8 capsules daily)
- Max EPA (six capsules daily)
- Pantothenic acid (250 mg daily)
- Taurine (500-1,000 mg daily)
- Zinc chelate (25-50 mg daily)
- Goldenseal root extract with no less than 5% hydrastine (250 mg twice daily)
- *Lactobacillus acidophilus* (one dry teaspoon, three times daily; if allergic to milk, use non-lactose *acidophilus*)

■ Dr. Braly also recommends supplementation with hydrochloric acid (HCl), the primary digestive acid in the stomach. He notes that aging, alcohol abuse, food allergies, and nutrient deficiencies create a lack of HCl in the stomach, which prevents food from being completely digested and permits *Candida* overgrowth. Supplementation, he says, helps restore the proper balance of intestinal flora. Dr. Braly typically recommends one capsule containing betaine hydrochloride and pepsin (a stomach enzyme) at the start of meals, increasing cautiously up to 2-4 capsules with each meal, if needed.

People who are taking nonsteroidal, anti-inflammatory drugs (NSAIDs), like cortisone or aspirin, should not take additional betaine hydrochloride, as it could cause ulcers. Hydrochloric acid supplementation should be done under medical supervision.

Enzyme Therapy—Lita Lee, Ph.D., an enzyme therapist based in Lowell, Oregon, uses plant enzyme supplements to treat yeast overgrowth. Many of her candidiasis patients come to her after unsuccessfully trying nystatin, probiotics, homeopathics, fatty acid supplementation, and various herbs. "Certain cellulose enzymes will digest the common kinds of yeast, whereas other yeasts sometimes yield to amylase enzymes," reports Dr. Lee. She uses a probiotic formula and cellulose enzymes to digest yeast and reestablish friendly bowel bacteria.

For **FOS** and **NutraFlora**, contact: Nutrition Company, 1400 W. 122nd Avenue, Suite 110, Westminster, CO 80234; tel: 303-254-8012; fax: 303-254-8201. For **UltraFlora Plus** and **Probioplex**, two FOS supplements contact: Metagenics APN, 4403 Vineland Road, Suite B10, Orlando, FL 32811; tel: 800- 647-6100.

Garlic—Garlic, a well-known folk remedy, is now formulated as an odorless extract called allicin. Allicin is the active ingredient in garlic, and has been found to be more potent than many other anti-fungal agents; a typical recommended dose is 4,000 mcg daily (equal to about one clove of fresh garlic). As an alternative to the garlic extract, you can also take either liquid garlic (available at health food stores) or fresh garlic cloves.

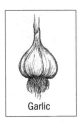

Garlic

Caprylic Acid—Caprylic acid is a naturally occurring fatty acid found in coconut oil that has been shown to be an effective anti-fungal. In one study, patients taking 3,600 mg of caprylic acid daily for two weeks completely eliminated their *Candida*.[24] Dr. Murray typically recommends a dosage of 1,000-2,000 mg daily, taken with meals.[25] Since caprylic acid is readily absorbed into the system, it should be taken in an enteric-coated or sustained-release form so that it is absorbed in the small intestines rather than the stomach. Other fatty acids derived from olives (oleic acid) and castor beans have also been found to be useful for treating candidiasis.

Chlorophyll— Chlorophyll is an excellent liver purifier that is also effective in reducing *Candida*. Naturopath Bernard Jensen, Ph.D., author of *Chlorella, Jewel of the Far East,* considers chlorella (a food algae) as the best source of chlorophyll. He indicates that chlorella can heal a toxic liver, soothe bowel tissue, and stimulate bowel function; a typical dose is 100 mg of chlorella daily.[26] Other sources of chlorophyll are barley juice, wheat grass juice, and spirulina (available at most health food stores).

Whey Globulin Extract— Whey globulin, a type of protein derived from milk, has an antibiotic effect that helps to eliminate yeast from the intestines. Taken orally, these proteins also help flush dead yeast organisms from the body by chemically binding to them so that they can be more easily eliminated.

Aloe Vera Juice— The juice and gel from this cactus-like plant has been used for centuries to treat a host of conditions and medical research is now confirming aloe's healing benefits. Studies have shown that aloe is helpful in detoxifying the bowel, neutralizing stomach acidity, and reducing populations of certain microorganisms, including yeasts.[27]

Herbal Medicine

Herbs are often used by alternative medicine practitioners to kill harmful yeasts and enhance immune function. They can be taken in teas, dried in capsules or tablets, or in suppository form. Dr. Murray recommends an anti-fungal agent consisting of a preparation of oregano, thyme, peppermint, and rosemary oils (0.2-0.4 ml twice daily between meals). Dr. Murray also recommends taking barberry (*Berberis vulgaris*) or Oregon grape (*Berberis aquifolium*). These herbs contain berberine, a natural antibiotic that acts against *Candida* overgrowth, normalizes intestinal flora, helps digestive problems, has antidiarrheal properties, and stimulates the immune system. He usually recommends taking these herbs three times daily as a tea (2-4 g), tincture (6-12 ml), fluid extract (2-4 ml), or powdered solid (250-500 mg).

Berberine-containing plants are generally nontoxic at recommended dosages, but high doses can interfere with vitamin B metabolism. They are not recommended for use by pregnant women.

For **SuperGarlic 3X** and **whey globulin** (in Probioplex; available only to health-care professionals), contact: Metagenics, Inc., 971 Calle Negocio, San Clemente, CA 92673; tel: 800-877-1703; fax: 949-366-0818. For **Caprylate Complex** (caprylic acid), contact: Progressive Labs, 1907 N. Britain Road, Irving, TX 75061; tel: 800-527-9512. For **Candimycin** (oregano, thyme, peppermint, and rosemary oils), contact: PhytoPharmica, P.O. Box 1745, Green Bay, WI 54305; tel: 800-376-7889 or 920-469-9099; fax: 920-469-4418. For **ADP** (another preparation of oregano, thyme, peppermint, and rosemary oils), contact: Biotics Research, P.O. Box 36888, Houston, TX 77236; tel: 800-231-5777; fax: 281-240-2304. For **Triple Yeast Defense** (pau d'arco and grapefruit seed extract), contact: Imhotep, Inc., P.O. Box 183, Main Street, Ruby, NY 12475; tel: 800-677-8577; fax: 914-336-5446.

Dr. Braly recommends goldenseal root extract, standardized to 5% or more of its active ingredient (hydrastine), at a dose of 250 mg twice daily. In a recent study, goldenseal worked better in killing off *Candida* than other common anti-*Candida* therapies, according to Dr. Braly. Pau d'arco is another herb that has long been used to treat infections and intestinal complaints and is reportedly an analgesic, antiviral, diuretic, and fungicide. This South American herb, also known as taheebo, is often prepared as a tea. Other anti-fungal and antibacterial herbs used to treat candidiasis include German chamomile, ginger, cinnamon, rosemary, licorice, and gentian.[28]

Ayurvedic Medicine

Ayurvedic medicine (SEE QUICK DEFINITION) considers candidiasis to be a condition caused by *ama*, the improper digestion of foods, according to Virender Sodhi, M.D. (Ayurveda), N.D., of Bellevue, Washington. As do other alternative physicians, Dr. Sodhi attributes this malfunction, and thus candidiasis, to the widespread use of antibiotics, birth-control pills and hormones, environmental stress, and society's addiction to sugar in the diet. "Ayurvedic medicine believes that these stresses on the system cause carbohydrates to be digested improperly," he says. "Furthermore, the immune system in the gut becomes worn down."

To address the *Candida* overgrowth and bolster immunity, Dr. Sodhi uses grapefruit seed oil and tannic acid, which act as anti-fungals and antibiotics, while *L. acidophilus* helps restore the balance of friendly bacteria in the intestines. Long pepper, ginger, cayenne, and the Ayurvedic herbs trikatu and neem, taken 30 minutes before meals, increase immune and digestive functions. He further recommends that his patients cleanse toxins from their systems using the pancha karma program, which involves herbs and dietary modification. With Dr. Sodhi's approach, candidiasis can usually be eliminated in four to six months.

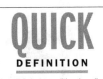

DEFINITION

Ayurveda is the traditional medicine of India, based on many centuries of empirical use. Its name means "end of the Vedas" (which were India's sacred texts), implying that a holistic medicine may be founded on spiritual principles. Ayurveda describes three metabolic, constitutional, and body types (*doshas*), in association with the basic elements of Nature in combination. These are *vata* (air and ether, rooted in intestines), *pitta* (fire and water/stomach), and *kapha* (water and earth/lungs). Ayurvedic physicians use these categories as the basis for prescribing individualized formulas of herbs, diet, massage, breathing, meditation, exercise, and detoxification techniques.

Virender Sodhi, M.D., N.D.: 2115 112th Avenue NE, Bellevue, WA 98004; tel: 425-453-8022; fax: 425-451-2670.

Eradicate Parasites

PARASITE INFECTIONS are often thought to cause weight loss, but the truth is that they can also be behind chronic obesity. Easily spread from person to person and through contaminated food and water, harmful parasites cause our bodies to lose their biological balance by secreting toxins and damaging vital organs. This invasion of parasites and subsequent imbalance throughout the body may lead to significant weight gain.

A complicating factor of a parasitic infection is that most people who have parasites don't know it. But what you don't know most definitely can hurt you. Parasites are probably much more common than you think and their invasion of the body may be a factor in a host of health problems, from cancer to chronic fatigue to weight problems. "Americans today are host to more than 130 different kinds of parasites," says nutritionist Ann Louise Gittleman, M.S., C.N.S., author of *Guess What Came to Dinner: Parasites and Your Health*. These parasites can range in size from microscopic single-cell protozoa to tapeworms up to 15 feet long. Although many may regard parasite infections as a problem of developing nations, the truth, according to the U.S. Centers for Disease Control, is that one in six Americans is host to a parasite.[1]

While such a high prevalence is news to most individuals, what is even less well-known is that parasites can also make you fat. In this chapter, we show the ways that parasites can contribute to weight problems. We look at the various ways you may be vulnerable to a parasite infection and what tests are useful to determine if you have parasites. Finally, we offer effective alternative treatments for eliminating the parasitic invaders from your body.

Success Story: Killing Parasites Reverses Weight Gain

"As I got older and less active, I started gaining weight," says George, 79. George's weight constantly fluctuated and, at one time, reached as high as 200 pounds. Dieting eventually helped him lose some weight, but even after losing weight, George still had a distended abdomen, which was firm to the touch. "I looked fat," he says, "even though I wasn't fat according to the scale."

George consulted nutritionist Gittleman with his concerns about his body shape. She immediately suspected parasites. Subsequent stool tests confirmed George was harboring a tapeworm in his intestines. George speculated that the infection may have been from eating sushi, as raw fish is a potential source of parasites. Gittleman prescribed a 4-week herbal anti-parasite program. She recommended a formula containing black walnut hulls, wormwood, *Cascara sagrada*, slippery elm, garlic, and cloves, designed to expel the parasites from the body. After two weeks, George's bloated stomach started to soften and, two weeks later, it disappeared completely.

"I never actually did see any worms," he says, "but I sure did see my gut melt away." After four weeks, George's waistline began to flatten and his weight stabilized at his normal level of 165 pounds.

> **Alternative Medicine Therapies for Eradicating Parasites**
>
> - Detoxification
> - Dietary Recommendations
> - Probiotics
> - Herbal Medicine
> - Traditional Chinese Medicine
> - Ayurvedic Medicine

Ann Louise Gittleman, M.S., C.N.S.: P.O. Box 255, Bozeman, MT 59771. For more on **herbal parasite formulas**, contact: Uni Key Health Systems, P.O. Box 7168, Bozeman, MT 59771; tel: 800-888-4353 or 406-586-9424.

How Parasites Pad Your Waistline

Parasite infections are often overlooked because they can cause a wide variety of health problems that mimic other diseases. Among the conditions that can be caused by parasites are fatigue, hypoglycemia, skin problems, arthritis-like symptoms, depression, upper respiratory tract infections, environmental illness, PMS, and gastrointestinal problems. Parasites can also be the cause behind chronic weight problems.[2]

Hormone Imbalance

One of the ways parasites lead to weight gain is by causing hormone imbalances. Hormones (SEE QUICK DEFINITION) regulate and control all of our bodily functions, from our metabolism (the rate at which we burn calories) to our mood. Too little or too much of any one hormone can seriously disrupt how the entire body functions and quickly lead to weight gain. Hermann Bueno, M.D., of New York City, an international authority on parasitic disease, says that parasites neutralize the action of hormones. "Parasites block the 'entryway' [the receptor site] where these hormones penetrate and interact with the cells of the target organ," he says. This blocking at the cellular level prevents hormones from stimulating the body's organs, which, in turn, can cause a myriad of illnesses. Several of these illnesses, such as hypoglycemia (low blood sugar) and hypothyroidism (a disease of the thyroid that lowers metabolism), are known to increase body weight.

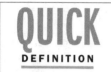

DEFINITION

Hormones are the chemical messengers of the endocrine system that impose order through an intricate communication system among the body's estimated 50 trillion cells. Examples include the male sex hormone (testosterone), the female sex hormones (estrogen and progesterone), melatonin (pineal), growth hormone (pituitary), and DHEA (adrenal).

For more about **hypoglycemia and insulin**, see Chapter 8: Strengthen Your Sugar Controls, pp. 184-201. For more about **hypothyroidism**, see Chapter 9: Overcome a Sluggish Thyroid, pp. 202-219. For more about **hormones and weight**, see Chapter 10: Restore Hormonal Balance, pp. 220-243.

Holistic health practitioner Suzanne Skinner, Ph.D., R.N.C., N.D., of Torrance, California, says that 90% of her patients have some type of parasite and most are not aware that they do. One of the more common infections she encounters is in the pancreas (an organ that helps regulate sugar levels in the blood by secreting the hormone insulin). The pancreas can become susceptible to parasites from eating too much junk food, which depletes its enzyme store, the pancreas' main defense against parasites. "When a person has used up their lifetime store of pancreatic enzymes from eating too much junk food, then the parasites invade the pancreas," explains Dr. Skinner. When the pancreas is infected with a parasite, one of the outcomes is hypoglycemia. Dr. Skinner says that "close to 75% of the cases of hypoglycemia that I see are linked to parasites in the pancreas."

Yeast Infection

Parasite infections can also contribute to the onset of candidiasis, an overgrowth of the yeast organism *Candida albicans* in the body.[3] This overgrowth is often found as a complication of giardiasis, an infection of the protozoan *Giardia lambia* (see "A Parasite Primer," pp. 316-317). Considered an opportunistic infection (one that develops when the body is compromised by other infections), candidiasis is the underlying cause of obesity in certain individuals. Both candidiasis and parasites are often the result of an excessive use of antibiotics or steroids, which kill off the beneficial bacteria that otherwise live in and protect the intestines. "The quickest way to deplete all the good, beneficial bacteria is to take a round of antibiotics," says Dr. Skinner. When these bacteria are destroyed, the intestines become fertile ground for harmful organisms.

Toxic Load

Parasites can cause weight gain by damaging the the body's detoxification system, particularly the liver and the lymphatic system (SEE QUICK DEFINITION). Some of the larger parasites can physically obstruct the bile ducts and other organs and parasites also dump their toxins into our bodies. The liver, colon, and lymphatic system are the body's chief defense against these harmful biological insults, but parasites and other factors can overload our capacity to eliminate them. "Toxicity is a primary cause of excessive weight, particularly in people who have problems losing weight and keeping it off," says nutritionist Jack Tips, N.D., Ph.D., of Austin, Texas.[4]

Food Allergies

Dr. Skinner has found that overweight people who complain of being bloated around the middle often have parasites in the intestinal tract (the bloating is caused by an inflammation of the intestinal lining). Over time, the inflammation weakens the intestines and can cause microscopic cracks to form in the lining, which then allows undigested food particles and bowel toxins to pass across the intestinal barrier and into the bloodstream. This condition, known as leaky gut syndrome, can lead to the development of food allergies, an underlying cause of many food cravings and addictions as well as weight gain.

Weakening the Immune System

The parasites themselves may also invade the bloodstream, causing the immune system (SEE QUICK DEFINITION) to channel much of its energy and resources to subduing them. Gary Kaplan, D.O., a family physician and president of the Medical

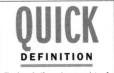

DEFINITION

The **lymphatic system** consists of lymph fluid and the structures (vessels, ducts, and nodes) involved in transporting it from tissues to the bloodstream. Lymph fluid occupies the space between the body's cells and contains plasma proteins, foreign particles, and cellular waste. Lymph nodes are clusters of immune tissue that work as filters or "inspection stations" for detecting and removing foreign and potentially harmful substances in the lymph fluid.

The **immune system** guards the body against foreign, disease-producing substances. Its "workers" are various white blood cells including one trillion lymphocytes and 100 million trillion antibodies produced and secreted by the lymphocytes. Lymphocytes are found in high numbers in the lymph nodes, bone marrow, spleen, and thymus gland.

For more about **yeast infections**, see Chapter 13: Eliminate Yeast Infections, pp. 294-309. For more about the **liver and body weight**, see Chapter 15: Cleanse the Liver, pp. 330-346. For more on the **lymph system**, see Chapter 16: Get the Lymph Flowing, pp. 348-363. For more about **food allergies**, see Chapter 11: Break Food Allergies and Addictions, pp. 244-270.

Acupuncture Research Foundation in Los Angeles, California, says that the body reacts to parasites that way it does to any antigen (SEE QUICK DEFINITION), "The immune system judges antigens to be foreign, undesirable particles and mounts an immune response to their presence."

Such an immune response can cause a variety of widespread, allergy-like symptoms. "I have found in a number of patients that parasite infestation can frequently produce an antigenic reaction that leads towards generalized joint pain and sometimes asthma," says Dr. Kaplan. Parasites cause a continuous immune response and, with time, an untreated parasite infection will severely weaken or exhaust the immune system, causing the body to become increasingly vulnerable to health problems, including obesity and cancer.[5] Many alternative practitioners recognize the relationship between parasites and chronic disease. "I am convinced that after dealing with patients for over eighteen years, that one of the major reasons for the chronic ill health we are seeing today is none other than parasites," says Gittleman.[6]

Sources of Parasites

You don't have to travel to an exotic tropical island to pick up a parasite. You may be exposing yourself to potential infection every day in your own home and surroundings. Parasites can be transmitted through contaminated food and water, foreign travel (particularly to countries with poor sanitary standards), and household pets or other animals.

Food—The U.S. food supply is commonly thought to be the safest in the world. Nevertheless, according to the U.S. Centers for Disease Control, up to 80 million illnesses occur in this country every year due to contaminated food supply. Approximately 9,000 of these reported illnesses result in death.[7]

Food contamination can happen in several ways. Raw or undercooked meats and fish pose a threat for parasite infestation. Beef and pork may contain tapeworms or the roundworm *Trichinella*. Raw fish (sushi or smoked salmon, for instance) may also contain tapeworms or anisakid worms. Fruits and vegetables, particularly from countries where parasites are prevalent or where human wastes may be used as fertilizer, may pose a risk of parasite contamination if they are not washed thoroughly before eating. Without adequate safeguards, both farming and processing practices may lead to contamination. Aquatic vegetables, such as watercress and bamboo shoots, may also contain parasitic cysts. Poor hygiene in the storage and preparation of food may lead to parasite infestation, in restaurants, nursing homes, day-care centers, or at home. Food handlers can contaminate the food they are preparing as can insects, such as flies or cockroaches.[8]

Water–"Don't drink the water" is the advice commonly given to travelers heading abroad. Unfortunately, this adage could readily apply in the U.S. as well—contaminated water is a common source of parasites in this country. Our drinking water comes from rivers, lakes, and reservoirs, all of which are threatened with contamination from agricultural runoff, waste products from farm animals, and human sewage.

Chlorination is no protection either. Two of the most common parasites, *Giardia* and *Cryptosporidium*, can survive in chlorinated water for up to 18 months. "Giardiasis [infestation with the *Giardia* parasite] may be a rampant problem in the U.S. today, since over 50% of our water supply is contaminated with it and, unlike bacteria, it is not killed by chlorination," says Steven Rochlitz, Ph.D., author of *Allergies and Candida*.[9] Water filtration systems may help remove *Giardia* from tap water, but few eliminate *Cryptosporidium*, which is so small that it simply passes through most filters. Many urban water systems have no filtration systems at all. Even springs and mountain streams are increasingly becoming contaminated with parasites from wild animals and human visitors.[10]

Foreign Travel–Dr. Bueno explains that, as international travel has increased, parasite infections have become more common in the U.S. "Parasites recognize no national borders," he says. "The world is getting smaller and parasites, generally associated with tropical diseases and third world countries, where climate and unsanitary living conditions encourage their growth, are now appearing in the United States." Dr. Bueno is not just talking about a case of traveler's diarrhea: some people return from their journeys carrying unsuspected parasitic infections, such as malaria, roundworms, or blood flukes.[11]

Pets–There are 240 diseases that can be transmitted from animals to humans (65 transmitted by dogs and 39 by cats), according to

A Parasite Primer

Parasites are organisms that survive by feeding off another living organism called the host, usually causing damage to the host. Protozoa, Trematodes (flukes), Cestoda (tapeworms), and Nematoda (roundworms and hookworms) are the four main types of parasites.

Protozoa:

Protozoa (microscopic, single-celled organisms) are the most common type of parasite found in the U.S. They reproduce rapidly in the intestinal tract and can migrate to other organs (liver, pancreas, heart, and lungs).

■ *Giardia*—a common parasite in the U.S., transmitted through contaminated water and food. *Giardia* infests the small intestine, incubating for up to three weeks before causing symptoms. Infection can damage the intestinal lining; symptoms include foul-smelling stools, cramps, bloating, headaches, and fatigue.

■ *Cryptosporidium parvum*—the most prevalent waterborne parasite in the U.S.; it can also be spread through contact with feces. Symptoms include diarrhea, nausea, cramps, and fever.

■ *Trichomonas vaginalis*—usually transmitted through sexual contact or from contaminated toilet seats, towels, or bath water. The infection is often symptom-less, but it can cause vaginal discharge, yeast infections, and painful urination in women or an enlarged prostate and urinary inflammation in men.

■ *Entamoeba histolytica*—spread through water or food, this protozoan may incubate for up to three months and then spread through the digestive tract; it can also migrate to other organs. Abdominal pain, bloating, and diarrhea are common symptoms. A high-carbohydrate diet can increase the severity of amebiasis.

■ *Toxoplasma gondii*—infection generally comes from cats; undercooked meats are another source. It may cause flu-like symptoms, such as fever, headache, swollen lymph nodes, and fatigue.

Flukes (Trematodes):

Flukes are leaf-shaped flatworms that attach to the host using two abdominal suckers. Flukes usually begin their life cycle in snails, then as larvae they infect fish, vegetation, or humans. Flukes can migrate to the lungs, intestines, heart, brain, and liver. Trematode eggs can cause inflammation in the body by releasing toxins that damage tissues.

■ Intestinal Fluke (*Fasciolopsis buski*)—contamination usually stems from eating infected water vegetables (water chestnuts, bamboo shoots, or watercress). The worms live in the small intestine, where they cause ulcerations and allergic reactions. Common symptoms are diarrhea, nausea, abdominal pain, and vomiting.

■ Sheep Liver Fluke (*Fasciola hepatica*)—fresh watercress is the most common source. This worm attaches itself in the gallbladder and bile ducts, causing inflammation and local trauma. Symptoms include jaundice, fever, coughing, vomiting, and abdominal pain.

■ Oriental Lung Fluke (*Paragonimus westermani*)—found mostly in Asian countries; spread by eating undercooked crabs and crayfish. The worms can penetrate the intestines and migrate to the lungs or brain. Symptoms include coughing fits and blood in the sputum.

■ Blood Flukes (*Schistosoma japonicum, Schistosoma mansoni,* and *Schistosoma haematobium*)—transmitted by swimming in contaminated water, blood flukes burrow into the skin and migrate to the heart, lungs, liver, or bladder. They can live inside the body for up to 30 years.

Tapeworms (Cestoda):

Tapeworms are flat, segmented, and ribbon-like and are the largest intestinal parasites, growing up to several feet in length. The most common source of infection is from eating undercooked meat or fish containing the larvae. The worms develop in the body and attach to the small intestine, surviving by absorbing nutrients from partially digested food. Often tapeworms produce no symptoms in their human host.

■ Beef Tapeworm (*Taenia saginata*)—enters the body in raw or undercooked beef; this tapeworm can live in the intestines for up to 25 years, growing to a length of eight feet. Symptoms include diarrhea, cramps, nausea, and loss of appetite. Long-term infection may lead to vitamin deficiencies.

■ Pork Tapeworm (*Taenia solium*)—undercooked pork, smoked ham, or sausage are common sources. The adult worms attach in the intestines, causing symptoms similar to those of the beef tapeworm. The larvae can infect the heart, liver, muscles, eyes, brain, and spine.

■ Fish Tapeworm (*Diphyllobothrium latum*)—infestations caused by eating undercooked or raw fish. It grows up to 15 feet in length and symptoms include vomiting, heartburn, diarrhea, and loss of appetite.

Roundworms and Hookworms (Nematoda):

These unsegmented worms multiply by producing eggs that require incubation time in the soil or another host before becoming infective to humans.

■ Roundworm (*Ascaris lumbricoides*)—one billion people may be infected with roundworm worldwide. The eggs are found on fruits and vegetables grown in contaminated soil, particularly in tropical and subtropical regions. They migrate through the liver, lungs, and intestines, causing inflammation and allergic reactions, abdominal pain, sleep disturbances, and fatigue.

■ Hookworm (*Necator americanus*)—hookworms burrow directly into the skin and are often found in people who go barefoot. They move into the blood, through the lungs, and to the intestines. Primary symptoms are blood loss and anemia, abdominal pain, diarrhea, and lack of energy.

■ Pinworm (*Enterobius vermicularis*)—infection is common in the U.S., primarily transmitted through contaminated food and water. The female lays eggs outside the anus, the worms then infect the large intestine and appendix. Common symptoms are anal itching and irritation, plus unusual symptoms such as hyperactivity, vision problems, and psychiatric disturbances.

■ Trichinella (*Trichinella spiralis*)—infections caused by eating undercooked pork. The worms migrate from the intestines and embed in muscle tissue in the chest, diaphragm, jaws, and upper arm. Symptoms include diarrhea, nausea, severe muscle pain, facial edema, difficulty breathing or chewing, and enlarged lymph glands.[12]

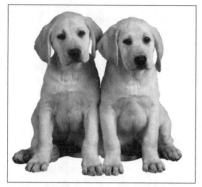

There are 240 diseases that can be transmitted from animals to humans, 65 transmitted by dogs and 39 by cats.

Gittleman. With an estimated 118 million pets in the U.S., it is easy to see how pets may be a major source for parasites. Roundworm, hookworm, and toxoplasmosis may be more common than most people think. "It is estimated that 50% of adult Americans may carry latent toxoplasmosis infections acquired from cats," according to Gittleman. Parasites are transmitted from animals to humans through contact with animal feces, fur containing parasite eggs, or infected fleas.[13]

Other Sources—Parasites can also be transmitted by insects (mosquitos, flies, cockroaches, and fleas), through sexual contact (common sexually transmitted parasites include *Giardia lamblia*, *Entamoeba histolytica*, and *Trichomonas vaginalis*), or even inhaled from the air. Day care centers are one of the primary sources for parasitic infections in children.[14]

Diagnosing a Parasite Infection

Symptoms and personal history are the first two things a physician should check when diagnosing a possible parasite infection. "I always begin with a detailed picture of the symptoms and then gather a complete history that will indicate if exposure to parasites should be factored in," says Leo Galland, M.D., author of *The Four Pillars of Healing*. "Red flags are things like a recent trip out of the country, extensive use of antibiotics (which weaken the immune system), or having a child in day care, where it's estimated 30% of staff are infected."

After determining whether a parasite infection may exist from a patient's symptoms and history, physicians generally confirm the diagnosis with various testing procedures. Different parasites require different formulations to kill them, so an accurate diagnosis is an important step in any treatment program. Unfortunately, parasite infections are often overlooked by mainstream physicians. Part of the problem is that they simply fail to use the right diagnostic test. According to David Casemore, M.D., of the Public Health Laboratories in Great Britain, parasitic infection "is almost certainly underdetected, possibly by a factor of ten or more."[15] A number of diagnostic tools can be useful in determining if you have parasites, including a purged stool test and mucus and blood tests.

Stool Analysis

Gittleman recommends using a purged stool test for parasites. This method differs from standard stool analysis—the patient ingests 1½ ounces of a high-sodium solution on an empty stomach to encourage more frequent and powerful bowel movements. These induced stool samples have greater levels of mucus, which provide higher numbers of organisms. Parasites generally begin to appear after the fourth bowel movement, but sometimes it may take as many as 12 bowel movements to dislodge them. The purged stool test may be more accurate than conventional stool analysis for diagnosing a parasite infection. The problem with a random stool sample is that parasites cling to the wall of the intestines and simply may not be present in the feces.[16]

CAUTION

A purged stool test is not recommended for individuals with high blood pressure as the high-sodium solution may exacerbate their problem, according to Gittleman. Pregnant women and those suffering from an intestinal obstruction or appendicitis should not take this test.

Uni Key Health Systems of Bozeman, Montana, makes a do-it-yourself purged stool test kit endorsed by Gittleman. You can do this test at home and send the sample to a parasitology laboratory for analysis. The test can detect 15 types of worms, more than a dozen types of protozoa, and yeasts like *Candida albicans*. The test results are sent to Gittleman's office and she will offer advice on treatment options.

Bueno-Parrish Test

Another test procedure recommended by alternative care practitioners is the Bueno-Parrish test. This test, developed by Dr. Bueno, involves the use of a rectal mucus swab to identify parasites. The procedure, technically called an anoscopy, involves taking a sample of mucus from inside the rectum with a cotton swab. A stain that makes even fragments of parasites visible is then applied to the swab material and examined with the help of a microscope. This procedure has helped identify parasite infections in patients who had previously been misdiagnosed.[17]

Blood Tests

Blood tests may be useful for diagnosing some parasitic infections. Elevated levels of a special white blood cell called an eosinophil may

For information on **stool analysis**, contact: Uni Key Health Systems, P.O. Box 7168, Bozeman, MT 59771; tel: 406-586-9424 or 800-888-4353. Great Smokies Diagnostic Laboratory, 63 Zillicoa Street, Asheville, NC 28801; tel: 828-253-0621 or 828-522-4762; fax: 828-252-9303. Meridian Valley Clinical Laboratory, 515 West Harrison Street, Suite 9, Kent, WA 98032; tel: 800-234-6825 or 253-859-8700; fax: 253-859-1135. For the **Bueno-Parrish test**, contact: Lexington Professional Center, 133 E 73rd Street, New York, NY 10021; tel: 212-988-4800. For **blood tests**, contact: Parasitic Disease Consultants Laboratory, 2177-J Flintstone Drive, Tucker, GA 30084; tel: 404-496-1370.

The signs of a parasite infection can occur almost immediately or develop months after exposure. Common symptoms include:

- Diarrhea, mucus or blood in a watery stool, or bowel movements with a fetid and offensive smell
- Stomach cramps
- Abdominal bloating and distention
- Severe gas
- Constipation
- Heartburn or nausea
- Headache
- Fatigue
- Joint pain
- Skin rashes
- Teeth grinding
- Sleep disturbances
- In children, a chronically itchy rectum and/or intense and persistent night terrors, which cause them to wake up screaming, could be signs that parasites are present. Hyperactivity may also be caused by parasites.
- An array of other psychological symptoms may be associated with parasitic infections, including moderate to severe depression, suicidal tendencies, irritability and mood swings, "spacey" feelings, changes in personality, decreased sex drive, and insomnia.[19]

indicate a parasite infection. Blood tests can also measure levels of antibodies to some parasites, including *Entamoeba histolytica*, most types of flukes, malaria, and *Trichinella*. Abnormal blood levels of some nutrients may indicate parasites. For example, low levels of iron, folic acid, and calcium may indicate the presence of *Giardia*.[18]

Alternative Medicine Therapies for Eradicating Parasites

Although antibiotics and other drugs are often used to treat parasitic infections, use of these drugs can pose a threat to overall health by upsetting the immune system. Those who already have a weakened immune system or are chronically ill should be especially careful. Naturopath Leon Chaitow, N.D., D.O., of London, England, points out that "in many cases, anti-parasitic prescriptive drugs have not proved to be effective. They may diminish symptoms for one or two months, but the symptoms later return with full force." Among the reasons for the return of symptoms is that these treatments have a very low effectiveness rate. According to Pavel Yutsis, M.D., of Brooklyn, New York, these conventional drug treatments (which are administered for 5-14 days) offer only a 50% cure rate.

In contrast, alternative medicine treatments like herbs have a gentler action and can be safely used for longer treatment cycles. "Successful therapy of chronic protozoal infection requires weeks or

Assessing Parasite Exposure

A medical history assessing the patient's potential exposure to parasites is crucial to getting an accurate diagnosis. Dr. Bueno and other alternative medicine practitioners typically ask patients the following questions to assess the likelihood of a parasite exposure:

■ What is your travel history (inside and outside the U.S.)?

■ What is the source of your drinking water? Have you ever drunk water from streams or rivers while camping?

■ Do you have pets in your household or are you in close contact with animals?

■ Do you frequently eat out, particularly at ethnic restaurants, sushi bars, or salad bars?

■ Do you like to eat raw fruits and vegetables?

■ Do you like raw or undercooked meat or fish?

■ Do you work in a hospital, day care center, sanitation department, around animals, or garden?

■ Do you engage in unprotected oral or anal sex?

■ Do you have some or all of these symptoms—dark circles under your eyes, distended abdomen, bluish lips, allergies, diarrhea or constipation, anemia, skin eruptions, anal itching, chronic fatigue, loss of appetite, insomnia, depression, or sugar cravings?[20]

months of treatment," says Dr. Yutsis. "For this reason we prefer to use herbal preparations, because the available drugs are generally too toxic to be recommended for extended periods of time."[21] Alternative treatments include detoxification, dietary recommendations, probiotics (friendly bacteria to support the intestines), herbal medicine, and Ayurvedic therapy.

CAUTION

Before beginning any parasite elimination program, consult a qualified health-care professional. This is especially important if you are pregnant.

Detoxification

Like other toxins, parasites can make it harder for the liver, kidneys, and intestines to detoxify and eliminate wastes from the body. If testing reveals that you have a parasitic infection, you may want to consider taking the following practical steps, recommended by William Lee Cowden, M.D., of Richardson, Texas, to rid your system of parasites:

For more information about **colon-cleansing programs**, see Chapter 12: Detoxify the Colon, pp. 272-293.

1) Cleanse the Intestines: Parasites tend to embed themselves in the intestinal wall, but over the course of several weeks, you can flush them out by using some of these natural substances (preferably in

combination): psyllium husks, agar-agar, citrus pectin, papaya extract, pumpkin seeds, flaxseeds, comfrey root, beet root, and bentonite clay (take bentonite only in combination with another substance, such as psyllium). You might also take extra vitamin C (minimum 2 g daily, but higher amounts up to individual bowel tolerance are more useful) to help flush out your intestines. Note, however, that vitamin C taken at the same time as wormwood (below) renders wormwood ineffective.

2) Do a Colon Irrigation: Irrigate the colon with 2-16 quarts of water via enema. To the water you may add black walnut tincture or extract, garlic juice, vinegar (two tablespoons per quart of water), blackstrap molasses (one tablespoon per quart of water), or organically grown coffee. Use filtered or distilled water for the enema; further sterilize it by boiling or ozonating it for 10-15 minutes before use, including before using it to prepare the coffee.

3) Prepare Your System: It is prudent to give your gallbladder and liver a week to prepare for the parasite program. To flush the gallbladder of its toxins, take lime juice in warm water or Swedish Bitters before each meal. Eliminate all refined and natural sugars, meats, and dairy products during the parasite program; even better, start cutting back on them during this preparatory week. Take barberry bark capsules, dandelion, or similar herbal extract to help cleanse the liver. The amount depends on health and the strength or composition of the specific substance used.

4) The Herbal Cleanout: Naturopathic physician Hulda Regehr Clark, N.D., Ph.D., recommends using a blend of three herbs to flush the parasites out of your system: black walnut hull tincture, wormwood capsules, and fresh ground cloves (to kill the parasites' eggs).

Dietary Recommendations

If you suspect a parasitic infection, you should eliminate all uncooked foods from your diet and cook all meats until well done; soak both organic and inorganic vegetables in salted water (one tablespoon per five cups) for a minimum of 30 minutes before cooking. It is also advisable to eliminate coffee, all sugars including fruits and honey, and all milk and dairy products, with the possible exception of raw goat's milk. Raw goat's milk contains secretory IgA and IgG immunoglobulins (SEE QUICK DEFINITION), types of antibodies that help strengthen the immune system. According to Steven Bailey, N.D., of Portland, Oregon, IgA and IgG are helpful in the treatment of parasites.

Gittleman says that the best diet for a parasite infection is one that "supports the host and starves the parasite." Specifically, she recommends against eating any sugar, white flour, or processed foods (such as prepackaged snack foods). Once inside the body, these foods provide ideal conditions for parasites to breed. She has found that a diet composed of 25% fat, 25% protein, and 50% complex carbohydrates (a type of starch found in vegetables and whole grains) is best for people with parasite infections.

Gittleman also advises limiting your intake of raw fruits and vegetables; instead, cook both fruits and vegetables. Sufficient levels of vitamin A are particularly important for preventing parasites, as this vitamin seems to increase resistance to penetration by larvae. Good dietary sources of vitamin A include properly cooked carrots, sweet potatoes, squash, and salad greens. A combination formula of digestive enzymes, taken between meals, may also be helpful for eliminating parasite larvae or eggs in the intestines.

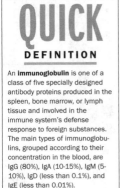

QUICK DEFINITION

An **immunoglobulin** is one of a class of five specially designed antibody proteins produced in the spleen, bone marrow, or lymph tissue and involved in the immune system's defense response to foreign substances. The main types of immunoglobulins, grouped according to their concentration in the blood, are IgG (80%), IgA (10-15%), IgM (5-10%), IgD (less than 0.1%), and IgE (less than 0.01%).

Certain foods are anti-parasitic, according to Gittleman, and you should incorporate more of these foods in your diet. These include pineapple and papaya, either as fresh juice or in supplement form, eaten in combination with pepsin (a stomach enzyme) and betaine hydrochloric acid (a supplement form of stomach acid). Avoid all meats and dairy products for at least one week at the beginning of therapy. You can also use pomegranate juice (four 8-ounce glasses daily), papaya seeds, fresh figs, finely ground pumpkin seeds (¼ cup to ½ cup daily), or two cloves of raw garlic daily. Because pomegranate juice can irritate the intestines, you should not drink it for more than four to five days at a time. Other anti-parasitic foods include onions, kelp, blackberries, raw cabbage, and ground almonds.[22]

Probiotics

Parasites can be fought with "friendly" bacteria or probiotics, such as *L. acidophilus*, *B. bifidum*, and *L. bulgaricus*. Dr. Chaitow recommends that any anti-parasitic protocol begin by using high dosage probiotics and treatment programs may last for as long as eight to 12 weeks. He reports an 80% success rate using this method in cases of seriously ill people afflicted with parasites.

A complementary approach is to supply the nutrients that directly feed the beneficial bacteria. Japanese researchers determined that a

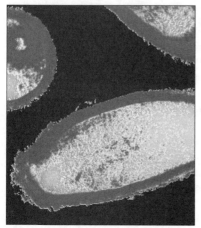

Friendly bacteria, or probiotics, refer to beneficial microbes inhabiting the human gastrointestinal tract where they are essential for proper nutrient assimilation. The human body contains an estimated several trillion beneficial bacteria comprising over 400 species, all necessary for health. Among the more well-known of these are *Lactobacillus acidophilus* (pictured here) and *Bifidobacterium bifidum*. Overly acidic bodily conditions, chronic constipation or diarrhea, dietary imbalances, consumption of highly processed foods, and the excessive use of antibiotics and hormonal drugs can interfere with probiotic function and even reduce the number of these microbes, setting up conditions for illness.

naturally occurring form of carbohydrate, called fructo-oligosaccharides (FOS), found in certain foods in minute amounts, could be a perfect food for *Bifidobacteria*. FOS selectively feeds the friendly microflora in the large intestine so that their numbers can increase. NutraFlora®, from GTC Nutrition in Westminster, Colorado, contains 95% pure FOS, in dry powder form or as a syrup, to be used as a dietary supplement. FOS is found in small amounts in garlic, honey, soybeans, asparagus, bananas, barley, and tomatoes.

Herbal Medicine

Herbal remedies have been used effectively for centuries for the treatment of parasitic infections. These remedies can also help prevent a parasitic infection when water or food conditions are questionable. According to Dr. Galland, it is advisable to continue any treatment regimen until at least two parasite tests, performed one month apart on purged stool specimens, are negative.

For more on **FOS** and **NutraFlora®**, contact: GTC Nutrition Company, 1400 West 122nd Avenue, Suite 110, Westminster, CO 80234; tel: 303-254-8012; fax: 303-254-8201.

Citrus Seed Extract—Citrus seed extract is highly active against protozoa, bacteria, and yeast, and has long been used in the treatment of parasitic infections. It is not absorbed into the tissue, is nontoxic and generally hypoallergenic, and can be administered for up to several months, a length of time which may be required to eliminate *Giardia* and the candidiasis that often accompanies it.

Artemisia annua—This is an herbal remedy of Chinese origin. Its antiprotozoal activity is especially effective against *Giardia*, but some caution is advisable—it can initially cause a worsening of symptoms, allergic reactions, and some intestinal irritation. *Artemisia annua* is often prescribed by Dr. Galland, along with citrus seed extract. It may be used with additional herbs known for their anti-parasitic activity and can also be used in conjunction with conventional drug therapy.

Artemisia absinthium—This is one of the oldest European medicinal plants. Known as "wormwood," it was highly prized by Hippocrates and is similar to the *Artemisia annua* of Chinese herbal tradition. *Artemisia absinthium* taken alone can be toxic, though, and therefore should be used in combination with other herbs to nullify its toxicity.

Other Anti-Parasitic Herbs—A number of other herbs (often found in combination formulas) may be useful in supporting the digestive tract and eliminating parasites:

■ Aloe vera: Known as "the potted physician," the aloe plant is filled with a clear gel that acts as a digestive tonic. Studies have shown that aloe can destroy bacteria, yeasts, and parasites in the intestines.[23]

■ Garlic (*Allium sativum*): Aside from its use in cooking, garlic is also an effective and well-researched medicinal herb, used in traditional medicines all over the world. Garlic and its preparations are known for their antibiotic, anti-fungal, and antiviral activity. It is effective against roundworms, tapeworms, pinworms, and hookworms.

■ Goldenseal (*Hydrastis canadensis*): One of the most widely used American herbs, goldenseal is considered to be a tonic remedy that stimulates immune response and is directly antimicrobial itself. Goldenseal's antimicrobial properties are due to berberine, an alkaloid that is effective against bacteria, fungi, and parasites, particularly *Giardia*.[24]

Before using any of the herbal remedies listed here, it is important that you first consult with a health-care professional who has been properly trained in their use. *Artemisia annua* should not be used during pregnancy. Garlic, if taken in too high a dose, may cause intestinal irritation.

For more on **herbal parasite formulas,** contact: Uni Key Health Systems, P.O. Box 7168, Bozeman, MT 59771; tel: 406-586-9424 or 800-888-4353. Allergy Research Group, 400 Preda Street, San Leandro, CA 94577; tel: 800-545-9960 or 510-639-4572; fax: 510-635-6730. Thorne Research, Inc., P.O. Box 25, Dover, ID 83825; tel: 800-228-1966 or 208-263-1337; fax: 208-265-2488. Tyler Encapsulations, 2204-8 N.W. Birdsdale, Gresham, OR 97030; tel: 800-869-9705 or 503-661-5401; fax: 503-666-4913.

Traditional Chinese Medicine

In traditional Chinese medicine (SEE QUICK DEFINITION), herbs are the primary treatment for parasites and the type used depends on the location of the parasites in the body, according to Maoshing Ni, D.O.M., Ph.D., L.Ac., of Yo San University of Traditional Chinese Medicine, in Santa Monica, California. For intestinal parasites, purgative herbs are usually used. Pumpkin and quisqualis seeds are two common remedies. The pumpkin seeds are eaten raw, while the quisqualis seeds are usually

QUICK
DEFINITION

Traditional Chinese medicine (TCM) originated in China over 5,000 years ago and is a comprehensive system of medical practice that heals the body according to the principles of nature and balance. A Chinese medicine physician considers the flow of vital energy (*qi*) in a patient through close examination of the patient's pulses, tongue, body odor, voice tone and strength, and general demeanor, among other elements. Underlying imbalances and disharmony in the body are described in terminology analogous to the natural world (heat, cold, dryness, or dampness). The concept of balance, or the interrelationship of organs, is central to TCM. In TCM, imbalances are corrected through the use of acupuncture, moxibustion, herbal medicine, dietary therapy, massage, and therapeutic exercise.

Maoshing Ni, D.O.M., Ph.D., L.Ac.: 1131 Wilshire Blvd., Suite 300, Santa Monica, CA 90401; tel: 310-917-2200; fax: 310-917-2267.

roasted. Both are taken every morning on an empty stomach, approximately 10-12 seeds each, for about two weeks. "Quisqualis and pumpkin seeds are mild and safe enough for adults and children to take daily as a preventative measure as well," says Dr. Ni.

Meliae seeds are much stronger than either pumpkin or quisqualis and should only be taken in more severe cases. The meliae seeds paralyze the parasites for approximately eight hours, allowing the body to eliminate them through the bowels. Betel nut is another typical treatment for intestinal parasites; the nut is chewed raw like chewing tobacco. "It can give a certain sense of euphoria, too, because it is slightly toxic," says Dr. Ni. "This is negligible, but some people might get diarrhea." Depending on the type of parasite, they may be able to get through the intestinal walls and into the bloodstream. "In situations like this you have to use some very strong antibiotic-like herbs," says Dr. Ni, "such as goldenseal and coptidis, which are anti-parasitic as well."

While eliminating the parasites with herbs, Dr. Ni also strengthens the immune system in order to get at the underlying cause of the parasitic infestation. He reports that proper nutrition and herbs such as ginseng, ligustri berries, and schisandra berries can accomplish this.

Ayurvedic Medicine

Ayurvedic medicine (SEE QUICK DEFINITION), a 5,000-year-old health-care tradition from India, has many natural remedies that address specific parasitic infections. According to Virender Sodhi, M.D. (Ayurveda), N.D., of Bellevue, Washington, the most effective herbs for *Giardia*, amoebas, *Cryptosporidium*, and other protozoal intestinal parasites are bilva, neem, and berberine, which can be taken in combination, he reports. He also recommends bitter melon, as well as such nutritional support as psyllium husk, turmeric, and *L. acidophilus* for the enhancement of the intestinal microflora. It may take several months to eliminate intestinal parasites.

CAUTION

Although the Ayurvedic remedies mentioned here are safe and easy to self-administer, Dr. Sodhi recommends consultation with a qualified practitioner before beginning any treatment protocol, to determine which of the various options will be best suited to individual needs and circumstances.

Important Reminders During Any Parasite Treatment

Whatever treatment you employ to rid your body of parasites, the following recommendations can help ensure that the program is a success:

■ If you have children and/or pets, they must be treated at the same time as the adults in the household to prevent re-infection.

■ Drink more pure water (not from the tap) than usual to help the body flush out the dead parasites from your system; at least 64 ounces of water per day for a 150-pound adult.

■ Sanitize your environment. When you have almost finished treatment, wash all pajamas, bed clothes, and sheets before using them again.

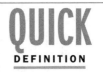

DEFINITION

Ayurveda is the traditional medicine of India, based on many centuries of empirical use. Its name means "end of the Vedas" (which were India's sacred texts), implying that a holistic medicine may be founded on spiritual principles. Ayurveda describes three metabolic, constitutional, and body types (*doshas*)—*vata*, *pitta*, and *kapha*—in association with the basic elements of Nature and uses them as the basis for prescribing individualized formulas of herbs, diet, massage, and detoxification techniques.

■ Although alternative medicine anti-parasitic therapies are milder than conventional treatments, no treatment program can successfully remove parasites from the body without causing some stress. This is because parasites create a toxic load in the body as they are killed off. Side effects of any treatment will often include intense and uncomfortable reactions, such as abdominal discomfort, joint pain, exhaustion, or flu-like symptoms. Consequently, an effective anti-parasite treatment program should include measures that will help strengthen the body's natural cleansing and detoxifying systems. Specifically, organs such as the liver, gallbladder, and intestines may need to undergo cleansing. The lymphatic system, the body's main waste disposal system, may also need to be cleansed, as it can become a reservoir of parasitic toxins.

How to Avoid Parasites

Several precautions can help you avoid parasites:

Food

■ Do not eat raw beef—it can be loaded with tapeworms and other parasites.

■ Do not eat raw fish or sushi—you are almost certain to get worms if you eat raw fish. (The Japanese eat horseradish as an anti-parasite measure.

■ Wash hands after handling raw meat or fish (including shrimp)—don't put your hands near your mouth without washing them first.

■ Use separate cutting boards for meat and for vegetables—spores from meat can seep into the board and contaminate vegetables or anything else you put on the board.

■ Wash utensils after cutting meat.

■ Wash vegetables and fruit thoroughly—particularly salad items, as they often harbor parasites. Wash in one teaspoon Clorox per one gallon of water; soak for 15-20 minutes. Then soak in fresh water for 20 minutes before refrigerating. Or substitute a few drops of grapefruit seed extract.

■ Do not drink from streams and rivers.

Pets

■ De-worm your pets regularly and keep their sleeping areas clean.

■ Do not sleep near your pets—they harbor many worms and other parasites.

■ Do not let pets lick your face.

■ Do not let pets eat off your dishes.

■ Do not walk barefoot around animals.

General

■ Always wash your hands after using the toilet.

■ Wash your hands after working in the garden—the soil can be contaminated with spores and parasites.

When Traveling

■ Don't drink the water.

■ Start taking Chinese herbs or other preventive medications two weeks before traveling and continue them while you travel.

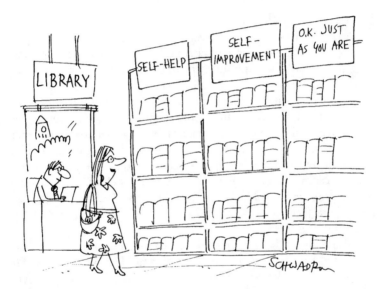

15 Cleanse the Liver

THE LIVER serves as a filter for the toxins that the body absorbs from food, air, and water. Unhealthy lifestyles, poor diet, and exposure to chemicals and pesticides can overload the liver with poisons, creating toxic conditions in the body that may cause a buildup of fat. Most people do not associate weight gain with exposure to toxic substances, but the truth is that the poisons that accumulate in our bodies can cause biochemical imbalances and damage organ systems, leading to a host of degenerative diseases. However, well before these diseases take hold, our bodies will begin to accumulate fat in response to the increased toxic burden. "Toxicity is a primary cause of excessive weight, particularly in people who have problems losing weight and keeping it off," says naturopath Jack Tips, N.D., Ph.D., of Austin, Texas, author of *Your Liver...Your Lifeline*.[1]

Although our bodies are equipped with mechanisms to eliminate toxins, modern life often overloads our innate cleansing capacity. The liver, in concert with the colon and lymphatic system, is the body's chief defense against harmful chemical and biological insults. These organs remove and destroy the toxic agents that enter our bodies, but these poisons can exceed the liver's capacity to eliminate them, creating toxicity in the body resulting in chronic illness.

Cleansing a toxic liver is always a difficult process. Nevertheless, for many it is absolutely necessary if they want to lose excess weight and restore their health. Dr. Tips estimates that most people suffer from some degree of liver toxicity.

"Unfortunately, only about one in 100,000 people has a truly healthy liver," he says.[2] Lindsey Duncan, C.N., a nutritionist based in Santa Monica, California, says, "I have found that in most overweight people, the liver is overloaded with pollutants, and its ability to do its job is impaired." In this chapter, we examine the ways an overburdened, toxic liver can lead to weight gain. We also delineate the sources of toxins that poison the body and how to test your liver function to see if this may be a factor in your weight problems. Finally, we offer several alternative medicine therapies for cleansing the liver and supporting its function.

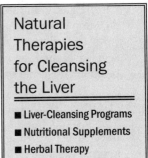

Natural Therapies for Cleansing the Liver

- Liver-Cleansing Programs
- Nutritional Supplements
- Herbal Therapy
- Flower Essence Therapy

Success Story: Flushing Away the Pounds

"I kept getting fatter and fatter, but I was starving to death," says George, a 34-year-old patient of Suzanne Skinner, N.D., Ph.D., R.N.C., a naturopath and nutritional consultant based in Torrance, California. George had been treated by a series of mainstream physicians, but none could help him with his weight problem. When he finally came to Dr. Skinner's office, George weighed more than 400 pounds.

One of the first things Dr. Skinner prescribed was an intensive liver and gallbladder flush. "I had to drink huge quantities of unrefined apple juice for days, do a short fast, and take doses of olive and lemon juice," he said. "It was not easy, especially forcing myself to drink the oil, but when the flush was done and I finally eliminated the contents of my gallbladder, I began to feel better and started losing weight."

Dr. Skinner also instructed George to take Ayurvedic (SEE QUICK DEFINITION) herbal supplements to support the liver and gallbladder cleansing process and digestive enzymes to support his pancreas. He was prohibited from eating any white flour and white sugar products, as well as cheese and chocolate. After only six months, George had lost 50

QUICK

DEFINITION

Ayurveda is the traditional medicine of India, based on many centuries of empirical use. Its name means "end of the Vedas" (which were India's sacred texts), implying that a holistic medicine may be founded on spiritual principles. Ayurveda describes three metabolic, constitutional, and body types (*doshas*), in association with the basic elements of Nature. These are *vata* (air and ether, rooted in the intestines), *pitta* (fire and water/stomach), and *kapha* (water and earth/lungs). Ayurvedic physicians use these categories (which also have psychological aspects) as the basis for prescribing individualized formulas of herbs, diet, massage, breathing, meditation, exercise, and detoxification techniques.

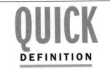

Suzanne Skinner, Ph.D., R.N.C., N.D., D.S.C.: 2204 Torrance Blvd., Torrance, CA 90501; tel: 310-518-4555.

pounds and felt hopeful for the first time in years. "I've improved incredibly. Besides losing so much weight, I'm no longer constipated and my digestion is better. I have more energy and feel stronger. I'm even able to swim or walk every day." The cleanse Dr. Skinner prescribed is very aggressive, and is best done with a professional's supervision, as part of a comprehensive and specially tailored cleansing program.

The Toxic Liver

Located between the lungs and the stomach, the liver is our largest internal organ, weighing 5-8 pounds, or about 2.5% of our total body weight. It serves as a kind of physiological ballast within the body, working to maintain stability and harmony among various biological systems. It functions as a nutrient warehouse and processing facility, supplying and regulating thousands of essential substances in the body. The liver is also specially equipped to dismantle the toxic compounds that enter our body everyday (see "How the Liver Handles Toxins," p. 335). When the liver becomes overloaded with toxins, it causes certain imbalances that lead to weight gain, including blood sugar imbalance, essential fatty acid deficiency, and slowed metabolism.

Blood Sugar Imbalance
Blood sugar, called glucose, is the body's primary fuel. When the body has more glucose in the bloodstream than it can use at a given moment, such as immediately following a meal, the liver converts the excess glucose into a starch called glycogen. Several hours after a meal, as blood glucose drops, the liver reconverts the stored glycogen back into glucose. In extreme emergencies, when the body's stores of glucose and glycogen have been exhausted, the liver resorts to transforming the body's protein stores (muscle mass and vital organs) into sugar.

When liver function is impaired, excess glucose in the blood does not get converted into glycogen; instead, it is converted into fat and stored. The proper functioning of the liver is thus vital to proper weight management. "When glycogen formation, storage, and release are inhibited by liver malfunction, the result is often fatigue and obesity," says Paul Yanick, Jr., Ph.D., a holistic health scientist from Woodbridge, New Jersey.[3]

Essential Fatty Acid Deficiencies
Deficiencies in certain fats called essential fatty acids (EFAs—SEE QUICK DEFINITION) often lead to weight gain. The liver plays a key role in

ensuring that the body receives an adequate supply of these vital nutrients. Ralph Golan, M.D., a holistic physician from Seattle, Washington, and author of *Optimal Wellness*, says, "Symptoms of nutrient or essential fatty acid deficiencies may not stem from dietary inadequacy, but from poor absorption due to problems in the liver and gallbladder."[4] Essential fatty acid deficiencies contribute to weight gain by increasing appetite and reducing energy levels, thereby making exercise more difficult. EFAs are also needed to boost the metabolic rate and increase energy production in the body.

The liver makes it possible for the body to absorb EFAs by producing bile. Bile is largely made up of wastes that the liver collects from the blood, specifically bilirubin, which is the by-product of spent red blood cells. Bile is manufactured in the liver and stored in the gallbladder, a small storage sac attached to the liver that empties into the small intestine. The gallbladder releases bile when fat is present in the intestine. Bile helps digest fat, breaking it up into microscopic droplets small enough to pass through the gastrointestinal wall. When the liver or gallbladder become clogged or overloaded with toxins, bile is not released into the intestines, resulting in poor digestion and absorption of EFAs. Studies show that individuals who are overweight frequently suffer from poor fat digestion and absorption.[5]

In addition, trans-fatty acids (SEE QUICK DEFINITION), substances found in fried or processed fatty foods, cause the liver to produce a thickened bile that is more difficult to expel. The result is congestion in the gallbladder, which can lead to the formation of hard crystals called gallstones. This congestion also impairs the digestion of fats, potentially leading to weight gain.

Slowing Metabolism

The thyroid gland (SEE QUICK DEFINITION) is one of the chief regulators of metabolism, the biological process by which energy (measured in calories) is extracted from food and used by the body. The thyroid is also very sensitive to toxic agents. When this gland is damaged by toxins, it does

QUICK DEFINITION

Essential fatty acids (EFAs) are unsaturated fats required in the diet. Omega-3 and omega-6 oils are the two principal types. The primary omega-3 oil is alpha-linolenic acid (ALA), found in flaxseed, canola, pumpkin, walnut, and soybeans. Fish oils contain the other principal omega-3 oils, DHA (docosahexaenoic acid) and EPA (eicosapentaenoic acid). Linoleic acid is the main omega-6 oil, found in most vegetable oils, including safflower, corn, peanut, and sesame. The most therapeutic form of omega-6 oil is gamma-linolenic acid (GLA), found in evening primrose, black currant, and borage oils.

A **trans-fatty acid** is a chemically and structurally altered hydrogenated vegetable oil (such as margarine), which is combined with hydrogen to lengthen shelf-life. It is estimated that Americans consume over 600 million pounds annually of TFAs in the form of frying fats. TFAs can increase the risk of heart disease by 27% when consumed as at least 12% of the total fat intake. TFAs reduce production of prostaglandins (hormones that control all cell-to-cell interactions) and interfere with fatty acid metabolism.

For more about **fatty acids and weight**, see Chapter 2: Healthy Eating, pp. 50-75. For more on the **thyroid and weight problems**, see Chapter 9: Overcome a Sluggish Thyroid, pp. 202-219.

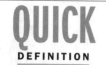

not produce or release the hormones that stimulate metabolism, causing fewer calories to get burned as fuel and more to be stored as fat.[6]

The liver helps to protect the thyroid from damage by eliminating toxins that enter the body. When the liver is overloaded with too many toxins, the thyroid is usually affected as well. Broda O. Barnes, M.D., Ph.D., a pioneer in thyroid research and author of over 100 research articles on this gland, was among the first to recognize the link between the thyroid and liver. Dr. Barnes discovered that many of his patients who suffered from an underactive thyroid (a condition called hypothyroidism) also had trouble converting glucose into glycogen, a task handled by the liver.[7] This and other indicators suggested to Dr. Barnes that liver and thyroid function were closely related.

What Poisons the Liver?

Virtually everything we take into our bodies gets filtered through the liver. This may include a lifetime of poor food choices, pesticides and chemicals, and residues of prescription drugs. Is it any wonder that this can overload the liver with toxins?

Human exposure to harmful chemical agents is far greater today than it was in previous generations. According to Dennis Crawford, D.C., of Fair Oaks, California, environmental toxins have increased 3,000 times over the last 50 years. Today, 69 million Americans live in areas that exceed smog standards and most drinking water contains over 700 harmful chemicals. Where do these toxins come from? The Environmental Protection Agency has identified more than 65,000 toxic chemicals that are released into the environment from industrial sources.[8] Agriculture also releases about one billion pounds of highly toxic pesticides into the environment each year. Not surprisingly, the residues of many of these pesticides end up in our food and our bodies. Exposure to these environmental toxins has a severe impact on the liver.

Other factors that strain the cleansing capacity of our livers are alcohol, tobacco, caffeine, recreational drug use and medications (particularly anabolic steroids, high-dose acetaminophen or aspirin, oral contraceptives, and chemotherapy).[9] In addition to being toxic themselves, some of these substances (particularly the medications) cause a decrease in the rate at which food moves through the intesti-

How the Liver Handles Toxins

The liver collects toxic waste from the blood, which flows through the organ at a rate of approximately 1½ quarts per minute. As the blood enters the liver, specialized immune cells called phagocytes remove and destroy harmful bacteria and other foreign matter. Acting in concert with the phagocytes are hepatocytes, cells that chemically break down toxins using special enzymes. The hepatocytes are able to manufacture new enzymes (SEE QUICK DEFINITION) for every new waste that enters the liver. This ability to "customize" enzymes is what makes the liver such a potent detoxifier.

"One can only marvel at the fact that hepatocytes will, on demand, fabricate the specific enzyme needed to metabolize a specific toxin," says Ralph Golan, M.D. In addition to harmful chemicals, the hepatocytes break down excess hormones, such as estrogen, cortisol, and adrenaline, that circulate in the blood. The hepatocytes' enzyme system works in a two-phase cycle. In

QUICK
DEFINITION

Enzymes are specialized living proteins fundamental to all living processes in the body, necessary for every chemical reaction and the normal activity of our organs, tissues, and cells. Enzymes are essential for the production of energy required to run cellular functions and enable the body to digest and assimilate food. Enzymes also assist in clearing the body of toxins and cellular debris.

phase I, the toxins are made less potent by a "deactivating" process (i.e., oxidation reduction, sulfoxidation, or hydrolysis). In phase II, the toxins are "packaged" in a molecular structure that allows them to dissolve in water. This packaging makes it easier for them to be excreted in the urine or feces.

When the liver is overloaded with toxins, this system malfunctions in a variety of ways. The liver tries to get rid of the toxic backlog by increasing the rate of the phase I cycle. Even though this processes a larger quantity of toxins, it is less effective in completely deactivating them. Along with increasing phase I, the liver may slow down the phase II cycle. Dr. Jack Tips describes individuals suffering from such a combined response as "pathological detoxifiers." The problem is that toxins are not being broken down in phase I and the slowdown in phase II makes it harder for the body to excrete them. This causes them to circulate in the blood and accumulate in fat and muscle tissue.[10]

---

nal tract, creating stagnant conditions favorable for harmful bacteria such as *Salmonella*, *Staphylococcus*, and *Clostridia*. These bacteria feed on fecal matter, producing toxic by-products in the colon. The toxins are then transferred to the liver, where they may decrease the liver's cleansing capacity.

Emotional stress can also have a toxic impact on the liver. In Chinese medicine, the liver is the seat of the emotions. "The emotional energy released by anger disrupts and depresses liver func-

For more on **the role of emotions in weight loss**, see Chapter 7: Heal Your Emotional Appetite, pp. 156-182.

tion," says Daniel Reid, author of *The Complete Book of Chinese Health and Healing*. Moreover, strong emotions, such as irritability and quick temper, can also be the symptoms of a diseased liver.[11]

Success Story: Detoxification Helps Asthma and Obesity

Brad, 54, was 5'11½" and weighed 260 pounds, but his chief goal in seeking the help of naturopath Kevin Davison, N.D., of Haiku, Hawaii, was to get control of his asthma. He'd had asthma for many years and suffered with frequent attacks, requiring that he use his inhaler three times a day as well as two to three doses of Allegra, a conventional antihistamine. He also complained of extreme fatigue, digestive problems (gas, diarrhea, and abdominal pain), swollen lower extremities and feet, lower back pain and bone pain, and excessive joint mobility causing frequent ankle sprains.

"He had exhausted all other possibilities in terms of getting control of his asthma," says Dr. Davison, "and he recognized that his weight was probably part of the problem." Dr. Davison first wanted to get a precise idea of Brad's body composition, that is, amounts of lean muscle, fat, and water. To do this, he used bio-impedence: a small electrical current is run through the body and differences in resistance can be calibrated to different types of body tissue. Brad, at 260 pounds, was 34% (or 88.4 pounds) healthy lean tissue, 28% (70.9 pounds) body fat, and 63.4 liters of water. Normal ranges would be 30%-42% lean tissue and 16%-20% body fat; water level is variable per individual. This put Brad significantly above the normal level of body fat.

Dr. Davison also wanted to assess Brad's thyroid function. He had Brad measure his basal (resting) body temperature, which involves taking underarm temperatures on consecutive mornings. Brad's average on his temperature test was 96.5° F, indicating depressed thyroid function (a normal average would be 97.8° F or higher). A blood test revealed that Brad's cholesterol level (223) and triglycerides (101) were both elevated. His blood level of high-density lipoproteins (HDLs, the "good" cholesterol) was 51 and low-density lipoproteins (LDLs, the so-called bad cholesterol) was 152; Dr. Davison was particularly concerned about the high levels of both total cholesterol and LDLs. For the final piece of the diagnostic puzzle, a saliva pH test revealed that Brad tended toward being acidic.

Because he felt food allergies were a factor, Dr. Davison started Brad on a modified elimination diet, which excluded yeast-derived products, caffeine, dairy, gluten-containing grains like wheat, refined carbohydrates, and food additives. He also recommended a macromineral supplement to help rebalance Brad's acid levels. Because of the depressed thyroid function, Dr. Davison recommended Metabolic Enhancer (two capsules, three times daily), a formula containing thyroid glandulars and nutrients to support the production of thyroid hormones, which helps increase the metabolic rate.

Brad lost seven pounds of water weight and 11 pounds of total weight in the first 12 days. Why did he lose so much water weight so quickly? Getting his pH balanced was the first factor. "If a person is too acidic, they tend to hold on to water because the body is trying to dilute metabolic waste products or toxins," says Dr. Davison. Reducing his exposure to allergenic foods was also important, according to Dr. Davison, because food allergies cause an inflammatory reaction that can lead to water retention. Increasing Brad's metabolism also helped burn off some weight.

Dr. Davison then started Brad on a liver detoxification program. He recommended a product called UltraClear, manufactured by Metagenics. UltraClear is a "medical food" based on rice protein to provide necessary nutrients to the body during the detoxification process. Brad was put on a diet of low-carbohydrate fruits and vegetables, large quantities of water, essential fatty acids (EFAs; sources include flaxseeds, pumpkin seeds, and walnuts), and protein from fresh ocean fish, free-range poultry, or legumes.

> ## Toxins That Can Poison the Liver
>
> - Pesticides, herbicides, and fungicides
> - Antibiotics and growth hormones used in food production
> - Vaccinations
> - Food additives and preservatives
> - Prescription drugs
> - Auto exhaust
> - Fluoride
> - Household cleaning fluids
> - Mercury amalgam fillings
> - Recreational drugs
> - Electromagnetic fields
> - X rays
> - Alcohol
> - Tobacco
> - Coffee
> - Hydrogenated fats
> - Fried foods
> - Cosmetics[12]

After four days, Dr. Davison moved Brad into the intensive clearing phase. He increased Brad's dose of UltraClear to five times per day, with a tablespoon of ground flaxseeds for EFAs. Brad's diet was to consist exclusively of a broth containing natural minerals to promote his body's alkalinity. The broth was made from equal amounts of celery, green beans, zucchini, spinach, and parsley, steamed, then blended with the water to form a puree (to be eaten at least twice per day). The

"Increased weight always increases the stress on organs and tissues, especially blood circulation to the kidneys and liver," explains Kevin Davison, N.D. "With obesity, the person is nutritionally starving but calorically over-loaded."

Kevin Davison, N.D., L.Ac.: 2310 Umi Place, Haiku, HI 96708; tel: 808-575-2328; fax: 808-575-2186. For **Metabolic Enhancer** (available to licensed health-care practitioners only), contact: Professional Health Products, 211 Overlook Drive, Suite 6, Sewickley, PA 15143; tel: 800-929-4133 or 412-741-6351; fax: 412-741-6372. For **UltraClear** and **UltraClear Sustain** (available to licensed health-care practitioners only), contact: Metagenics, Inc., 971 Calle Negocio, San Clemente, CA 92673; tel: 800-692-9400; fax: 949-366-0818.

combination of UltraClear and the diet "are very good for cleaning out the hardware of the system and all the bile channels of the liver," explains Dr. Davison. He had Brad take a buffered vitamin C supplement as well, to help reduce any detoxification symptoms. After one week, the swelling in Brad's feet and ankles had reduced by 70%, his bowel movements normalized, and he was able to reduce his asthma medication by 80%.

Two months after his first visit to Dr. Davison, Brad had lost 45 pounds. He was then put on UltraClear Sustain, a "pre-biotic" formula to help rebuild his intestinal lining, and started reintroducing foods into his diet, noting any allergic responses that might arise. Brad took a multivitamin/mineral formula for nutritional support and Dr. Davison also used acupuncture treatments to increase liver circulation and bile flow. "Increased weight always increases the stress on organs and tissues, especially blood circulation to the kidneys and liver," explains Dr. Davison. "With obesity, the person is nutritionally starving but calorically over-loaded."

After five months, Brad's weight was down to 195, healthy lean tissue was at 37%, his body fat was down to 20% (he'd lost about 12 pounds of fat), and water was at 51 liters. His cholesterol was a healthier 157, triglycerides were 93, and his level of LDL cholesterol had dropped to 100. Most importantly, Brad felt great and he was completely off his asthma medication.

Diagnosing Liver Function

Standard liver function tests used by most mainstream physicians can detect serious liver disorders such as hepatitis, viral infections, or cirrhosis. However, most of these tests are not as precise in detecting earlier, more subtle stages of liver toxicity. "Laboratory tests may be completely normal, even when serious liver symptoms exist," says Dr. Golan.[13]

Dr. Golan recommends using a testing procedure called the Functional Liver Detoxification Profile, created by Jeffrey Bland, Ph.D., of Gig Harbor, Washington, which examines the liver's ability to carry out its function of filtering toxins. After an overnight fast, the patient is given two challenge substances, caffeine and sodium benzoate (a common preservative), to test the liver's ability to clear them from the body. Saliva samples are taken to measure caffeine clearance and a urine sample measures for the breakdown products of sodium benzoate. Adequate levels of these substances should appear in the body fluids of individuals with healthy livers. These levels can be used to precisely diagnose problems in both phase I (the caffeine challenge) and phase II (the sodium benzoate challenge) of the liver's detoxification processes.

Jeffrey Bland, Ph.D., is CEO of HealthComm, Inc., a company that supplies nutritional products to health-care professionals. HealthComm also maintains a practitioner referral database. For more information, contact: HealthComm, Inc., 5800 Soundview Drive, Gig Harbor, WA 98335; tel: 800-245-9076. For the **Functional Liver Detoxification Profile**, contact: Great Smokies Diagnostic Laboratory, 63 Zillicoa Street, Asheville, NC 28801; tel: 800-522-4762 or 704-253-0621; fax: 704-252-9303.

Look for the Warning Signs—As mentioned above, emotional outbursts may also reflect a liver problem, especially if tantrums are accompanied by headaches, dizziness, blurred vision, and mental confusion. "If you are feeling fatigued, cranky, or nervous, and you get frequent headaches, this could be your liver's way of informing you that it needs to be cleansed," according to Dr. Yanick.[14]

A constipated bowel can also be caused by a toxic liver. Higher fat content tends to slow the movement of food through the intestines and colon, a condition which occurs when the body produces too little bile. When the liver and gallbladder are producing and releasing adequate bile, the fat is broken up and better absorbed by the body. One of the easiest ways to check the fat content of your stool—and thus your liver function—is to see whether your stools float or sink after a bowel movement. If the stool floats instead of sinks, it means you are not properly breaking down and absorbing fat in your intestines. This could mean either a gallbladder infection or a defect in how your liver's phase II process is breaking down fat.

Natural Therapies for Cleansing the Liver

A number of alternative therapies can help alleviate the toxic load of the liver, including cleansing the liver using natural substances, nutrients and herbs, and flower essence therapy.

Liver-Cleansing Programs
Appropriate cleansing treatments for the liver vary depending on the extent of the toxic overload. In general, mild toxicity can be corrected by consuming ample quantities of fresh fruit, vegetables, whole grains, and a limited amount of high-quality proteins. It is important to stop

eating and drinking harmful substances, such as alcohol, caffeine, and saturated fats. Periodic liver-cleansing treatments can also help prevent an excess buildup of liver toxins. One of the hallmarks of natural medicine is attention to the condition of the internal organs, especially the liver and gallbladder, and it is surprisingly easy to use herbs and nutrients to safely and effectively cleanse these organs. Many holistic practitioners, in fact, recommend such an organ cleansing on a yearly basis as a disease prevention and health maintenance strategy.

A Natural Liver Flush—The healthy and efficient functioning of the liver is central to well-being and disease prevention, which explains why it's advisable to periodically flush the organ clean using natural substances, says master herbalist and acupuncturist Christopher Hobbs, L.Ac. "Liver flushes are used to stimulate elimination of wastes from the body, to open and cool the liver, to increase bile flow, and to improve overall liver functioning," says Dr. Hobbs. "I have taken liver flushes for many years now and can heartily recommend them." Here are Dr. Hobbs' instructions for preparing and administering a liver flush:[16]

- Citrus Juice—Squeeze enough fresh lemons or limes to produce one cup of juice, says Dr. Hobbs. A small amount of distilled or spring water may be added to dilute the juice, but the more sour it tastes, the better it will perform as a liver cleanser. Orange and grapefruit juices may also be used, provided they are blended with some lemon or lime juice.

- Garlic and Ginger—To the citrus juice mixture add the juice of 1-2 cloves of garlic, freshly-squeezed in a garlic press, and a small amount of freshly grated raw ginger juice, Dr. Hobbs advises. Grate the raw ginger on a cheese or vegetable grater then put the shreds into a garlic press and squeeze out the juice.

- Olive Oil—Add one tablespoon of high-quality olive oil (such as extra virgin) to the citrus, garlic, and ginger juice. Either blend or shake the ingredients to guarantee complete mixing.

- Taking the Flush—The liver flush is best taken in the morning, preferably after some stretching and breathing exercises, says Dr.

Symptoms of a Toxic Liver

- Overweight
- Food allergies
- High cholesterol
- Fatigue
- Jaundice
- Hormonal imbalances
- Headaches or dizziness
- Constipation and bloating
- Skin problems (acne, eczema, psoriasis)
- Hypoglycemia
- Nausea
- Eye problems
- Memory difficulties[15]

CAUTION

Consult a qualified health professional before you begin any detoxification program.

Hobbs. Do not eat any foods for one hour following the flush, he adds.

■ Cleansing Herbal Tea—After an hour has elapsed, Dr. Hobbs recommends taking two cups of an herbal blend he calls "Polari Tea." It consists of dry portions of fennel (1 part), flax (1 part), burdock (¼ part), fenugreek (1 part), licorice (¼ part), and peppermint (1 part). Simmer the herbs (except the peppermint) for 20 minutes, then add the peppermint and allow to steep for ten minutes. For convenience, you may prepare several quarts of the tea in advance.

■ Continuing the Flush—Dr. Hobbs suggests doing the liver flush twice yearly, in the spring and fall, for two full cycles each. A cycle consists of ten consecutive days of taking the flush ingredients, followed by three days off, then another ten days on. "I have never seen anyone experience negative side effects from this procedure."

A Liver and Gallbladder Clean-Out—This liver and gallbladder flush procedure comes from Keith DeOrio, M.D., director of the DeOrio Medical Group in Santa Monica, California. The clean-out program, which calls for apple juice or cider, Epsom salts, and olive oil, works as a detoxifying agent to restore normal function to the liver and gallbladder. The acids in the apple juice help to soften gallstones, the magnesium in the Epsom salts relaxes the sphincters of the gallbladder and bile duct, and the olive oil produces contractions in the liver and gallbladder that help in the excretion of stored waste materials, says Dr. DeOrio. To do the flush, Dr. DeOrio typically advises following these steps:

■ Days 1-5—Follow your usual diet. Drink as much apple juice or cider (preferably organic) as possible on these days, diluting the juice

Coffee Enema to Purge the Liver

A coffee enema can be a useful option for detoxifying the liver. It causes the blood vessels in the large intestine to expand, helping to purge the liver and colon of accumulated toxins, dead cells, and waste products. The enema is prepared by brewing organic caffeinated coffee and letting it cool to body temperature, then delivering it via an enema bag. Coffee contains choleretics, substances that increase the flow of toxin-rich bile from the gallbladder. The coffee enema may be among the only pharmaceutically effective choleretics noted in the medical literature that can be safely used many times daily without toxic effects. "The coffee enema is capable of purging toxins because it dilates the bile ducts and stimulates enzymes capable of removing toxins from the blood," says Etienne Callebout, M.D., a London-based physician and homeopath. Caffeine also stimulates dilation of blood vessels and relaxation of smooth muscles, which further increases bile flow; this effect does not happen when the coffee is consumed as a beverage.[17]

Keith DeOrio, M.D.:
The DeOrio Medical Group, 1821 Wilshire Blvd., Suite 100, Santa Monica, CA 90403; tel: 310-828-3096; fax: 310-453-1918. For **Phosfood**, contact: Standard Process, P.O. Box 1289, Alameda, CA 94501; tel: 800-662-9134 or 510-865-4322; fax: 510-865-4335. For **lipotropic products**, contact: Enzymatic Therapy, 825 Challenger Drive, Green Bay, WI 54311; tel: 800-783-2286 or 920-469-1313; fax: 920-469-4444. Solgar, 500 Willow Tree Road, Leonia, NJ 07605; tel: 800-645-2246 or 201-944-2311; fax: 201-944-7351. Metagenics, Inc., 971 Calle Negocio, San Clemente, CA 92673; tel: 800-692-9400; fax: 714-366-0818.

with an equal amount of water. While individual tolerances vary, Dr. DeOrio recommends drinking at least ½ gallon of the diluted juice each day. Add one ounce of Phosfood (a product that helps dissolve gallstones) to each gallon of juice before it is diluted.

■ Day 6—Eat lunch as usual at noon. At 3 p.m., dissolve two teaspoons of Epsom salts in two ounces of hot water and drink. To offset the unpleasant taste, Dr. DeOrio suggests following this with a little freshly squeezed orange juice. Before bed, lightly heat ½ cup of cold-pressed olive oil and then drink the oil, followed by a small glass of orange juice. (Alternatively, you may blend the olive oil with the juice and drink the mixture.) Immediately afterward, get into bed and lie on your right side with your right knee pulled up to your chest. This ensures that the liver, located on the right side of the body at the base of the rib cage, receives the full benefit of the olive oil/orange juice mixture. Maintain this position for 30 minutes, then sleep normally.

■ Day 7—One hour before eating breakfast, dissolve two teaspoons of Epsom salts in two ounces of hot water and drink.

Dr. DeOrio cautions that some people experience mild nausea or, in rare cases, vomiting when using the olive oil and orange juice mixture. Though momentarily uncomfortable, these symptoms are actually a good sign, confirming that the flush is working, Dr. DeOrio says. The nausea is due to the release of stored toxins from the gallbladder and liver. Both nausea and vomiting should pass after a few hours, according to Dr. DeOrio. If one experiences pain in your upper right abdomen following the flush, Dr. DeOrio usually suggests drinking another two teaspoons of Epsom salts dissolved in hot water. If pain persists for more than four to six hours, consult a physician.

Nutritional Supplements

Lipotropics are substances that naturally prevent excess fat from accumulating in the liver. They help cleanse the liver by promoting the flow of fat and bile into the gallbladder, and stimulate the growth of phagocyte cells (the bacteria-eating cells in the liver).[18] Naturopath Michael Murray, N.D., author of *Natural Alternatives for Weight Loss*, notes that nutritionists commonly prescribe a lipotropic agent to treat hepatitis or cirrhosis of the liver.

Lipotropic Vitamins—Betaine and inositol (two B vitamins) along with choline (a B-complex co-factor) are common lipotropic agents. You can obtain these substances from dietary sources. Betaine is found primarily in beets; beet root supplements (in capsule form) and ox bile extracts are used to ease bile congestion and improve bile flow to the small intestine. Inositol is found in fruits, meats, milk, and whole grains. Choline is present in high amounts in egg yolks, meat, milk, whole grains, and soybeans. Choline can chemically react with both water and fat, making it particularly suited for helping to transport fat-soluble toxins found in the liver to the kidneys, where they are excreted out of the body. Dr. Murray recommends taking a daily supplement that includes betaine, inositol, choline, and the amino acid methionine, at the combined dosage of 1,000 mg.[19]

Amino Acids—The amino acid methionine helps stimulate the flow of fats from the liver. Glutathione and carnitine are two other amino acids that help cleanse the liver. Glutathione, a critical antioxidant (SEE QUICK DEFINITION), reduces free radical damage to cells, prevents depletion of other antioxidants, and activates certain immune cells.

Glutathione is manufactured in the liver from glutamic acid and the amino acid N-acetyl-cysteine (NAC). Jay Lombard, M.D., recommends NAC (1 g daily on an empty stomach), lipoic acid (200 mg daily with food), and selenium (no more than 200 mcg daily with food) to raise glutathione levels.[20]

Carnitine is manufactured in the liver from the amino acids methionine and lysine with the aid of vitamin C. The body uses carnitine to transport fats into the mitochondria (the energy centers of cells) for combustion and energy production. When liver function is impaired, both glutathione and carnitine levels may become low. Carnitine supplements can also help cleanse weak livers of accumulated toxins. The typical recommended dose is 300 mg daily.

Another amino acid, taurine, is needed by the liver in order to manufacture bile acids for the digestion of fats. If the synthesis of bile acids is impaired, it can result in an elevation of cholesterol levels. Taurine is also necessary for the liver's detoxification process, particularly in removing

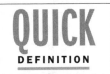

QUICK DEFINITION

An **antioxidant** (meaning "against oxidation") is a natural biochemical substance that protects living cells against damage from harmful free radicals. Antioxidants work against the process of oxidation—the robbing of electrons from substances. If unblocked or left uncontrolled, oxidation can lead to cellular aging, degeneration, arthritis, heart disease, cancer, and other illnesses. Antioxidants in the body react readily with oxygen breakdown products and free radicals, and neutralize them before they can damage the body. Antioxidant nutrients include vitamins A, C, and E, beta carotene, selenium, coenzyme Q10, pycnogenol (grape seed extract), L-glutathione, superoxide dismutase, and bioflavonoids. Plant antioxidants include *Ginkgo biloba* and garlic. When antioxidants are taken in combination, the effect is stronger than when they are used individually.

environmental chemicals (such as chlorine and petroleum solvents) from the body. A typical dosage is 200-500 mg daily.[21]

Chlorophyll—Chlorophyll is a liver purifier and healer. Naturopath Bernard Jensen, Ph.D., author of *Chlorella, Jewel of the Far East*, considers chlorella, a food algae, as the best source of chlorophyll. He indicates that chlorella is able to help a toxic, mineral-deficient liver by cleansing and soothing bowel tissue, stimulating bowel function, and contributing to the repair and rejuvenation of liver cells.[22] A typical recommended dose of chlorella is 100 mg daily. Other sources of chlorophyll include sprouted barley juice and wheat grass juice (available at most health food stores).

Psyllium Husk—Psyllium is an excellent source of soluble fiber and has been shown to be effective in lowering cholesterol levels, thus helping those with compromised liver function metabolize fat. Typical recommended dose is 3-4 grams mixed with water or juice, three times daily. Drinking this mixture before meals may help with appetite control.[23] Drink extra water when taking psyllium.

Herbal Supplements
Certain herbs have a mild detoxifying effect on the liver. Taken regularly, they can be used to prevent liver disease and maintain healthy function.

Milk Thistle—Milk thistle (*Silybum marianum*) grows primarily in Europe, where it is often prescribed to treat and protect the liver. As far back as the 17th century, this herb was known as "a friend to liver and blood." The active ingredient in milk thistle is silymarin, a substance that prevents inflammation and protects against the harmful effects of free radicals. It also stimulates liver cell growth and the production of bile. Milk thistle seeds can be used to make a tea or powdered seeds can be taken in capsule form. To make a tea, steep one teaspoon of seeds in ½ cup of water; drink one to 1½ cups of tea daily. For the powdered form of milk thistle, typically take one capsule (approximately one teaspoon) with water five times per day.

For **herbal liver formulas** (available only to health-care professionals), contact: Apple-A-Day, 4201 Bee Caves Road, Suite C-212, Austin, TX 78746; tel: 512-328-3996; fax: 512-328-0812.

Dandelion Root—"Dandelion root (*Taraxacum officinale*) is regarded as one of the finest liver remedies, both as food and as medicine," according to naturopaths Michael Murray, N.D., and Joseph Pizzorno, Jr., N.D., authors of *A*

Textbook of Natural Medicine.[24] The common dandelion has been used for centuries as a liver remedy and weight-loss aid. Its ability to stimulate the production and secretion of bile was first noted by researchers in 1875. Dandelion is also a potent diuretic, meaning it promotes the excretion of urine, which helps flush toxins from the body. Drs. Murray and Pizzorno typically suggest taking four grams of dried root (available in capsule form) or 4-8 ml of dandelion extract, three times daily.

Oregon Grape Root–Oregon grape root (*Berberis aquifolium*) is considered a gentle stimulant for the liver and gallbladder. It helps improve overall liver function as well as its detoxification processes. Because of its bitter taste, Oregon grape root is generally taken as a tea: mix one part Oregon grape root with one part dandelion root and ¼ part fennel seed.[25]

Globe Artichoke–Globe artichoke (*Cynara scolymus*) is a tonic herb that is liver protective. Research indicates that it may lower cholesterol levels as well as reducing amounts of metabolic waste products in the blood. Globe artichoke is available in capsule form or as a dried herb; typical recommended dose is 300-500 mg daily.[26]

Dietary Support
Certain dietary recommendations will help support the liver during the detoxification process. Try to avoid fats from animal sources (meats and dairy) and limit the overall amount of animal foods you eat. Incorporate more chlorophyll-rich foods (particularly dark leafy greens) and raw vegetables into your diet. [27]

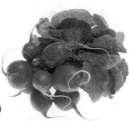

When the liver becomes toxic, more water is required to help flush impurities from the liver out through the kidneys. You should drink eight large glasses of pure water daily to bring your liver back to health; the best source is distilled water. Dr. Skinner considers distilled water to be the only form of water that is truly pure. She says that even filtered and spring water are not as good as distilled water, as the former contain fine mineral particles, which can clog the circulatory system and liver and add to the body's toxic burden. Although minerals are important to nutritional health, the type of minerals present in water are inorganic—a chemical form that is not biologically active and cannot be used by the body. Dr. Skinner also says that, contrary to what other health and nutrition experts claim, distilled water does not leach minerals from the body. "It only collects and removes inorganic minerals that have already been refused and rejected by the cells," she says. "No liquid can leach out organic minerals once they have become integrated in the body."[28]

Flower Essence Therapy

In traditional Chinese medicine, the liver is closely related to the emotions of anger, irritability, resentment, and jealousy. Resolving these emotional problems can help restore the health of the liver. "Bringing repressed anger to the surface where it can be dealt with frees the liver from some of its toxic burden," says David Kamnitzer, D.C., of the Center for Well-Being in Campbell, California. One way to resolve emotional issues is through flower essence therapy, an alternative treatment frequently used to treat psychological and spiritual issues. Flower essences are made by floating fresh blossoms in spring water and letting them sit in the sun for a few hours. The blossoms are removed, leaving the essence of the flower, which is then diluted to a dosage level. Drops of the essences are placed under the tongue, ingested in a tonic, or diluted in a bath. Although you can administer a flower essence treatment yourself, a trained practitioner can help tailor a treatment program specific to your needs and offer counseling as you work through emotional issues.

For information on **flower remedies**, contact: Flower Essence Society, P.O. Box 1769, Nevada City, CA 95959; tel: 800-548-0075 or 916-265-9163; fax: 916-265-6467.

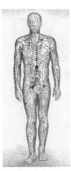

The lymph system is part
of the body's internal plumbing, helping it dispose of
wastes and debris generated by muscles and
other body tissues. A variety of factors can cause lymph
fluid to become heavy and thick, which restricts its
flow and causes it to back-up in the body.
Such blockages not only cause excess body weight
but a number of other serious diseases.

16 Get the Lymph Flowing

THE LYMPH SYSTEM is part of the body's internal plumbing, helping it dispose of wastes and debris generated by muscles and other body tissues. A variety of factors can cause lymph fluid to become heavy and thick, which restricts its flow and causes it to back-up in the body. Such blockages not only cause excess body weight but a number of other serious diseases.

You may have never heard of the lymphatic system or be aware of the important role it has in maintaining your health. The lymph system serves as the body's central drainage system, channeling cellular wastes and toxic materials away from cells, then eliminating them from the body. This waste disposal mechanism is why the lymphatic system has been called "the metabolic garbage can of the body."[1]

However, if this "garbage can" is not emptied often enough, serious problems can result as the body becomes overburdened with toxins. The lymph fluid, normally clear, can become heavy and thick and the lymph nodes and channels can stagnate with toxins. This accumulation of wastes in the lymph puts an added burden on the other detoxification organs, particularly the liver and kidneys. Eventually, these organs can also become weakened by the constant flow of toxins from the polluted lymph nodes and channels, leading to a cascade of health problems, including an accumulation of excess weight.

Unclogging the lymph can make the difference for many overweight individuals. Unfortunately, mainstream medicine tends to ignore the lymph's role in maintaining a healthy body weight. Few conventional doctors examine or treat the lymph and rarely even mention or discuss it with their patients. "The action of the lymph system is basic to everything else that happens in the body, but mainstream medicine has overlooked its vital importance," says Marika von Viczay, N.D., Ph.D., of Asheville, North Carolina. Getting heavy stagnant lymph moving again, and preventing its future build-up, is possible with the right treatment. The result may be not only a trimmer body but a healthier one as well. In this chapter, we look at how stagnant lymph can lead to excess weight. We examine the potential causes of a sluggish lymph system and ways to determine if this may be a factor in your weight problem. Finally, we offer a variety of alternative medicine techniques for getting the lymph flowing again.

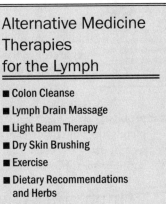

Alternative Medicine Therapies for the Lymph

- Colon Cleanse
- Lymph Drain Massage
- Light Beam Therapy
- Dry Skin Brushing
- Exercise
- Dietary Recommendations and Herbs
- Herbal Wraps
- Acupressure and Reflexology

Marika von Viczay, N.D., Ph.D.: 85 Tunnel Road, Suite 12-A264, Asheville, NC 28805; tel: 704-253-8371; fax: 704-258-1350.

Success Story: Unclogging the Lymph, Losing Weight

"My legs were severely swollen and I had a double chin," says Colette, 55, whose weight fluctuated between 180 pounds and 200 pounds on her 5'6" frame. On a friend's recommendation, Colette went to see naturopathic physician Dr. von Viczay. From her exam of Colette, Dr. von Viczay recognized the symptoms of stagnant and toxic lymph (see "Your Lymph System at a Glance," p. 352) and immediately recommended a program for Colette to get her lymph fluid moving again.

"My legs seemed to be full of fluid, so I thought I had circulation problems," Colette remarks. "I'd never even heard of the lymphatic system. I just knew I was uncomfortable and needed help." Fluid retention is a common result when the body is overwhelmed with toxins. Dr. von Viczay's program was intended to restore Colette's lym-

For more about **the liver and its role in detoxifying the body**, see Chapter 15: Cleanse the Liver pp. 330-346.

phatic system to normal functioning and move toxic wastes out of the body. She started Colette on lymph drain massage, a special massage technique that works gently to induce lymph flow. She also recommended a light beam generator, a flashlight-sized device that uses mild stimulation from light energy (photons) to unclog the lymph.

After a few sessions, Colette noticed that her appearance had changed as her system became unclogged and ended her problems with fluid retention. "My double chin disappeared completely after the first treatment," she says. "Now I eat normally and my weight stays between 145 pounds and 150 pounds. Unclogging my lymph system turned my body around."

Lymph and Weight Gain

A clogged lymphatic system can affect the entire body. The symptoms associated with blocked lymph include edema (swelling of the hands and feet), bursitis (a painful condition involving the arm sockets and shoulders), bunions, joint stiffness, dry flaking skin, bad breath, body odors, lethargy, and depression. When the lymph system becomes overburdened, toxins build up in the tissues creating an environment conducive to the development of chronic diseases such as cancer and arthritis. There are also specific ways that it can have a detrimental effect on body weight.

Cellulite—Among the places that fat accumulates in our bodies is directly beneath the skin. In some regions, such as the upper hips, thighs, arms, and buttocks, pockets of fat can give the overlying skin a dimpled texture. This dimpled skin, which looks a little like orange rind and is commonly referred to as cellulite, is a sign that waste discharged from the body's cells is pooling beneath the surface. This build-up of waste is often due to a blockage in the body's lymph system. Although the lymph is generally not a very viscous fluid, it can become thick and gooey when it is forced to carry too many wastes. There is a direct correlation between decreased lymphatic flow and the development of cellulite.[2] Dr. von Viczay explains that when the lymph is congested, "the fluid develops a cottage cheese–like consistency. You can see this in the cellulite deposits just under the skin."

Slows Metabolism—Clogged lymph can also cause a drop in metabolism (the rate at which the body burns calories), which further increases the likelihood of weight gain. In order to lose weight, you must be able to release stored toxins as well as the normal by-products of digestion that build up in the body. These substances move through your body via the lymph system. Retaining these toxins slows down your metabolism, meaning that you may start gaining weight or have to work harder just to maintain your weight.

Fluid Retention—"Many cases of overweight, in my opinion, are nothing more than retention of stagnant fluid that comes about when protein molecules couple with water in the body and block the lymph system," says Courtland Reeves, M.S., director of ELF Labs, a lymph treatment research firm in St. Francisville, Illinois. In contrast to the organized patterns of proteins that make up our muscles and other body structures, protein molecules in the lymph are disorganized and loose, attaching to one another in random clumps. Like logs floating in a river, these clumps tend to accumulate in areas where the lymph vessels narrow or are pinched, causing jams that affect fluids in whole regions of the body.

What Clogs the Lymph?

A number of factors can contribute to clogging the lymphatic system:

■ Not getting sufficient exercise is a major factor in lymph problems. Exercise moves the muscles and creates pressure within the lymph vessels, forcing the fluid to flow. When the muscles are not exercised, the lymph is not put under this pressure and begins to stagnate.

■ Overexposure to environmental chemicals or other toxins can interfere with the smooth flow of lymph fluid.

■ Stress leads to a stagnant lymph by creating tension in the body that can lead to structural misalignment in the neck, which pinches the lymph vessels.

■ Intestinal problems, such as chronic constipation, also adversely affect the lymph system. The walls of the colon serve as an outlet for the lymph and thus cannot be plugged up with mucus or fecal matter. In order to effectively release lymphatic material, the inner lining of the colon needs to be healthy.

For more on the **colon's influence on body weight**, see Chapter 12: Detoxify the Colon, pp. 272-293.

■ Some dietary practices can inhibit lymph flow, particularly too many mucus-producing foods such as dairy, fatty foods (especially those containing hydrogenated oils), highly processed foods, and allergenic foods.

Your Lymph System at a Glance

The lymphatic system is the body's master drain. It includes a vast network of capillaries that transport the lymph, a series of nodes throughout the body (primarily in the neck, groin, and armpits) that collect the lymph, and three organs (the tonsils, spleen, and thymus) that produce white blood cells (lymphocytes) to scavenge for toxins and microbes.

Lymph is the fluid that fills the spaces between cells in the body. This fluid contains nutrients to be delivered to cells and cellular debris (bacteria, dead cells, heavy metals, and waste products) to be removed. The purpose of the lymphatic system is to carry toxins away from the cells by collecting and filtering the lymph, neutralizing and disposing of bacteria or other invaders, and returning its contents to the bloodstream.

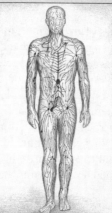

The lymph flows slowly through the body to the abdomen and chest (at the rate of three quarts per day), where it drains into the bloodstream through large ducts. Once in the blood, the toxins carried by the lymph are transported to the liver and kidneys, where they are broken down and excreted. Some of the lymph also empties directly into the colon, where it is eliminated with the feces. Unlike blood circulation, the lymphatic system does not have a pump (like the heart) to move it along. Rather, its movement depends on muscle contractions, general body activity, massage and other forms of compression, and gravity. The lymph system becomes most active during times of illness such as the flu, when the nodes (particularly at the throat) visibly swell with collected waste products.

- Structural misalignments, particularly in the neck and shoulder area, can contribute to sluggish lymph circulation.
- Medications.
- Impaired blood circulation due to chronic conditions such as diabetes or atherosclerosis may also interfere with lymph flow.
- Some surgical procedures (such as breast or abdominal surgery) require the removal of adjacent lymph nodes, which can disrupt the lymphatic system. Radiation therapy can have the same effect.
- Hormonal imbalances.
- Infections or traumatic injuries.
- Since they are absorbed through the skin, antiperspirants can slow the lymph by closing down the lymph nodes located in the underarm area.[3]

■ Tight-fitting clothing, such as the type people often wear for exercise or even women's bras, pinches the lymph vessels.

Diagnosing Lymph Problems

Alternative medicine practitioners use a variety of diagnostic tools to determine if the lymphatic system has become sluggish or clogged, including urine analysis, darkfield microscopy, electrodermal screening, and iridology.

Urine Analysis

Many alternative health-care professionals rely on a 24-hour urine analysis to assess a patient's digestive function and associated health conditions. Developed by Howard F. Loomis, Jr., D.C., a chiropractor and expert on urinalysis in Madison, Wisconsin, the test looks at an individual's total urine output over a 24-hour period. This enables a physician to see how the concentrations of various substances in the urine change over time.[4] The test assesses organ function indirectly by examining what by-products the body is discarding in the urine.

For more about **urinalysis** or to reach **Howard F. Loomis, Jr., D.C.**, contact: 21st Century Nutrition, 6421 Enterprise Lane, Madison, WI 53719; tel: 800-662-2630; fax: 608-273-8110.

For assessing potential lymph dysfunction, the 24-hour urine test can show if a person has kidney-lymphatic stress. Allergens (substances that produce an allergic reaction) and toxins build up in the bloodstream and the kidneys become exhausted from trying to cleanse the blood. The lymphatic system then becomes stressed by working to neutralize these allergens. Urine volume (the total output over the 24-hour period) in relationship to specific gravity (density of the urine compared to water) shows whether the person's kidneys and lymph system are stressed. A normal or low urine volume with a low specific gravity indicates a kidney-lymphatic stress pattern.

Also, the indican value on the urinalysis indicates colon toxicity and the degree to which digestion is malfunctioning. Indican is a group of toxic compounds that are formed when undigested protein is decomposed by pathogenic bacteria in the small intestine. The level of urinary indican is a general indicator of the inability to digest food. Indican that is not excreted in the feces is absorbed into the blood, detoxified by the liver, returned to the blood, and passed through the kidneys to be eliminated in the urine. This process causes particular stress to the liver and lymphatic system, so a high level of indican in the urine may indicate an overburdened lymph system.

Darkfield Microscopy

Darkfield microscopy is a way of studying living whole blood cells under a specially adapted microscope that projects the dynamic image, magnified 1,400 times, onto a video screen. The skilled practitioner can detect early signs of illness in the form of abnormalities in the blood known to produce disease. Relevant technical features in the blood include color, blood components, and the size of certain immune cells. The amount of time the blood cell stays viable indicates the overall health of the individual. Darkfield microscopy reveals distortions of red blood cells (which indicate nutritional status), possible undesirable bacterial or fungal life forms, and blood ecology patterns indicative of health or illness. In cases of lymph stagnation, the blood cells will appear to be coagulating or sticking together excessively, which makes the blood viscous. This may indicate an overburdened lymph system.

Electrodermal Screening

Electrodermal screening (EDS) is a form of computerized information gathering which is based on physics, not chemistry. A blunt, non-invasive electric probe is placed at specific points on the patient's hands, face, or feet, corresponding to acupuncture points at the beginning or end of energy meridians. Minute electrical discharges from these points serve as information signals about the condition of the body's organs and systems, useful for the physician in evaluation and

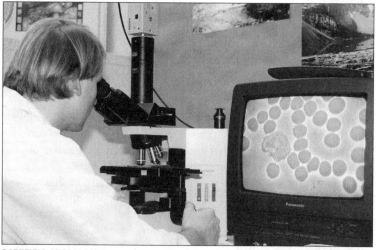

DARKFIELD MICROSCOPY.

developing a treatment plan. The trained EDS practitioner conducts an "interview" with the patient's organs and tissues, gathering information about the status of those systems and their energy pathways. In EDS testing, there are specific points which will indicate impaired functioning or blockage of the lymphatic system.

Iridology

Iridology examines the iris of the eye in order to diagnose dysfunction in the body. It was first developed in the 19th century by a Hungarian physician named Ignatiz von Peckzely and was popularized in the U.S. in the 1950s by Bernard Jensen, D.C. Iridology considers the iris to be a map of the entire body, with areas of the iris reflecting specific areas of the body. A problem or illness in the body appears as a spot, streak, or discoloration in the iris. An iridologist can thus discover the location of specific areas of weakness by examining the eyes. A toxic lymph system will appear as a discoloration of a particular area of the iris called the lymph ring.

Success Story: Detoxification Unclogs the Lymph

Ian, 45, was 5'8" and weighed 180 pounds. While this is hardly an excess of weight, Ian was at the point in his life where he was motivated to do something about his middle-age bulge. He came to see holistic chiropractor Richard Richman, D.C., who practices kinesiology (SEE QUICK DEFINITION) in Alameda, California. Dr. Richman first determined Ian's body type. He used Dr. Elliot Abravanel's body-typing system, which determines type according to a dominant endocrine gland (thyroid, adrenal, pituitary, or gonadal) indicating the individual's metabolic rate. Ian was an adrenal type, meaning that he tended to be thick and stocky, gaining weight around the midsection and the entire torso.

Ian's urine analysis and blood tests revealed nothing clinically out of the ordinary. This didn't surprise Dr. Richman. "Many times people will have problems and go to see their doctor, who will look at blood tests and say things are 'OK' when clearly everything isn't OK," says Dr. Richman. "There

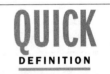

QUICK DEFINITION

Applied kinesiology, first developed by George Goodheart, D.C., of Detroit, Michigan, is the study of the relationship between muscle dysfunction (weak muscles) and related organ or gland dysfunction. Applied kinesiology employs a simple strength resistance test on a specific indicator muscle that is related to the organ or part of the body that is being tested. If the muscle tests strong (maintaining its resistance), it indicates health. If it tests weak, it can mean infection or dysfunction.

For more on **body typing**, see Chapter 1: Individualize Your Diet, pp. 34-49. For more on **dry skin brushing**, see this chapter, pp. 359-361.

could be a number of things that are borderline gray. While medical doctors do a great job of crisis care, when they try to move that type of care into subclinical conditions, it just doesn't work." When Dr. Richman ordered a darkfield exam of Ian's blood, it revealed that he was toxic. Darkfield microscopy studies blood cells under a specially adapted microscope that projects the magnified image onto a video screen, where the practitioner can detect early signs of illness. Dr. Richman says that, examining Ian's blood, he could see "waste products between the blood cells needed to be cleaned out."

He started Ian on a detoxification program to stimulate his lymph system and eliminate toxins from his body. Dr. Richman had Ian begin with a combination of dry skin brushing and Epsom salt baths or sessions in a sauna. Dry skin brushing stimulates the lymphatic system and the saunas or baths open up the skin pores and cause the body to sweat more, which also eliminates toxins. Dr. Richman encouraged Ian to drink more water (particularly before each sauna), to start on a colon-cleansing program, and to take a trace mineral formula for support during the detoxification process.

After a week of these therapies, Dr. Richman put Ian on a fast to help his body detoxify even further. The fast proceded along the following schedule:

- Day 1 (Wednesday): fresh, organic non-starchy vegetables (such as red or yellow bell peppers, tomatoes, cabbage, leafy green vegetables, squash, daikon, and root vegetables) along with healthy juices
- Day 2 (Thursday): fruits only
- Day 3 (Friday): juices, either fruit or vegetable
- Day 4 (Saturday): distilled water only; if this proves too difficult, stick with the juices from day 3
- Day 5 (Sunday): juices only
- Day 6 (Monday): fruits only
- Day 7 (Tuesday): fresh, organic non-starchy vegetables along with healthy drinks

Richard Richman, D.C.: Alameda Holistic Institute, 1505 Webster, Alameda, CA 94501; tel: 510-523-2120.

CAUTION

A fast should be done only under the proper supervision of a qualified health-care practitioner.

After one week, Ian could return to normal eating patterns, emphasizing clean, organic proteins (nuts and seeds) and fresh, organic fruits and vegetables. Dr. Richman recommends food combining for his patients—that they not eat protein and starches together, as these are difficult for the body to digest in combination, according to Dr. Richman. He also recommends avoiding all saturated fats.

Ian also started an exercise program. Dr. Richman encourages daily aerobic activity (but no less than 20 minutes three times per week) to stimulate the lymph system and burn calories. Walking and swimming are excellent choices for just about anyone, according to Dr. Richman, or simply try incorporating more physical activity into your daily life: ride your bike to work, walk to the store instead of driving, take the stairs instead of the elevator.

As part of his program, Dr. Richman tries to increase people's awareness of what and how they're eating. "People aren't very conscious of what they're putting into their mouth or the rate they're putting it in their mouth," he says. Slowing down and allowing your digestive system to register the amount of food you've eaten and paying greater attention to meals can help you lose weight. He offers a number of "table techniques" to increase awareness of your eating patterns:

- Before eating, let go of the day's activities and focus on what you're doing.
- Say a prayer, give thanks, or acknowledge the food according to your personal beliefs.
- Don't watch TV and eat at the same time.
- Take smaller food portions and leave a little on your plate.
- Cut your food into small pieces and chew each bite (15-20 times) thoroughly.
- Put down your knife and fork between bites.
- Have a good conversation with a dinner companion. "This slows down your consumption so that you are more aware of getting full and less likely to overeat," explains Dr. Richman.

With the help of this detoxification program, Ian returned to his normal weight within three months. Dr. Richman encouraged him to repeat the cleansing fast three times per year as a maintenance therapy. Ian is happy with his slimmer waistline and has adopted the new eating and lifestyle changes without any problems, according to Dr. Richman.

Alternative Medicine Therapies for the Lymph

Unclogging the lymph system is an important part of any detoxification strategy and should be part of any comprehensive approach to weight loss. "I have not seen a person who could not benefit from lymph therapy," states Dr. von Viczay. "Detoxification in this way, by reestablishing free lymphatic circulation throughout the body, is a vital part of the healing process." Techniques that can help unclog the lymph include colon cleansing, manual lymph drain massage, light beam therapy, dry skin brushing, exercise, dietary recommendations and herbs, herbal wraps, acupressure, and reflexology.

Colon Cleanse

Cleansing the colon can help stimulate the flow of lymph. "The first step in cleansing the lymphatic system is to cleanse the colon," says nutritionist Robert Gray, of San Francisco, California, author of *The Colon Health Handbook*. Gray reports that treatments that stimulate and unclog the lymph will eventually produce lymph residues in the stools. "[The lymph's] general appearance [in the stool] is like petroleum jelly, although it may vary in color from practically clear to dark brown," he says. This jelly-like lymph could harden and become stuck in the colon, causing constipation and a host of other ailments. To ensure that this material is eliminated from the body, a colon cleanse is necessary.[5]

W. Lee Cowden, M.D., an alternative medicine practitioner based in Richardson, Texas, recommends a 5-month colon-cleansing treatment program. The program includes a diet high in fiber and eliminates dairy products and refined white flour products (such as pastas, bread, and pastries). In addition to dietary changes, he recommends herbal supplements and increased fiber intake—the goal is to have 2-3 bowel movements daily. The herbs, which include slippery elm, *Cascara sagrada*, papain, cayenne, and ginger, also help to clear debris that can accumulate on the walls of the intestines over time.

For more about **colon cleansing**, see Chapter 12: Detoxify the Colon, pp. 272-293.

Lymph Drain Massage

Danish scientist Emil Vodder, Ph.D., developed a technique for lymph massage in the 1930s called manual lymph drainage. The technique employs gentle stationary circles on the lymph nodes, palpating with the tips or the entire length of the fingers. Using these light circular pumping and draining movements, the entire lymph system or particular points can be massaged, depending on the condition of the patient and the location of blockages. Manual lymph drain massage manipulates the lymphatic channels, located just beneath the surface of the skin, to stimulate lymphatic flow and enhance the release of toxins and fluids. The technique uses no oil nor is pressure or kneading of muscles used, as in other types of massage. Lymph drain massage is a commonly prescribed technique in Europe, especially in Germany, Austria, France, and Scandinavia. The technique has recently gained increased attention in North America,

CAUTION

Lymph drain massage should not to be confused with conventional massage techniques, as it relies on gentle and directed manipulations designed to induce lymph flow. The lymph should only be massaged lightly, as too much pressure can cause it to thicken.

with about 160 therapists certified in the Vodder method currently practicing in Canada and the United States.

Light Beam Therapy

Light can be used as part of a detoxification program for unclogging the lymphatic system. Among the devices used to break up viscous lymph are the Light Beam Generator™ and the Lymph-Pro Laser™. The light beam generator resembles a flashlight with a long, extensible housing. Practitioners use this hand-held device to focus energy on blocked lymph areas. The energy from the generator breaks the electrical bonds that hold clusters of lymph protein molecules together, thus unclogging blockages. "Light beam therapy can be used anywhere on the body where there is a problem," says Robert Jacobs, N.M.D., D.Hom. (Med), of London, England, "and because of its deep penetration, it can help heal organs and structures deep within the body, as well as skin problems." Dr. Jacobs also points out that since healthy cells are in a stable energetic state, there are no adverse effects when the device is used in 30-45 minute sessions.[7]

Light beam therapy is often used to augment the benefits of massage. Dr. von Viczay says that the combination "enhances manual drainage techniques and works much faster than lymphatic massage alone." Some therapists using the device have found that they can accomplish in one session what would normally take eight sessions of manual lymph drainage alone. "I have seen cellulite eliminated in a week with a combination Vodder lymph massage and 30-40 minutes of light beam treatments two times per day," says Courtland Reeves, M.S.

Dry Skin Brushing

The skin is the largest eliminative organ of the body, which is why it is sometimes called "the third kidney." The skin can eliminate more

Do-At-Home Lymph Massage

While not intended as a substitute for lymph drain massage, a self-massage technique may be helpful in stimulating the flow of lymph. Doing one leg at a time, elevate the leg and gently massage from your ankle, around your knee, and up toward your hip, massaging the front and back of your leg. This technique moves lymph fluid in the direction it should naturally flow. The ideal time to perform this type of massage is at night or at the end of the day's activities.[6]

For **referrals to certified Vodder therapists**, contact: North American Vodder Association of Lymphatic Therapy, 11526 Coral Hills Drive, Dallas, TX 75229; tel: 214-243-5959; fax: 214-243-3227. For **referrals to manual lymph drainage therapists**, contact: National Lymphedema Network, 2211 Post Street, Suite 404, San Francisco, CA 94115; tel: 800-541-3259; website: www.hooked.net/users/lymphnet.

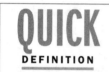

QUICK

DEFINITION

Acupuncture meridians are specific pathways in the human body for the flow of life force or subtle energy, known as *qi* (pronounced *CHEE*). In most cases, these energy pathways run up and down both sides of the body, and correspond to individual organs or organ systems, designated as Lung, Small Intestine, Heart, and others. There are 12 principal meridians and eight secondary channels. Numerous points of heightened energy, or *qi*, exist on the body's surface along the meridians and are called acupoints. There are more than 1,000 acupoints, each of which is potentially a place for acupuncture treatment.

than a pound of waste products in the form of sweat throughout the day. It is also an absorptive organ, capable of absorbing oxygen, vitamins, minerals, even protein; but it can also absorb toxic substances (through air and water contact), which can find their way into internal organs.

Dry skin brushing is based on concepts from acupuncture (SEE QUICK DEFINITION), which states that there are an estimated three million nerve points spread over the surface of the skin, 1,000 of which are nodal, meaning they can serve as treatment nodes in acupuncture. Dry skin brushing, by applying friction to the acupuncture points, can take advantage of these energy connections, stimulating and invigorating the entire nervous system, so that every organ, gland, muscle, and ligament benefits. Dry skin brushing, if done in the correct fashion (see "How to Perform a Dry Skin Brush," p. 361), helps to physically move toxic lymph fluid through the lymph vessels. It also improves the skin's ability to eliminate toxins, oxygenates the tissues, and reduces cellulite. One session of light, but brisk, stimulation of the skin is equivalent to 20 minutes of exercise for encouraging the healthy movement of fluid through the lymphatic channels.

Exercise

Exercise is one of the most effective treatments for unclogging the lymph and restoring its flow. "The lymphatic [flow] becomes very active during exercise," says Arthur C. Guyton, M.D., Chairman of the Department of Physiology and Biophysics at the University of Mississippi School of Medicine and author of *Basic Human Physiology*. "During exercise the rate of lymph flow can increase to as high as 14 times normal because of the increased activity."[8]

While just about any type of exercise will improve lymph flow, light bouncing on a mini-trampoline, also called a rebounder, is especially effective in helping to restore the lymph. The mini-trampoline used for rebounding has a flexible jumping surface, measuring 28"-36" in diameter and set 6"-9" off the ground. When you land on the rebounder, you land with twice the force of gravity, which affects every muscle and cell of the body. Rebounding is gentle, playful, and very effective in stimulating the lymph. The changes in gravitational force can dislodge the clumps in the lymph and stimulate the flow of stag-

How to Perform a Dry Skin Brush

To perform a dry skin brush, you will need a moderately soft, natural vegetable fiber, bristle brush, preferably with a removable wooden handle. Nylon or synthetic fibers build up undesirable static electromagnetic energy, in addition to being too sharp and possibly hurting the skin. When starting, you will need to brush gently; however, within a few days, your skin should become conditioned.

Begin at the fingertips and work your way up the inner and outer surfaces of each arm, towards the heart, using short brisk strokes. Then, start at the feet and brush upwards towards the groin, one leg at a time. Include the top and the sole of each foot, the front and back of the leg, the pelvis, the belly, the buttocks, and the lower back; avoid the head and neck. The strokes should not irritate but be brisk enough to color the skin pink and cause a tingling sensation. Dry skin brushing is best done before a shower or bath. As you become accustomed to dry brushing, the process should take no more than ten minutes daily. It would be a good idea to brush your skin daily for three months, then twice weekly as a lifetime practice. Every two weeks or so, wash your brush with soap and water and dry it in the sun or in a warm place, as your brush will rapidly fill with impurities and need to be washed regularly. For hygienic reasons, each person should have a separate brush.

---

nant fluid; during the rebounding exercise, the lymph ducts expand and lymph flow increases.

Rebounding is also effective for burning off calories. For example, a 150-pound person spending one hour on a rebounder will burn 410 calories; the same person jogging for one hour (at five miles per hour) will burn only 355 calories. Unlike a regular trampoline, the rebounding device is not meant for bouncing high or performing gymnastic tricks. Because it is so gentle, a rebounder can be safely used by almost anyone.[9]

For information on **rebounders**, check your local fitness and sporting goods store, or contact: Best of Health, Unit #1758 W.E. Mail 8770-170st, Edmonton, Alberta T5T-4J2, Canada; tel: 800-561-1513 or 403-487-7898; fax: 403-444-1048.

Dietary Recommendations and Herbal Supplements

In general, it is important to include ample quantities of fresh fruits and vegetables in your diet to ensure the health of the lymph. Certain vegetables and fruits, such as cabbage, pineapple, grapes, papaya, and melons, have a particularly strong effect on the lymph. These foods contain enzymes that break down excess or stagnant proteins in the lymphatic channels. You should also avoid fatty foods, particularly those made from hydrogenated oils, such as margarine, which contain high quantities of trans-fatty acids (SEE QUICK DEFINITION), substances that block the proper digestion of fat in the body. Heavily processed foods, including all products made from refined white flour, should also be avoided,

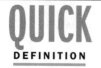

as should any food product high in chemical additives. These foods slow the digestive process and add to the body's toxic load.

Nutritionist Robert Gray identifies bayberry bark, acacia gum, aloe, bladderwrack, couchgrass, Irish moss, lemon balm, lobelia, oatstraw, and red clover as herbs that thin the consistency of the lymph. Not only will this improve lymph flow, but it will also enhance your overall immune function. "Thinning the lymph by using lymph-purifying herbs can greatly improve the mobility and disease-fighting effectiveness of the white blood cells," according to Gray.

Many of these lymph-purifying herbs will, as a result of the detoxification process, tend to increase the toxicity of the blood. Gray recommends taking a blood-purifying herb along with a lymph-purifying herb, so that "the blood will be simultaneously purified rather than made more toxic." Blood-purifying herbs include garlic, rosemary, and yellowdock root. Cabbage and iceberg lettuce are also considered to have blood-purifying effects. Lymphatic cleansing formulations containing these cleansing herbs are available in health food stores. Gray also recommends taking the herbs in conjunction with dry skin brushing treatments, as he considers the combination to be "the most effective lymphatic cleanser."[10]

Herbal Wraps

Lymph can be stimulated by using body wraps or lotions containing essential oils made from herbs. Certain herbs, such as rosemary, eucalyptus, sage, and juniper, are known to stimulate circulation, thus helping to move stagnant lymph. "The idea is to get more blood to the area," explains Rob McCaleb, president of the Herb Research Foundation in Boulder, Colorado. "The metabolic activity is increased and fat is decreased." Body wraps are prepared by diluting the essential oil with vegetable oils such as sunflower and almond or gels such as

aloe and seaweed. The mixture is applied to the skin, then the area is covered (comfortably, not tightly) in plastic wrap. You should relax during the wrap, leaving it in place for about 45 minutes.[11] Precautions: Never leave a wrap on overnight and wraps are not recommended for pregnant women.

Herbologist and nutritionist Graydon Collins, based in Snohomish, Washington, has developed an herbal wrap designed to help reduce cellulite called Body Essence Gel. It includes Irish moss, aloe powder, buckthorn, ginger, bayberry, seaweed, white oak bark, sea minerals, myrrh, cider vinegar, eucalyptus, senna, and sarsaparilla. Collins suggests soaking in a bath of herbs and sea salt prior to using the gel in order to relax the body and open the pores. His Bath Velvet formula includes Epsom salts, calcium, seaweed, sea salt, ginger, and buckthorn. Soak in a hot bath containing five ounces of the formula for 12-17 minutes; the baths should not be done more often than every 2-3 days.

Acupressure and Reflexology

Acupressure and acupuncture, used by Chinese medical practitioners, are effective for stimulating lymphatic activity. Chiropractic adjustment can enhance lymph function and alleviate structural misalignments of the spine that may be impeding lymph flow. Reflexology, a therapy that stimulates organs of the body through gentle pressure applied to the foot, is also effective in inducing lymph flow. According to Inge Dougans, a Danish reflexologist and educator, massaging in areas between and around the toes will help stimulate lymph drainage. He explains that "in the webs between the toes are the reflexes for lymph drainage in the neck and chest region of the body. Lymph reflexes for the groin area are linked to the reproductive system and run across the top of the foot from the inner ankle bone to the outer ankle bone."[13]

Lymph Exercise for the Office

Sitting behind a desk for long periods can make for a sluggish lymph system. To give your lymph a lift, raise your arms up over your head for a few minutes several times a day. This can help open the axillary (underarm) lymph nodes. Also, sit with your feet elevated in front of you whenever you can, as this helps the lymph drain up through the legs into the groin area. Deep breathing is another easy and effective technique. Jack Shields, M.D., a lymphologist from Santa Barbara, California, has researched the cleansing effects that deep breathing has on the lymphatic system. He found that deep breathing created a vacuum effect that sucked lymph into the bloodstream, which increased the rate of toxic elimination by as much as 15 times the normal rate.[12]

Endnotes

Introduction: Not Just Another Diet Book

1 Philip Elmer-DeWitt. "Fat Times." *Time* 145:3 (January 16, 1995).

2 Carol J.G. Ward. "Weighty Resolution: Be Wary of Fad Dieting." *The Arizona Republic* (January 4, 1999), D3.

3 Robert J. Kuczmarski, Dr.PH., R.D., et al. "Weight Gain on the Rise in the United States." *Journal of the American Medical Association* 272:3 (1994), 205-211. F. Xavier Pi-Sunyer, M.D. "The Fattening of America." *Journal of the American Medical Association* 272:3 (1994), 238.

4 Lisa Grunwald. "Discovery: Do I Look Fat to You? 28 Questions (and All the Answers) About Our National Obsession." *Life* (February 1, 1995), 58.

5 Peggy Olivero. "Obesity: The Next Generation." *Nourish* (February/March 1996, 8.

6 Michael T. Murray, N.D. *Natural Alternatives for Weight Loss* (New York: William Morrow, 1996), viii.

7 Michael Fumento. *The Fat of the Land* (New York: Viking, 1997), 11.

8 J.E. Manson et al. "Body Weight and Mortality Among Women." *New England Journal of Medicine* 333:11 (1995), 677-685.

9 T.B. Van Itallie. "Health Implications of Overweight and Obesity in the United States." *Annals of Internal Medicine* 103:6 Part 2 (1985), 983-988.

10 K.M. Rexrode et al. "A Prospective Study of Body Mass Index, Weight Change, and Risk of Stroke in Women." *Journal of the American Medical Association* 277:19 (1997), 1539-1545.

11 M.A. Denke, C.T. Sempos, and S.M. Grundy. "Excess Body Weight: An Underrecognized Contributor to High Blood Cholesterol Levels in White American Men." *Archives of Internal Medicine* 153:9 (1993), 1093-1103.

12 L. Garfinkel. "Overweight and Cancer." Annals of Internal Medicine 103:6 Part 2 (1985), 1034-1036. F.X. Pi-Sunyer. "Health Implications of Obesity." *American Journal of Clinical Nutrition* 53:6 Suppl. (1991), 1595S-1603S.

13 "Obesity." Nutrition Week (July 28, 1995).

14 JoAnne E. Manson et al. "Body Weight and Mortality Among Women." *New England Journal of Medicine* 333:11 (1995), 677-685.

15 Jill Kelly, Ph.D. "Obesity: Nondiet Approaches for What's Eating Your Patients." *Alternative & Complementary Therapies* (October 1997), 326-332.

16 Lisa Grunwald. "Discovery: Do I Look Fat to You? 28 Questions (and All the Answers) About Our National Obsession." *Life* (February 1, 1995), 58.

17 Ibid.

18 "America's Weight Problem Continues." Calorie Control Council press release (May 11, 1998). For more information, contact the Calorie Control Council at 404-252-3663.

19 Lisa Grunwald. "Discovery: Do I look Fat to You? 28 Questions (and All the Answers) About Our National Obsession." *Life* (February 1, 1995), 58.

20 National Institute of Diabetes and Digestive and Kidney Diseases. *Understanding Adult Obesity NIH Publication No. 94-3680* (Washington, DC: National Institutes of Health, 1998).

21 Susan McQuillan, M.S., R.D., with Edward Saltzman, M.D. *Complete Idiot's Guide to Losing Weight* (New York: Alpha Books, 1998), 29.

22 Lisa Grunwald. "Discovery: Do I Look Fat to You? 28 Questions (and All the Answers) About Our National Obsession." *Life* (February 1, 1995), 58.

23 Paula Derrow. *Weight Watchers Magazine* (July 1993), 14.

24 Carol Simontacchi, C.C.N., M.S. *Your Fat Is Not Your Fault* (New York: Jeremy P. Tarcher/Putnam, 1997), 32.

25 "Controlling Weight No Longer Considered Dieting." Calorie Control Council press release (May 11, 1998). For more information, contact the Calorie Control Council at 404-252-3663.

26 "Rating the Diets." *Consumer Reports* (June 1993), 353-357.

27 Susan McQuillan, M.S., R.D., with Edward

Saltzman, M.D. *Complete Idiot's Guide to Losing Weight* (New York: Alpha Books, 1998), 11.

28 Michael Fumento. *The Fat of the Land* (New York: Viking, 1997).

29 "New Strategies to Achieve Your Healthiest Weight: Health After 50." *Johns Hopkins Medical Letter* 7:1 (1995), 4.

30 "Increasing Prevalence of Overweight Among U.S. Adults: The National Health and Nutrition Examination Surveys, 1960 to 1991." *Journal of the American Medical Association* 272 (1994), 205-207.

31 Cynthia Dohrmann, Ph.D. "The Anatomy of Fat." *Let's Live* (January 1996), 29-32. S.P. Walker et al. "Body Size and Fat Distribution as Predictors of Stroke Among U.S. Men." *American Journal of Epidemiology* 144:12 (1996), 1143-1150.

32 Lisa Grunwald. "Discovery: Do I Look Fat to You? 28 Questions (and All the Answers) About Our National Obsession." *Life* (February 1, 1995), 58.

33 Daniel B. Mowrey, Ph.D. *Fat Management: The Thermogenic Factor* (Lehi, UT: Victory Publications, 1994), 40-41.

Chapter 1: Individualize Your Diet

1 Barry Sears, Ph.D. *The Zone* (New York: HarperCollins, 1995), 30.

2 Ralph Golan, M.D. *Optimal Wellness* (New York: Ballantine, 1995), 400.

3 Ann Louise Gittleman, M.S., with James Templeton and Candelora Versace. *Your Body Knows Best* (New York: Pocket Books, 1996), 37.

4 Ibid., 17.

5 Jane Kirby, R.D. "Carbs vs. Protein." *Fitness* (January/February 1997), 66.

6 Ann Louise Gittleman, M.S., with James Templeton and Candelora Versace. *Your Body Knows Best* (New York: Pocket Books, 1996), 37.

7 Monika Klein, C.C. N. "Eating by the Book." *Nutrition Science News* (November 1999), 516.

8 Ann Louise Gittleman, M.S., with James Templeton and Candelora Versace. *Your Body Knows Best* (New York: Pocket Books, 1996), 109.

9 Monika Klein, C.C.N. "Eating by the Book." *Nutrition Science News* (November 1999), 516.

10 Ibid.

Chapter 2: Healthy Eating

1 "Alterations in Metabolic Rate After Weight Loss in Obese Humans." *Nutrition Reviews* 43:2 (1985), 41-42.

2 Robert Garrison, Jr., M.A., R.Ph., and Elizabeth Somer, M.A., R.D. *Nutrition Desk Reference* (New Canaan, CT: Keats, 1995), 27.

3 H. Trowell, D. Burkit, and K. Heaton. *Dietary Fibre, Fibre-Depleted Foods and Disease* (New York: Academic, 1985).

4 M.H. Davidson et al. "The Hypocholesterolemic Effects of Beta-Glucan in Oatmeal and Oat Bran: A Dose-Controlled Study." *Journal of the American Medical Association* 265:14 (1991), 1833-1839. J.W. Anderson and C.A. Bryant. "Dietary Fiber: Diabetes and Obesity." *American Journal of Gastroenterology* 81:10 (1986), 898-906.

5 A. Kendell et al. "Weight Loss on a Low-Fat Diet: Consequences of the Imprecision of the Control of Food Intake in Humans." *American Journal of Clinical Nutrition* 53:5 (1991), 1124-1129.

6 Y. Schutz et al. "Failure of Dietary Fat to Promote Fat Oxidation: A Factor Favoring the Development of Obesity." *American Journal of Clinical Nutrition* 50:2 (1989), 307-314.

7 J.P. Flatt. "Body Weight, Fat Storage, and Alcohol Metabolism." *Nutrition Reviews* 50:9 (1992), 267-270.

8 Ibid.

9 Eric R. Braverman, M.D. "Dieting, Weight Loss, and Eating Disorders." *P.A.T.H. Wellness Manual* (Princeton, NJ: Princeton Associates for Total Health, 1995), 127.

10 A.C. Ross. "Vitamin A Status: Relationship to Immunity and the Antibody Response." *Proceedings of the Society for Experimental Biology and Medicine 200:3* (1992), 303-320. G. Dennert. "Retinoids and the Immune System: Immunostimulation by Vitamin A." In: M.B. Sporn et al., ed. *The Retinoids* (Orlando, FL: Academic, 1984), 373-390. B.E. Cohen et al. "Reversal of Postoperative Immunosuppression in Man by Vitamin A." *Surgery, Gynecology and Obstetrics* 149:5 (1979), 658-662.

11 Dean Ornish. *Diet and Your Heart* (New York: Holt, Rinehart, and Winston, 1982), 1983.

12 American Dietetic Association. "Vegetarian Diets." *ADA Reports: Journal of the American Dietetic Association* 88:3 (1988), 351-355.

13 David S. Ludwig, M.D., Ph.D., et al. "Dietary Fiber, Weight Gain, and Cardiovascular Disease Risk Factors in Young Adults." *Journal of the American Medical Association* 282:16 (1999), 1539-1546.

14 R.L. Walford et al. "The Calorically Restricted Low-Fat Nutrient-Dense Diet in Biosphere 2 Significantly Lowers Blood Glucose, Total Leukocyte Count, Cholesterol, and Blood Pressure in Humans." *Proceedings of the National Academy of Sciences* 89:23 (1992), 11533-11537.

15 Linda Lizotte, R.D., C.D.N. "Healthy Eating Basics." Available from: Designs for Health, 211 Pondway Lane, Trumbull, CT 06611; tel: 203-371-4383; fax: 530-618-6730.

16 R.L. Walford and M. Crew. "How Dietary Restriction Retards Aging: An Integrative Hypothesis." *Growth, Development, and Aging* 53:4 (1989), 139-140.

17 Linda Lizotte, R.D., C.D.N. "Healthy Eating Basics." Available from: Designs for Health, 211 Pondway Lane, Trumbull, CT 06611; tel: 203-371-4383; fax: 530-618-6730.

18 Walter C. Willett, M.D., et al. Letter to David Kessler, M.D., Commissioner, U.S. Food and Drug Administration (November 23, 1995).

19 Ann Louise Gittleman, M.S. *Beyond Pritikin* (New York: Bantam, 1996), 23, 39-40.

20 Ibid., 18.

21 E.A. Mascioli et al. "Medium-Chain Triglycerides and Structured Lipids as Unique Nonglucose Energy Sources in Hyperalimentation." *Lipids* 22:6 (1987), 421-423.

22 Stephen E. Langer, M.D., with James F. Scheer. *Solved: The Riddle of Illness* (New Canaan, CT: Keats Publishing, 1995), 25. C.F. Lim et al. "Influence of Nonesterified Fatty Acid and Lysolecithins on Thyroxine Binding to Thyroxine-Binding Globulin and Transthyretin." *Thyroid* 5:4 (1995), 319-324.

23 S. Ikemoto et al. "High-Fat Diet–Induced Hyperglycemia." *Proceedings of the National Academy of Sciences* 92 (195), 3096-3099.

24 Ralph Golan, M.D. *Optimal Wellness* (New York: Ballantine, 1995), 47.

25 Ann Louise Gittleman, M.S. *Beyond Pritikin* (New York: Bantam, 1996), 40.

26 Susan Herrmann Loomis. "Paradox? What Paradox? The French Are Finally Getting Fat." *The New York Times* (September 9, 1998).

27 Burton Goldberg and the Editors of *Alternative Medicine Digest*. *Alternative Medicine Guide to Heart Disease* (Tiburon, CA: Future Medicine Publishing, 1998), 30.

28 Ann Louise Gittleman, M.S. *Beyond Pritikin* (New York: Bantam, 1996), 69.

29 Ralph Golan, M.D. *Optimal Wellness* (New York: Ballantine, 1995), 173.

30 Jeffrey S. Bland, Ph.D. "What's All The Fuss About Hydrogenated Oils?" *Delicious!* (January/February 1993), 44-45. Gloria Bucco. "The Margarine Myth." *Delicious!* (January/February 1993), 38.

31 William Campbell Douglass, M.D. *The Milk Book: How Science is Destroying Nature's Nearly Perfect Food* (Dunwoody, GA: Second Opinion Publishing, 1993), 103-110.

32 B. Hennig. "Dietary Fat and Macronutrients: Relationships to Artherosclerosis." *Journal of Optimal Nutrition* 1:1 (1992), 21-23.

33 Ann Louise Gittleman, M.S. *Beyond Pritikin* (New York: Bantam, 1996), 30.

34 Paul Theroux. "Under the Spell of the Trobriand Islanders." *National Geographic* 182:1 (July 1992), 117-136. Ann Louise Gittleman, M.S. *Beyond Pritikin* (New York: Bantam, 1996), 71.

35 F. Berschauer et al. "Nutritional-Physiological Effects of Dietary Fats in Rations for Growing Pigs. 4. Effects of Sunflower Oil and Coconut Oil on Protein and Fat Retention, Fatty Acid Pattern of Back Fat and Blood Parameters in Piglets." *Archiv fur Tierernahrung* 34:1 (1984), 19-33. J. Yazbech et al. "Effects of Essential Fatty Acid Deficiency on Brown Adipose Tissue Activity in Rats Maintained at Thermal Neutrality." *Comparative Biochemistry and Physiology A: Comparative Physiology* 94:2 (1989), 273-276. I. Liscum and N.K. Dahl. "Intracellular Cholesterol Transport." *Journal of Lipid Research* 33 (1992), 1239-1254.

36 F. Berschauer et al. "Nutritional-Physiological Effects of Dietary Fats in Rations for Growing Pigs 4: Effects of Sunflower Oil and Coconut Oil on Protein and Fat Retention, Fatty Acid Pattern of Back Fat and Blood Parameters in Piglets." *Archiv fur Tierernahrung* 34:1 (1984), 19-33. J. Yazbech et al. "Effects of Essential Fatty Acid Deficiency on Brown Adipose Tissue Activity in Rats Maintained at Thermal Neutrality." *Comparative Biochemistry and Physiology A: Comparative Physiology* 94:2 (1989), 273-276.

37 Sheldon Margen, M.D., and the Editors of the University of California at Berkeley Wellness Letter. *The Wellness Encyclopedia of Food*

and Nutrition (New York: Rebus, 1992),
498. Udo Erasmus. *Fats That Heal, Fats
That Kill* (Burnaby, British Columbia,
Canada: Alive Books, 1993), 237.

Chapter 3: Supplements for Weight Loss

1 Hazel Parcells, N.D., D.C., Ph.D. "The
Challenge To Stay Healthy." *Parcells Letter*
1:2 (February 1996), 1-2.

2 E.M. Pao and S. Mickle. "Problem Nutrients in
the United States." *Food Technology*
(September 1981), 58-79.

3 Judith A. DeCava, B.S., C.N.C., C.W.C.
Overcoming Overweight (Columbus, GA:
Brentwood Academic, 1994), 29-30.

4 Sherry A. Rogers, M.D. *Wellness Against All
Odds* (Syracuse, NY: Prestige, 1994), 145-
150.

5 "Totally Misleading." *Tufts University Diet &
Nutrition Letter* 13:1 (March 1995), 1.

6 Paul Bergner. *The Healing Power of Minerals:
Special Nutrients and Trace Minerals*
(Rocklin, CA: Prima, 1997), 68-75.

7 Judith A. DeCava, B.S., C.N.C., C.W.C.
Overcoming Overweight (Columbus, GA:
Brentwood Academic, 1994), 32.

8 Mark Mayell. *Off-the-Shelf Natural Health* (New
York: Bantam, 1995), 371-372.

9 Stephen E. Langer and James F. Scheer.
Solved: The Riddle of Illness (New Canaan,
CT: Keats Publishing, 1995), 31.

10 L.J. Machlin and A. Bendich. "Free Radical
Tissue Damage: Protective Role of
Antioxidant Nutrient." *FASEB Journal* 1:6
(1987), 441-445.

11 Katherine F. Adams. *Nutritive Value of
American Foods in Common Units
Agriculture Handbook No. 456* (Washington,
DC: U.S. Department of Agriculture, 1975).

12 K.J. Rothman et al. "Teratogenecity of High
Vitamin A Intake." *New England Journal of
Medicine* 333 (1995), 1369-1373.

13 J.R. DiPalma and W.S. Thayer. "Use of Niacin
as a Drug." *Annual Review of Nutrition 11*
(1991), 169-187.

14 P.J. Bingley et al. "Nicotinamide and Insulin
Secretion in Normal Subjects." *Diabetiologia*
36 (1993), 675-677.

15 M.R. Werbach, M.D. *Nutritional Influences on
Illness* (Tarzana, CA: Third Line Press, 1993).

16 Mark Mayell. *Off-the-Shelf Natural Health*
(New York: Bantam, 1995), 371-372.

17 D.S. Gridley et al. "In Vivo and In Vitro
Stimulation of Cell-Mediated Immunity by
Vitamin B6." *Nutrition Research* 8:2 (1988),
201-207.

18 J. Martineau et al. "Vitamin B6, Magnesium,
and Combined B6-Magnesium: Therapeutic
Effects in Childhood Autism." *Biological
Psychiatry* 20 (1985), 467-468.

19 M. Cohen and A. Bendich. "Safety of
Pyridoxine: A Review of Human and Animal
Studies." *Toxicology Letters* 34 (1986), 129-
139.

20 Mark Mayell. *Off-the-Shelf Natural Health*
(New York: Bantam, 1995), 371-372.

21 Elson M. Haas, M.D. *Staying Healthy With
Nutrition* (Berkeley, CA: Celestial Arts, 1992),
137.

22 Stephen Langer, M.D., with James F. Scheer.
"Stress, Adrenal Glands, and Weight Loss."
Solved: The Riddle of Weight Loss (Rochester,
VT: Healing Arts Press, 1989), 67.

23 Stephen E. Langer, M.D., with James F.
Scheer. *Solved: The Riddle of Illness* (New
Canaan, CT: Keats Publishing, 1995), 32.

24 Frank Murray. "Advanced New Form of
Vitamin C: Ester C." *Better Nutrition for
Today's Living* (January 1993).

25 Michael T. Murray, N.D. *Encyclopedia of
Nutritional Supplements* (Rocklin, CA: Prima
Publishing, 1996), 438.

26 Tamas Decsi, M.D., Ph.D., et al. "Obese Kids
Can Lack Antioxidants." *Journal of
Pediatrics* 130 (1997), 653-655.

27 Betty Kamen, Ph.D. *The Chromium
Connection* (Novato, CA: Nutrition
Encounter, 1992), 118.

28 W.W. Campbell and R.A. Anderson. "Effects
of Aerobic Exercise and Training on the
Trace Minerals Chromium, Copper, and
Zinc." *Sports Medicine* 4 (1987), 9-18.

29 Jeffrey S. Bland, Ph.D. "Take Your Vitamins."
Delicious! 8:7 (October 1992), 61.

30 Lavon Dunne. *The Nutrition Almanac* (New
York: McGraw Hill, 1990).

31 Gail Darlington and Linda Gamlin. *Diet and
Arthritis* (London, England: Vermilion, 1996).

32 W.R. Ghent et al. "Iodine Replacement in
Fibrocystic Disease of the Breast." *Canadian
Journal of Surgery* 36 (1993), 453-460.

33 Michael A, Schmidt, D.C., C.N.S. and Jeffrey
Bland, Ph.D. "Thyroid Gland as Sentinel:
Interface Between Internal and External
Environment." *Alternative Therapies* 3:1
(January 1997), 78-81

34 John Beard, Myfanwy Borel, and Francis J. Peterson "Changes in Iron Status During Weight-Loss with Very-Low-Energy Diets." *American Journal of Clinical Nutrition* 66 (1997), 104-110.

35 V. Gordeuk et al. "Iron Overload: Causes and Consequences." *Annual Review of Nutrition* 7 (1987), 485-508. P. Biemond et al. "Intra-articular Ferritin-Bound Iron in Rheumatoid Arthritis." *Arthritis and Rheumatism* 29 (1986), 1187-1193. J.T. Salonen et al. "High Stored Iron Levels are Associated With Excess Risk of Myocardial Infarction in Eastern Finnish Men." *Circulation* 86 (1992), 803-811.

36 Michael A. Schmidt, D.C., C.N.S. and Jeffrey Bland, Ph.D. "Thyroid Gland as Sentinel: Interface Between Internal and External Environment." *Alternative Therapies* 3:1 (January 1997), 78-81.

37 L. Kiremidjian-Schumacher et al. "Supplementation With Selenium and Human Immune Cell Functions; II, Effect on Cytotoxic Lymphocytes and Natural Killer Cells." *Biological Trace Element Research* 41 (1994), 115-127.

38 O. Andersen and J.B. Nielsen. "Effects of Simultaneous Low-Level Dietary Supplementation with Inorganic and Organic Selenium on Whole-Body, Blood, and Organ Levels of Toxic Metals in Mice." *Environmental Health Perspectives* 102:Suppl. 3 (1994), 321-324.

39 U.S. Centers for Disease Control. "Selenium Intoxication." *Morbidity and Mortality Weekly Report* 33 (1984), 157.

40 Eric R. Braverman, M.D. P.A.T.H. *Wellness Manual* (Princeton, NJ: Princeton Associates for Total Health, 1995), 124.

41 "Greater Health and Longevity: Chlorella, the Green Algae Superfood, May Be the Answer." *Alternative Medicine Digest* 12 (1996), 56.

42 Bernard Jensen, D.C., Ph.D. *Chlorella, Jewel of the Far East* (Escondido, CA: Bernard Jensen International, 1992), 40-46.

43 Joseph B. Marion. *The Anti-Aging Manual* (South Woodstock, CT: Information Pioneers, 1996), 237.

44 Mark Mayell. *Off-the-Shelf Natural Health* (New York: Bantam, 1995), 369.

45 M.F. McCarthy. "Hypothesis: Sensitization of Insulin-Dependent Hypothalamic Glucoreceptors May Account for the Fat-Reducing Effects of Chromium Picolinate." *Journal of Optimal Nutrition* 21 (1993), 36-

53. Michael T. Murray, N.D. *Encyclopedia of Nutritional Supplements* (Rocklin, CA: Prima Publishing, 1996), 306.

Chapter 4: Enzymes and Weight Loss

1 Burton Goldberg and the Editors of *Alternative Medicine Digest. Alternative Medicine Guide to Chronic Fatigue, Fibromyalgia, and Environmental Illness* (Tiburon, CA: Future Medicine Publishing, 1998), 214.

2 Burton Goldberg Group. *Alternative Medicine: The Definitive Guide* (Tiburon, CA: Future Medicine Publishing, 1993), 215.

3 Ralph Golan, M.D. *Optimal Wellness* (New York: Ballantine, 1995), 143.

4 D.A. Lopez, M.D., R.M. Williams, M.D., Ph.D., and K. Miehlke, M.D. *Enzymes: The Fountain of Life* (Charleston, SC: Neville Press, 1994), 107-109.

5 Maile Pouls Ph.D. "Digestive Problems." *Alternative Medicine Digest* 18 (May/June 1997), 40.

6 Ralph Golan, M.D. Optimal Wellness (New York: Ballantine, 1995), 151. Anthony J. Cichoke, D.C. *Enzyme & Enzyme Therapy* (New Canaan, CT: Keats, 1994), 6. E. Howell. *Enzyme Nutrition: The Food Enzyme Concept* (Garden City Park, NY: Avery, 1987), 130.

7 Anthony J. Cichoke, D.C. *Enzyme & Enzyme Therapy* (New Canaan, CT: Keats, 1994), 35-38.

8 Maile Pouls Ph.D. "Digestive Problems." *Alternative Medicine Digest* 18 (May/June 1997), 40.

9 Lita Lee, Ph.D. "The 24-Hour Urinalysis According to Loomis." *Earthletter* 4:2 (Summer 1994), 2.

10 Howard Loomis, D.C. "Muscle Contraction and Body Distortions: How to Recognize Disease." 21st Century Nutrition seminar, San Francisco, California (April 4, 1998).

11 C.B. Beal and J.E. Brown. "A Simple Screening Test for Gastric Achlorhydria." *American Journal of Digestive Diseases* 13 (1968), 133. Ralph Golan, M.D. *Optimal Wellness* (New York: Ballantine, 1995), 173.

12 Ralph Golan, M.D. *Optimal Wellness* (New York: Ballantine, 1995), 148-149.

13 Anthony J. Cichoke, D.C. *Enzyme & Enzyme Therapy* (New Canaan, CT: Keats, 1994), 86.

14 Ibid., 87.

15 E. Howell, M.D. *Food Enzymes for Health and Longevity* (Woodstock Valley, CT: Omangod

Press, 1980).

16 Lita Lee, Ph.D., and Lisa Turner, with Burton Goldberg. *The Enzyme Cure* (Tiburon, CA: Future Medicine Publishing, 1998), 25-27.

17 Anthony J. Cichoke, D.C. *Enzyme & Enzyme Therapy* (New Canaan, CT: Keats, 1994), 17.

18 Burton Goldberg Group. *Alternative Medicine: The Definitive Guide* (Tiburon, CA: Future Medicine Publishing, 1993), 217.

19 Mary Wagner, R.D., and Mark Hewitt, M.D. "Oral Satiety in the Obese and Nonobese." *Journal of the American Dietetic Association* 67:4 (October 1975), 344-346.

20 Burton Goldberg Group. *Alternative Medicine: The Definitive Guide* (Tiburon, CA: Future Medicine Publishing, 1993), 643.

21 Howard Loomis, D.C. *Enzyme Replacement Therapy* (Madison, WI: 21st Century Nutrition).

22 E. Howell, M.D. *Enzyme Nutrition: The Food Enzyme Concept* (Garden City Park, NJ: Avery, 1987).

23 Maile Pouls Ph.D. "Digestive Problems." *Alternative Medicine Digest* 18 (May/June 1997), 40.

24 Ralph Golan, M.D. *Optimal Wellness* (New York: Ballantine, 1995), 149-150.

Chapter 5: Optimize Your Calorie Burning

1 Stephen Langer, M.D., with James F. Scheer. *Solved: The Riddle of Weight Loss* (Rochester, VT: Healing Arts Press, 1989), 143.

2 Daniel B. Mowrey, Ph.D. "The Major Scientific Breakthrough of the '90s: Reducing Body Fat Through Thermogenics." *Health Store News* 11:5 (October/November 1994).

3 M. Laville et al. "Decreased Glucose-Induced Thermogenesis at the Onset of Obesity." *American Journal of of Clinical Nutrition.* 57 (1993), 851-856. Carol Ezzell. "Getting the Skinny on Obesity." *Journal of NIH Research* (April 1994), 72-75. Daniel B. Mowrey, Ph.D. *Fat Management: The Thermogenic Factor* (Lehi, UT: Victory Publications, 1994), 90-92.

4 M. Laville et al. "Decreased Glucose-Induced Thermogenesis at the Onset of Obesity." *American Journal of Clinical Nutrition* 57:6 (1993), 851-856.

5 Ann Louise Gittleman, M.S. *Beyond Pritikin* (New York: Bantam, 1996), 30.

6 Michael T. Murray, N.D., and Joseph Pizzorno, N.D. *Encyclopedia of Natural Medicine* (Rocklin, CA: Prima, 1998), 685.

7 Carol Simontacchi, C.C.N., M.S. *Your Fat Is Not Your Fault* (New York: Jeremy P. Tarcher/Putnam, 1997), 68-70.

8 Daniel B. Mowrey, Ph.D. "Thermogenesis: The Whole Story." *Let's Live* (November 1995), 61-93. Daniel B. Mowrey, Ph.D. *Fat Management: The Thermogenic Factor* (Lehi, UT: Victory Publications, 1994), 17.

9 Ann Louise Gittleman, M.S. *Beyond Pritikin* (New York: Bantam, 1996), 30. Michael T. Murray, N.D. *Natural Alternatives for Weight Loss* (New York: William Morrow, 1996), 12.

10 Eleanor Noss Whitney and Marie A. Boyle. *Understanding Nutrition* 4th ed. (St. Paul, MN: West Publishing, 1987), 259.

11 Stephen Langer, M.D., with James F. Scheer. *Solved: The Riddle of Weight Loss* (Rochester, VT: Healing Arts Press, 1989), 142.

12 Burton Goldberg Group. *Alternative Medicine: The Definitive Guide* (Tiburon, CA: Future Medicine Publishers, 1993), 762.

13 Carol Simontacchi, C.C.N., M.S. *Your Fat Is Not Your Fault* (New York: Jeremy P. Tarcher/Putnam, 1997), 70.

14 Daniel B. Mowrey, Ph.D. *Fat Management: The Thermogenic Factor* (Lehi, UT: Victory Publications, 1994), 29.

15 Ann Louise Gittleman, M.S. *Beyond Pritikin* (New York: Bantam, 1996), 30.

16 Maggie Greenwood-Robinson, Ph.D. *Natural Weight Loss Miracles* (New York: Perigee/Berkley Publishing, 1999), 89-90.

17 T.B. Seaton et al. "Thermic Effect of Medium-Chain and Long-Chain Triglycerides in Man." *American Journal of Clinical Nutrition* 44 (1986), 630-634.

18 Michael T. Murray, N.D., and Joseph Pizzorno, N.D. *Encyclopedia of Natural Medicine* (Rocklin, CA: Prima, 1998), 692.

19 Daniel B. Mowrey, Ph.D. *Fat Management: The Thermogenic Factor* (Lehi, UT: Victory Publications, 1994), 32.

20 Daniel B. Mowrey, Ph.D. *Fat Management: The Thermogenic Factor* (Lehi, UT: Victory Publications, 1994), 19.

21 P.A. Daly et al. "Ephedrine, Caffeine, and Aspirin: Safety and Efficacy for Treatment of Human Obesity." *International Journal of Obesity* 17:1 (1993), S73-S78. C.M. Colker et al. "Ephedrine, Caffeine, and Aspirin Enhance Fat Loss Under Nonexercising Conditions." *Journal of the American College of Nutrition* 16:5 (1997), 501.

22 Michael T. Murray, N.D., and Joseph Pizzorno,

N.D. *Encyclopedia of Natural Medicine* (Rocklin, CA: Prima, 1998), 688. Daniel B. Mowrey, Ph.D. *Fat Management: The Thermogenic Factor* (Lehi, UT: Victory Publications, 1994), 38, 199.

23 Daniel B. Mowrey, Ph.D. *Fat Management: The Thermogenic Factor* (Lehi, UT: Victory Publications, 1994), 241.

24 For a good summary of the scientific research, see: Larry S. Hobbs. "Ephedrine + Caffeine = The Ideal Diet Pill." *Townsend Letter for Doctors and Patients* (June 1996), 62-74.

25 Y. Oi et al. "Garlic Supplementation Enhances Norepinephrine Secretion, Growth of Brown Adipose Tissue, and Triglyceride Catabolism in Rats." *Journal of Nutritional Biochemistry* 6 (1995), 250-255.

26 Daniel B. Mowrey, Ph.D. *Fat Management: The Thermogenic Factor* (Lehi, UT: Victory Publications, 1994), 259.

27 Mark Mayell. *Off-the-Shelf Natural Health* (New York: Bantam, 1995), 362.

28 Stephen Fulder, Ph.D. *The Ginseng Book: Nature's Ancient Healer* (Garden City Park, NY: Avery, 1996), 65.

29 Lester A. Mitscher, Ph.D., and Victoria Dolby. *The Green Tea Book: China's Fountain of Youth* (Garden City Park, NY: Avery, 1998), 14-16.

30 John Anderson. "Trade in Your Latte for Yerba Maté, South America's Green Tea." *Alternative Medicine* 27 (December 1998/January 1999), 78-82.

31 Maggie Greenwood-Robinson, Ph.D. *Natural Weight Loss Miracles* (New York: Perigee/Berkley Publishing, 1999), 107-114.

32 Robert Crayhon, M.S. *The Carnitine Miracle* (New York: M. Evans, 1998), 74, 213.

33 Beth M. Ley and Richard N. Ash, M.D. *DHEA: Unlocking the Secrets to the Fountain of Youth* (Aliso Viejo, CA: BL Publications, 1997), 66.

Chapter 6: Start Exercising

1 "Majority of Americans Spend Leisure Time Inactively." *Let's Live* (March 1996), 12. H.R. Yusuf. "Leisure-Time Physical Activity Among Older Adults." *Archives of Internal Medicine* 156: 12 (June 24, 1996), 1321-1326.

2 JoAnn Manson et al. "Body Weight and Mortality Among Women." *New England Journal of Medicine* (September 1995), 677-685.

3 Jack Tips, N.D., Ph.D., *Your Liver...Your Lifeline* (Ogden, UT: Apple-A-Day Press, 1995), 41.

4 The President's Council on Physical Fitness and Sports, 200 Independence Avenue SW, Room 738-H, Washington, DC 20201; tel: 202-690-9000; fax: 202-690-5211; website: www.surgeongeneral.gov/ophs/pcpfs.htm.

5 Pam Grout. *Jumpstart Your Metabolism* (New York: Fireside, 1998), 21.

6 Burton Goldberg and the Editors of *Alternative Medicine Digest. Alternative Medicine Guide to Heart Disease* (Tiburon, CA: Future Medicine Publishing, 1998), 61.

7 Kathryn Woolf-May et al. "Effects of an 18-Week Walking Programme on Cardiac Function in Previously Sedentary or Relatively Inactive Adults." *British Journal of Sports Medicine* 31 (1997), 48-53.

8 Ann Louise Gittleman, M.S. *Beyond Pritikin* (New York: Bantam, 1996), 33.

9 Ibid., 112.

10 *Journal of the American Medical Association* 275:18 (May 8, 1996).

11 The President's Council on Physical Fitness and Sports, 200 Independence Avenue SW, Room 738-H, Washington, DC 20201; tel: 202-690-9000; fax: 202-690-5211; website: www.surgeongeneral.gov/ophs/pcpfs.htm. The Cooper Institute for Aerobic Research, 12330 Preston Road, Dallas, TX 75230; tel: 800-635-7050; fax: 972-341-3224; website: www.cooperinst.org.

12 R. Pate et al. "Physical Activity and Public Health: A Recommendation From the Centers for Disease Control and Prevention and the American College of Sports Medicine." *Journal of the American Medical Association* 65 (1995), 312-318.

13 John M. Jakicic, Ph.D., et al. "Effects of Intermittent Exercise and Use of Home Exercise Equipment on Adherence, Weight Loss, and Fitness in Overweight Women, A Randomized Trial." *Journal of the American Medical Association* (October 27, 1999), 1554.

14 Abby C. King and Diane L. Tribble. "The Role of Exercise in Weight Regulation in Non-Athletes." *Sports Medicine* (May 1991), 331-349.

15 Jack H. Wilmore. "Body Composition in Sport and Exercise: Directions for Future Research." *Medicine and Science in Sports and Exercise* (1983), 21-31.

16 K.N. Pavlou et al. "Exercise as an Adjunct to

Weight Loss and Maintenance in Moderately Obese Subjects." *American Journal of Clinical Nutrition* (May 1989), 1115-1123.

17 Richard Rafoth, M.D. *Bicycling Fuel* (Osceola, WI: Bicycle Books, 1988). Gary Robertson. "Exercise Goes High-Tech." *Richmond Times Dispatch* (February 6, 1997).

18 The President's Council on Physical Fitness and Sports, 200 Independence Avenue SW, Room 738-H, Washington, DC 20201; tel: 202-690-9000; fax: 202-690-5211; website: www.surgeongeneral.gov/ophs/pcpfs.htm.

19 Paul Dunphy. "Heal Thyself." *Natural Health* (September/October 1992), 32-33.

20 Steven L. Wolf, Ph.D., P.T., et al. "Exploring the Basis for Tai Chi Chuan as a Therapeutic Exercise Approach." *Archives of Physical Medicine and Rehabilitation* (1997), 886-892.

21 Sophia Delza. *Tai Chi-Chuan: Body and Mind in Harmony* (Albany, NY: SUNY Press, 1985), 1,3,6.

22 Philip S. Lansky, M.D., and Yu Shen, M.D. "The Swimming Dragon." *Health World* (July/August 1990), 47.

23 Ibid.

Chapter 7: Heal Your Emotional Appetite

1 John P. Foreyt and G. Ken Goodrick. "Factors Common to Successful Therapy for the Obese Patient." *Medicine and Science in Sports and Exercise* 23:3 (1991), 292-297.

2 E.M. Webber. "Psychological Characteristics of Bingeing and Nonbingeing Obese Women." *Journal of Psychology* 128:3 (1994), 339-351.

3 V.J. Felitti. "Childhood Sexual Abuse, Depression, and Family Dysfunction in Adult Obese Patients: A Case Control Study." *Southern Medical Journal* 86:7 (1993), 732-736.

4 K. Raikkonen et al. "Anger, Hostility, and Visceral Adipose Tissue in Healthy Postmenopausal Women." *Metabolism* 48:9 (1999), 1146-1151. T.P. Carmody, R.L. Brunner, and S.T. St. Jeor. "Hostility, Dieting, and Nutrition Attitudes in Overweight and Weight-Cycling Men and Women." *International Journal of Eating Disorders* 26:1 (1999), 37-42. A.J. Hill, C.F. Weaver,

and J.E. Blundell. "Food Craving, Dietary Restraint, and Mood." *Appetite* 17:3 (1991), 187-197.

5 Elizabeth Somer, M.A., R.D. *Food and Mood* (New York: Henry Holt, 1995), 260.

6 M. Scofield. *Work Site Health Promotion* (Philadelphia: Hanley & Belfus, 1990), 459.

7 Timothy D. Schellhardt. "Company Memo to Stressed-Out Employees: 'Deal With It'." *The Wall Street Journal* (October 2, 1996).

8 Stephen Langer, M.D., with James F. Scheer. *Solved: The Riddle of Weight Loss* (Rochester, VT: Healing Arts Press, 1989), 67.

9 "Obesity May Be Linked to Poor Management of Stress, Interview With Maria Simonson, Ph.D., ScD." *Obesity 90 Update* (September/October 1990), 3.

10 Hara Estroff Marano. "Chemistry & Craving." *Psychology Today* (January/February 1993), 74.

11 Kathleen A. Pichola, Ph.D. "Preventing Eating Disorders: Promoting Healthy Body Image." (Unpublished seminar materials). For more information, contact: Kathleen A. Pichola, Ph.D., 12429 Cedar Road, Suite 18, Cleveland Heights, OH 44106.

12 Stephen Langer, M.D., with James F. Scheer. *Solved: The Riddle of Weight Loss* (Rochester, VT: Healing Arts Press, 1989), 63-66.

13 Shad Helmsetter, Ph.D. *What to Say When You Talk To Yourself* (Scottsdale, AZ: Grindle Press/Audio, 1986).

14 J. Acheterberg. "Ritual: The Foundation for Transpersonal Medicine." *Revision* 14:3 (1992), 158-164.

15 R. Kellner et al. "Changes in Chronic Nightmares After One Session of Desensitization or Rehearsal Instructions." *American Journal of Psychiatry* 149:5 (May 1992), 659-663. J.S. House, K.R. Landis, and D. Umberson. "Social Relationships and Health." *Science* 241:4865 (July 1988), 540-545. J. Acterberg. *Imagery in Healing: Shamanism and Modern Medicine* (Boston: Shambhala, 1985).

16 Christine Northrup, M.D. *Women's Health: A Special Supplement to Health Wisdom for Women* (January 1996), 15.

17 The Burton Goldberg Group. *Alternative Medicine: The Definitive Guide* (Tiburon, CA: Future Medicine Publishing, 1993), 245.

18 R. Dilts and T. Hallbom. *Beliefs: Pathways to Health and Well-Being* (Portland, OR:

Metamorphous Press, 1990), 1-2.

19 Russel J. Reiter and J. Robinson. *Melatonin: Your Body's Natural Wonder Drug* (New York: Bantam Books, 1995), 131-145.

20 J.E. Blundell. "Serotonin and Appetite." *Neuropharmacology* 23:128 (1984), 1537-1551.

21 "Increase Serotonin With 5-HTP." *Life Enhancement Special Issue* (1998), 3-7. Elson M. Haas, M.D. Staying Healthy With Nutrition (Berkeley, CA: Celestial Arts, 1992), 45-46. Robert C. Atkins, M.D. *Dr. Atkins' Health Revelations* (March 1998), 6-7. "With a Little Help From Serotonin." *NutriCology In Focus* (February 1998), 3-5, 13. C. Cangiano et al. "Eating Behavior and Adherence to Dietary Prescriptions in Obese Adult Subjects Treated With 5-Hydroxytryptophan." *American Journal of Clinical Nutrition* 56:5 (1992), 863-867.

22 R.H. Bannerman et al., eds. "Hypnosis." *Traditional Medicine and Health Care Coverage* (Geneva, Switzerland: World Health Organization, 1983).

23 R. A. Chalmers et al., eds. *Scientific Research on Maharishi's Transcendental Meditation and TM-Sidih Program: Collected Papers*, Vol. 2-4 (Vlodrop, Netherlands: Maharishi Vedic University Press, 1989).

24 R.K. Wallace et al. "Physiological Effects of Transcendental Meditation." *Science* 167 (1970), 1751-1754. M.C. Dillbeck et al. "Physiological Differences between TM and Rest." *American Physiologist* 42 (1987), 879-881.

25 R. W. Cranson et al. "Transcendental Meditation and Improved Performance on Intelligence-Related Measures: A Longitudinal Study." *Personality and Individual Differences* 12 (1991), 1105-1116.

26 D.H. Shapiro and R.N. Walsh. *Meditation: Classic and Contemporary Perspectives* (New York: Aldine, 1984).

27 P. Huard and M. Wong. *Chinese Medicine* (New York: World University Library/McGraw Hill, 1968).

28 Lei Zhenping. "Treatment of 42 Cases of Obesity With Acupuncture." *Journal of Traditional Chinese Medicine* 8:2 (June 1988), 125-126.

29 J.F. Quinn. "Therapeutic Touch as Energy Exchange: Testing the Theory." *Advances in Nursing Science* 6:2 (January 1984), 42-49. D. Krieger. *Therapeutic Touch: How to Use Your Hands to Help or Heal* (Englewood Cliffs, NJ: Prentice Hall, 1979).

30 Beryl Bender Birch. *Power Yoga* (New York: Simon & Schuster, 1995), 44-45.

31 Personal communication from Beryl Bender Birch.

32 Joel Kramer. "Yoga as Self-Transformation." (Unpublished manuscript), 4.

33 Patricia Kaminski and Richard Katz. *Flower Essence Repertory* (Nevada City, CA: The Flower Essence Society, 1994), 118-119.

34 Ibid.

35 G.H. Dodd. *Receptor Events in Perfumery: The Psychology and Biology of Fragrance* (London: Chapman and Hall, 1988).

36 Jeanne Rose. *The Aromatherapy Book: Applications and Inhalations* (Berkeley, CA: North Atlantic Books, 1992), 73, 92, 106, 118, 121, 139.

37 William Lee, D.Sc., R.Ph., and Lynn Lee, C.N. *The Book of Practical Aromatherapy* (New Canaan, CT: Keats, 1992), 58, 59, 67, 68.

Chapter 8: Strengthen Your Sugar Controls

1 "Weight: What Have You Got To Lose?" *Consumer Reports on Health* (September 1995), 97-100.

2 A.F. Heini et al. "Divergent Trends in Obesity and Fat Intake Patterns: the American Paradox." *American Journal of Medicine* 102 (March 1997), 259-264. Michael Fumento. *The Fat of the Land* (New York: Penguin Books, 1997), 83.

3 Barry Sears, Ph.D. *The Zone* (New York: HarperCollins, 1995), 29.

4 D. Porte, Jr., and S.C. Woods. "Regulation of Food Intake and Body Weight by Insulin." *Diabetologiag* 20 Suppl. (March 1981), 274-280. Jeffrey Moss, D.D.S., C.N.S., C.C.N. "Hyperinsulinemia and Insulin Resistance—A Missing Link in Obesity and Cardiovascular Disease." *Townsend Letter for Doctors and Patients* (May 1977), 125-129.

5 Jeffrey Moss, D.D.S. "Hyperinsulinemia and Insulin Resistance—A Missing Link in Obesity and Cardiovascular Disease." *Townsend Letter for Doctors and Patients* (April 1996), 87-91.

6 Joseph E. Pizzorno, Jr., N.D., and Michael T. Murray, N.D. *A Textbook of Natural Medicine* Vol. II (Seattle, WA: John Bastyr College Publications, 1988), 6-7.

7 Stephen Langer, M.D., with James F. Scheer. *Solved: The Riddle of Weight Loss* (Rochester, VT: Healing Arts Press, 1989), 39.

8 Ralph Golan, M.D. *Optimal Wellness* (New York: Ballantine, 1995), 193.

9 Kathleen DesMaisons, Ph.D. *Potatoes Not Prozac* (New York: Simon & Schuster, 1998), 54-56.

10 Elliot D. Abravanel, M.D., and Elizabeth King. *Dr. Abravanel's Anti-Craving Weight Loss Diet* (New York: Bantam, 1990), 53-57.

11 Kathleen DesMaisons, Ph.D. *Potatoes Not Prozac* (New York: Simon & Schuster, 1998), 87-94.

12 Stephen Langer, M.D., with James F. Scheer. *Solved: The Riddle of Weight Loss* (Rochester, VT: Healing Arts Press, 1989), 37-47.

13 William Mauer, D.O. *Low Blood Sugar Clinical Practice Patient Pamphlet* (Arlington Heights, IL: Kingsley Medical Center), 6.

14 Ralph Golan, M.D. *Optimal Wellness* (New York: Ballantine, 1995), 189-191. Kathleen DesMaisons, Ph.D. *Potatoes Not Prozac* (New York: Simon & Schuster, 1998), 95-136.

15 Ann Louise Gittleman, M.S., C.N.S. "Perimenopause—When Signs of 'The Change' Come Too Early." *Alternative Medicine* 26 (October/November 1998), 84-92.

16 Richard N. Podell, M.D., F.A.C.P., and William Proctor. *The G-Index Diet* (New York: Warner, 1993).

17 Ann Louise Gittleman, M.S. *Supernutrition for Women* (New York: Bantam, 1991), 68.

18 Betty Kamen, Ph.D. *The Chromium Connection* (Novato, CA: Nutrition Encounter, 1992), 118.

19 W.W. Campbell and R.A. Anderson. "Effects of Aerobic Exercise and Training on the Trace Minerals Chromium, Copper, and Zinc." *Sports Medicine* 4 (1987), 9-18.

20 M.F. McCarthy. "Hypothesis: Sensitization of Insulin-Dependent Hypothalamic Glucoreceptors May Account for the Fat-Reducing Effects of Chromium Picolinate." *Journal of Optimal Nutrition* 21 (1993), 36-53.

21 Betty Kamen, Ph.D. *The Chromium Connection* (Novato, CA: Nutrition Encounter, 1992), 187.

22 "Aid for Diabetes and Its Complications." *Alternative Medicine Digest* 16 (January/February 1997), 66-67.

23 Ralph Golan, M.D. *Optimal Wellness* (New York: Ballantine, 1995), 191-192.

24 Reader's Digest. *Healing Power of Vitamins, Minerals, and Herbs* (Pleasantville, NY: Reader's Digest Association, 1999), 369.

25 Michael Tierra, L.Ac., O.M.D. *The Way of Herbs* (New York: Pocket Books, 1998), 143-144. Maggie Greenwood-Robinson, Ph.D. *Natural Weight Loss Miracles* (New York: Perigee/Berkley Publishing Group, 199), 142-143.

26 Michael Tierra, L.Ac., O.M.D. *The Way of Herbs* (New York: Pocket Books, 1998), 196-197.

27 Lester A. Mitscher, Ph.D., and Victoria Dolby. *The Green Tea Book: China's Fountain of Youth* (Garden City Park, NY: Avery Publishing Group, 1998), 120-121.

28 Richard N. Podell, M.D., F.A.C.P., and William Proctor. *The G-Index Diet* (New York: Warner, 1993), 36.

29 Ibid.

Chapter 9: Overcome a Sluggish Thyroid

1 Stephen Langer, M.D., and James F. Scheer. *Solved: The Riddle of Illness* (New Canaan, CT: Keats Publishing, 1995), 185.

2 Ibid., 186-189.

3 Ibid., 188-189.

4 Daniel B. Mowrey, Ph.D. *Fat Management: The Thermogenic Factor* (Lehi, UT: Victory Publications, 1994), 173.

5 Ralph Golan, M.D. *Optimal Wellness* (New York: Ballantine, 1995), 383.

6 Lita Lee, Ph.D. "Hypothyroidism: A Modern Epidemic." *Earthletter* (Spring 1994), 1. Michael A. Schmidt, D.C., C.N.S., and Jeffrey Bland, Ph.D. "Thyroid Gland as Sentinel: Interface Between Internal and External Environment." *Alternative Therapies* 3:1 (January 1997), 78-81.

7 Lita Lee, Ph.D. "Hypothyroidism: A Modern Epidemic." *Earthletter* (Spring 1994), 1.

8 Burton Goldberg and the Editors of *Alternative Medicine Digest*. *Chronic Fatigue, Fibromyalgia, and Environmental Illness* (Tiburon, CA: Future Medicine Publishing, 1998), 198-199. Ralph Golan, M.D. *Optimal Wellness* (New York: Ballantine, 1995), 381.

9 Tom Valentine. "If You Eat Soy, Watch Your Thyroid Function: New Study." *True Health* (Autumn 1997), 1-3. R.L. Divi et al. "Anti-Thyroid Isoflavones From Soybean: Isolation, Characterization, and Mechanisms of Action." *Biochemical Pharmacology* 54:10 (November 15, 1997), 1087-1096. Stephen E. Langer, M.D., with James F. Scheer. *Solved: The Riddle of Illness* (New Canaan,

CT: Keats Publishing, 1995).

10 Stephen Langer, M.D., with James F. Scheer. *Solved: The Riddle of Weight Loss* (Rochester, VT: Healing Arts Press, 1989), 15-17.

11 Lynne McTaggart and Harald Gaier. "Thyroid Disease: Overactive Medicine." *What Your Doctors Don't Tell You* 7:7 (October 1996), 2-5.

12 Jorge H. Mestman, M.D. "Perinatal Thyroid Dysfunction: Prenatal Diagnosis and Treatment." *Medscape Women's Health* 2:7 (1997).

13 Lita Lee, Ph.D. "Hypothyroidism: A Modern Epidemic." *Earthletter* (Spring 1994), 2.

14 E. Denis Wilson. *Wilson's Syndrome* (Orlando, FL: Cornerstone, 1993), 38.

15 Ibid.

16 Ann Louise Gittleman, M.S. *Super Nutrition for Menopause* (New York: Simon and Schuster, 1993), 124-129.

17 William G. Crook, M.D. "Thyroid and Adrenal Hormones." *The Yeast Connection and the Woman* (Jackson, TN: Professional Books, 1995), 547-557.

18 Burton Goldberg Group. "Candidiasis." *Alternative Medicine: The Definitive Guide* (Tiburon, CA: Future Medicine Publishing, 1993), 588.

19 Stephen Langer, M.D., and James F. Scheer. *Solved: The Riddle of Weight Loss* (Rochester, VT: Healing Arts Press, 1989), 15-18.

20 Raphael Kellman, M.D. "Energizing Chronic Fatigue." *Alternative Medicine Digest* 19 (August/September 1997), 60-64. Richard Leviton. "Reviving the Thyroid." *Alternative Medicine Digest* 22 (February/March 1998), 54-59.

21 Stephen Langer, M.D., and James F. Scheer. *Solved: The Riddle of Illness* (New Canaan, CT: Keats Publishing, 1995), xiv.

22 Michael A. Schmidt, D.C., C.N.S., and Jeffrey Bland, Ph.D. "Thyroid Gland as Sentinel: Interface Between Internal and External Environment." *Alternative Therapies* 3:1 (January 1997), 78-81.

23 Stephen Langer, M.D., and James F. Scheer. *Solved: The Riddle of Illness* (New Canaan, CT: Keats Publishing, 1995), 31.

24 Ibid., 32.

25 Stephen Langer, M.D., and James F. Scheer. *Solved: The Riddle of Weight Loss* (Rochester, VT: Healing Arts Press, 1989), 15-17.

26 Michael A. Schmidt, D.C., C.N.S., and Jeffrey Bland, Ph.D. "Thyroid Gland as Sentinel:

Interface Between Internal and External Environment." *Alternative Therapies* 3:1 (January 1997), 78-81.

27 Y.B. Tripathi et al. "Thyroid-Stimulatory Action of Z-Guggulsterone: Mechanism of Action." *Planta Medica* 54 (1988), 271-277.

28 B. Saunier et al. "Cyclic AMP Regulation of Gs Protein: Thyrotropin and Forskolin Increase the Quantity of Stimulatory Guanine Nucleotide-Binding Proteins in Cultured Thyroid Follicles." *Journal of Biological Chemistry* 265 (1990), 19942-19946. P.P. Roger et al. "Regulation of Dog Thyroid Epithelial Cell Cycle by Forskolin: An Adenylate Cyclase Activator." *Experimental Cell Research* 172 (1990), 282-292. B. Haye et al. "Chronic and Acute Effects of Forskolin on Isolated Thyroid Cell Metabolism." *Molecular and Cellular Endocrinology* 43 (1990), 41-50.

Chapter 10: Restore Hormonal Balance

1 John R. Lee, M.D., with Virginia Hopkins. *What Your Doctor May Not Tell You About Menopause* (New York: Warner Books, 1996), 34.

2 John R. Lee, M.D., with Virginia Hopkins. *What Your Doctor May Not Tell You About Menopause* (New York: Warner Books, 1996), 131. John R. Lee, M.D., Jesse Hanley, M.D., and Virginia Hopkins. *What Your Doctor May Not Tell You About Premenopause* (New York: Warner Books, 1999), 184.

3 Theresa L. Crenshaw, M.D. *The Alchemy of Love and Lust* (New York: G.P. Putnam's Sons, 1996), 205.

4 K.T. Khaw and E. Barrett-Connoe. "Lower Endogenous Androgens Predict Central Adiposity in Men." *Annals of Epidemiology* 2:5 (1992), 675-682. P. Marin, M. Krotkiewski, and P. Bjorntorp. "Androgen Treatment of Middle-Aged, Obese Men: Effects on Metabolism, Muscle and Adipose Tissues." *European Journal of Medicine* 1:6 (1992), 329-336.

5 G. Tibblin et al. "The Pituitary-Gonadal Axis and Health in Elderly Men: A Study of Men Born in 1913." *Diabetes* 45:11 (1996), 1605-1609.

6 Eugene Shippen, M.D., and William Fryer. *The Testosterone Syndrome* (New York: M. Evans, 1998), 91.

7 Theo Colborn, Dianne Dumanoski, and John

Peterson Myers. *Our Stolen Future* (New York: Dutton/Penguin Group, 1996).

8 Betty Kamen, Ph.D. "Thyroid and Stress Connections." *Hormone Replacement Therapy: Yes or No?* (Novato, CA: Nutrition Encounter, 1993), 196.

9 A.W. Meikle et al. "Effects of a Fat-Containing Meal on Sex Hormones in Men." *Metabolism* 39:9 (1990), 943-946.

10 C.D Hunt et al. "Effects of Dietary Zinc Depletion on Seminal Volume and Zinc Loss: Serum Testosterone Concentrations and Sperm Morphology in Young Men." *American Journal of Clinical Nutrition* 56:1 (1992), 148-157.

11 Joseph Pizzorno, N.D. *Total Wellness* (Rocklin, CA: Prima, 1996), 244.

12 Eugene Shippen, M.D., and William Fryer. *The Testosterone Syndrome* (New York: M. Evans, 1998), 49.

13 S.J. Brown. "Environmental Doctors Take Up Pollution Prevention Cause." *Family Practice News* (January 1, 1995), 6.

14 J. Yeh and A.J. Friedman. "Nicotine and Cotinine Inhibit Rat Testis Androgen Biosynthesis in vitro." *Journal of Steroid Biochemistry* 33:4A (1989), 627-630.

15 Joseph Pizzorno, N.D. *Total Wellness* (Rocklin, CA: Prima, 1996), 242.

16 Ibid., 236-237.

17 John R. Lee, M.D., with Virginia Hopkins. *What Your Doctor May Not Tell You About Menopause* (New York: Warner Books, 1996), 300.

18 Michael Murray, N.D., and Joseph Pizzorno, N.D. *Encyclopedia of Natural Medicine* 2nd Ed. (Rocklin, CA: Prima, 1998), 636.

19 E.H. Brown and L.P. Walker, Pharm.D., M.Ac., D.H.M. "Diet, Exercise and Hormone Balance." *Menopause and Estrogen* (Berkeley, CA: Frog Ltd., 1996), 111-119.

20 John R. Lee, M.D., with Virginia Hopkins. *What Your Doctor May Not Tell You About Menopause* (New York: Warner Books, 1996), 317.

21 Ann Louise Gittleman, M.S., C.N.S. "Perimenopause—When Signs of 'The Change' Come Too Early." *Alternative Medicine* (October/November 1998), 84-92.

22 John R. Lee, M.D., with Virginia Hopkins. *What Your Doctor May Not Tell You About Menopause* (New York: Warner Books, 1996), 279-317.

23 John R. Lee, M.D. *Natural Progesterone: The Multiple Roles of a Remarkable Hormone* (Sebastopol, CA: BLL Publishing, 1993), 41.

24 John R. Lee, M.D., with Virginia Hopkins. *What Your Doctor May Not Tell You About Menopause* (New York: Warner Books, 1996), 263-278.

25 Betty Kamen, Ph.D. "Thyroid and Stress Connections." *Hormone Replacement Therapy: Yes or No?* (Novato, CA: Nutrition Encounter, 1993), 35-36.

26 Jill Stansbury. "Fortifying Fertility With Vitamins and Herbs." *Nutrition Science News* 2:12 (December 1997), 606-612.

27 Linda Ojeda, Ph.D. *Menopause Without Medicine* (Alameda, CA: Hunter House, 1995), 101.

28 Kathleen A. Head, N.D. "Premenstrual Syndrome: Nutritional and Alternative Approaches." *Alternative Medicine Review* 2:1 (1997), 12-25.

29 L. Slaven and C. Lee. "Mood and Symptom Reporting Among Middle-Aged Women: The Relationship Between Menopausal Status, Hormone Replacement Therapy, and Exercise Participation." *Health Psychology* 16 (1997), 203-208.

30 Arthur Schwartz, M.D., and M.P. Cleary. "The Effect of Dehydroepiandrosterone on Body Weight Gain." *Journal of Nutrition* 117:2 (February 1987), 406-407.

31 Eugene Shippen, M.D., and William Fryer. *The Testosterone Syndrome* (New York: M. Evans, 1998), 190-193.

32 "Staying Sexually Fit During Male Menopause." *Alternative Medicine Digest* 10 (1995), 10-13. Sandra Cabot, M.D. *Smart Medicine for Menopause* (Garden City Park, NY: Avery, 1995).

33 Julian Whitaker, M.D. "A Hormone Replacement Program for Men." *Health and Healing* 8:2 (February 1998), 1-4. Available from: Philips Publishing, Inc., 7811 Montrose Road, Potomac, MD 20854; tel: 800-539-8219; 12 issues/$69 in the U.S.

34 M.S. Fahim et al. "Effect of Panax ginseng on Testosterone Level and Prostate in Male Rats." *Archives of Andrology* 8:4 (1982), 261-263.

35 James A. Duke, Ph.D. *The Green Pharmacy* (Emmaus, PA: Rodale, 1997), 192.

36 Gary S. Ross, M.D. "Men's Health Issues in Clinical Practice: Andropause." *Biomedical Therapy* XV:3 (June 1997), 94-95.

Chapter 11: Break Food Allergies and Addictions

1 James Braly, M.D. *Dr. Braly's Food Allergy and Nutrition Revolution* (New Canaan, CT: Keats Publishing, 1992), 61.

2 Stephen Langer, M.D., with James F. Scheer. *Solved: The Riddle of Weight Loss* (Rochester, VT: Healing Arts Press, 1989), 52.

3 Burton Goldberg Group. *Alternative Medicine: The Definitive Guide* (Tiburon, CA: Future Medicine Publishing, 1993), 512.

4 Arthur Winter, M.D., F.I.C.S., and Ruth Winter, M.S. *Smart Food* (New York: St. Martin's Griffin, 1999), 77.

5 Stephen Langer, M.D., with James F. Scheer. *Solved: The Riddle of Weight Loss* (Rochester, VT: Healing Arts Press, 1989), 51.

6 M. Lessner, M.D. *Nutrition and Vitamin Therapy.* (Berkeley, CA: Parker House, 1982).

7 Stephen Langer, M.D., with James F. Scheer. *Solved: The Riddle of Weight Loss* (Rochester, VT: Healing Arts Press, 1989), 52.

8 Ralph Golan, M.D. *Optimal Wellness* (New York: Ballantine Books, 1995).

9 Ibid.

10 James Braly, M.D. *Dr. Braly's Food Allergy and Nutrition Revolution* (New Canaan, CT: Keats Publishing, 1992), 60.

11 S. van Toller and G.H. Dodd, eds. *Receptor Events in Perfumery: The Psychology and Biology of Fragrance* (London: Chapman and Hall, 1988).

12 Roberta Wilson. *Aromatherapy for Vibrant Health & Beauty* (Garden City Park, NY: Avery Publishing, 1994), 99.

Chapter 12: Detoxify the Colon

1 Robert Gray. *The Colon Health Handbook* (Reno, NV: Emerald Publishing, 1990), 12.

2 Ibid., 18.

3 Burton Goldberg Group. *Alternative Medicine: The Definitive Guide* (Tiburon, CA: Future Medicine Publishing, 1995), 144.

4 Richard Anderson, N.D., N.M.D. *Cleanse and Purify Thyself* (Mt. Shasta, CA: Arise & Shine, 1988), 34.

5 Bernard Jensen, D.C., Ph.D., and Sylvia Bell. *Tissue Cleansing Through Bowel Management* (Escondido, CA: Bernard Jensen International, 1981), 23.

6 Ralph Golan, M.D. *Optimal Wellness* (New York: Ballantine, 1995), 160.

7 Elaine Gottschall, M.S. *Breaking the Vicious Cycle* (Kirkton, Ontario, Canada: Kirkton Press, 1994), 18-20, 26.

8 Robert Gray. *The Colon Health Handbook* (Reno, NV: Emerald Publishing, 1990), 7.

9 Ralph Golan, M.D. *Optimal Wellness* (New York: Ballantine, 1995), 160.

10 James L. D'Adamo, N.D. *The D'Adamo Diet* (Toronto, Ontario, Canada: McGraw-Hill Ryerson, 1989), 172.

11 Michael Murray, N.D. "The Importance of Dietary Fiber." *Phyto-Pharmica Review* 4:1 (1990), 1-4.

12 W.H. Turnbull and H.G. Thomas. "The Effect of Plantago Ovata Seed Preparation on Apetite Variables, Nutrient, and Energy Intake." *International Journal of Obesity* 19 (1995), 338-342.

13 Michael Murray, N.D. "The Importance of Dietary Fiber." *Phyto-Pharmica Review* 4:1 (1990), 1-4.

14 Clare Maxwell-Hudson. *Massage: The Ultimate Illustrated Guide* (New York: DK Publishing, 1999), 148-149.

15 Inge Dougans. *The Complete Illustrated Guide to Reflexology* (Rockport, ME: Element Books, 1996), 40.

Chapter 13: Eliminate Yeast Infections

1 William G. Crook, M.D. *The Yeast Connection and the Woman* (Jackson, TN: Professional Books, 1995), 25. Simon Martin. *Candida: The Natural Way* (Boston, MA: Element Books, 1998), 7.

2 Stephen Langer, M.D., with James F. Scheer. *Solved: The Riddle of Weight Loss* (Rochester, VT: Healing Arts Press, 1989), 26.

3 Jack Tips, N.D., Ph.D. *Conquer Candida and Restore Your Immune System* (Austin, TX: Apple-A-Day Press, 1995), 36, 125.

4 Burton Goldberg Group. *Alternative Medicine: The Definitive Guide* (Tiburon, CA: Future Medicine Publishing, 1993), 587.

5 Jack Tips, N.D., Ph.D. *Conquer Candida and Restore Your Immune System* (Austin, TX: Apple-A-Day Press, 1995), 126. Dennis W. Remington, M.D., and Barbara Higa Swasey, R.D. *Back To Health* (Provo, UT: Vitality House International, 1989), 100.

6 Dennis W. Remington, M.D., and Barbara Higa Swasey, R.D. *Back To Health* (Provo, UT: Vitality House International, 1989), x. Jack

Tips, N.D., Ph.D. *Conquer Candida and Restore Your Immune System* (Austin, TX: Apple-A-Day Press, 1995), 17.

7 Stephen Langer, M.D., with James F. Scheer. *Solved: The Riddle of Weight Loss* (Rochester, VT: Healing Arts Press, 1989), 25-27.

8 Orian C. Truss, M.D. *The Missing Diagnosis* (Birmingham, AL: The Missing Diagnosis, 1985), x, 3. Jack Tips, N.D., Ph.D. *Conquer Candida and Restore Your Immune System* (Austin, TX: Apple-A-Day Press, 1995), 126.

9 Dennis W. Remington, M.D., and Barbara Higa Swasey, R.D. *Back To Health: Yeast Control* (Provo, UT: Vitality House International, 1989), 16

10 Jack Tips, N.D., Ph.D. *Conquer Candida and Restore Your Immune System* (Austin, TX: Apple-A-Day Press, 1995), 59-60.

11 Ann Louise Gittleman, M.S. *Supernutrition for Women* (New York: Bantam, 1991), 79.

12 Jack Tips, N.D., Ph.D. *Conquer Candida and Restore Your Immune System* (Austin, TX: Apple-A-Day Press, 1995), 60-61.

13 William G. Crook, M.D. *The Yeast Connection and the Woman* (Jackson, TN: Professional Books, 1995), 83. Ralph Golan, M.D. *Optimal Wellness* (New York: Ballantine, 1995), 214. John R. Lee, M.D. *What Your Doctor May Not Tell You About Menopause* (New York: Warner, 1996), 34.

14 Ralph Golan, M.D. *Optimal Wellness* (New York: Ballantine, 1995), 214.

15 William G. Crook, M.D. *The Yeast Connection and the Woman* (Jackson, TN: Professional Books, 1995), 83.

16 Stephen Langer, M.D., with James F. Scheer. *Solved: The Riddle of Weight Loss* (Rochester, VT: Healing Arts Press, 1989), 24.

17 Burton Goldberg Group. *Alternative Medicine: The Definitive Guide* (Tiburon, CA: Future Medicine Publishing, 1993), 588.

18 Simon Martin. *Candida: The Natural Way* (Boston, MA: Element Books, 1998), 10-11. This information is adapted from a Candida questionnaire developed by William Crook, M.D., and included in his book, *The Yeast Connection Handbook* (Jackson, TN: Professional Books, 1996), pp. 15-19.

19 Stephen Langer, M.D., with James F. Scheer. *Solved: The Riddle of Weight Loss* (Rochester, VT: Healing Arts Press, 1989), 24.

20 Jack Tips, N.D., Ph.D. *Conquer Candida and Restore Your Immune System* (Austin, TX:

Apple-A-Day Press, 1995), 68-69.

21 Michael T. Murray, N.D. "Chronic Candidiasis: A Natural Approach." *American Journal of Natural Medicine* 4:4 (May 1997), 17-19.

22 M. Rosenbaum, M.D., and M. Susser, M.D. *Solving the Puzzle of Chronic Fatigue Syndrome* (Tacoma, WA: Life Sciences Press, 1992), 131.

23 Jacqueline Young. *Cystitis: The Natural Way* (Rockport, MA: Element Books, 1997), 68.

24 W.J. Crinnion. "Clinical Trial Results on Neesby's Capricin." (Unpublished manuscript). Available from: Probiologic, Inc., 1803 132nd Avenue NE, Bellevue, WA 98005.

25 Michael T. Murray, N.D. "Chronic Candidiasis: A Natural Approach." *American Journal of Natural Medicine* 4:4 (May 1997), 17-21.

26 Bernard Jensen, D.C., Ph.D. *Chlorella, Jewel of the Far East* (Escondido, CA: Bernard Jensen International, 1992), 40-46.

27 John Anderson. "The Potted Physician: 13 Ways Aloe Vera Can Help You." *Alternative Medicine* 28 (February/March 1999), 56-62.

28 Leon Chaitow. *Post-Viral Fatigue Syndrome* (London: Dent, 1989).

Chapter 14: Eradicate Parasites

1 Ann Louise Gittleman, M.S. *Guess What Came To Dinner: Parasites and Your Health* (Garden City Park, NY: Avery Publishing Group, 1993), 1, 9. J.M. Mansfield, ed. *Parasitic Diseases* (New York: Marcel Dekker, 1981).

2 Ann Louise Gittleman, M.S. *Guess What Came To Dinner: Parasites and Your Health* (Garden City Park, NY: Avery Publishing Group, 1993), 2-3. Hermann Bueno, M.D. *Uninvited Guests* (New Canaan, CT: Keats: 1996), 18-19.

3 William G. Crook, M.D. *The Yeast Connection Handbook* (Jackson, TN: Professional Books, 1996), 187.

4 Hermann Bueno, M.D. *Uninvited Guests* (New Canaan, CT: Keats: 1996), 18-19. Jack Tips, N.D., Ph.D. *Your Liver...Your Lifeline* (Ogden, UT: Apple-A-Day Press, 1995), 90.

5 W. John Diamond, M.D., and W. Lee Cowden, M.D., with Burton Goldberg. *Alternative Medicine Definitive Guide to Cancer* (Tiburon, CA: Future Medicine Publishing, 1997), 625.

6 Hermann Bueno, M.D. *Uninvited Guests* (New

Canaan, CT: Keats: 1996), 19. Ann Louise Gittleman, M.S. *Guess What Came To Dinner: Parasites and Your Health* (Garden City Park, NY: Avery Publishing Group, 1993), 4.

7 Sheldon Margen, M.D., and Dale A. Ogar. "Is Meat Safe to Eat." *Your Health* 36:25 (December 9, 1997), 34.

8 Hermann Bueno, M.D. *Uninvited Guests* (New Canaan, CT: Keats: 1996), 13.

9 Ann Louise Gittleman, M.S. *Guess What Came To Dinner: Parasites and Your Health* (Garden City Park, NY: Avery Publishing Group, 1993), 12.

10 Hermann Bueno, M.D. *Uninvited Guests* (New Canaan, CT: Keats: 1996), 12.

11 Hermann Bueno, M.D. *Uninvited Guests* (New Canaan, CT: Keats: 1996), 15.

12 Ann Louise Gittleman, M.S. *Guess What Came To Dinner: Parasites and Your Health* (Garden City Park, NY: Avery Publishing Group, 1993), 37-56. Hermann Bueno, M.D. *Uninvited Guests* (New Canaan, CT: Keats: 1996), 20-32.

13 Ann Louise Gittleman, M.S. *Guess What Came To Dinner: Parasites and Your Health* (Garden City Park, NY: Avery Publishing Group, 1993), 15-16. Hermann Bueno, M.D. *Uninvited Guests* (New Canaan, CT: Keats: 1996), 14.

14 Ann Louise Gittleman, M.S. *Guess What Came To Dinner: Parasites and Your Health* (Garden City Park, NY: Avery Publishing Group, 1993), 9-19.

15 D. Casemore, M.D. "Foodborne Protozoal Infection." *The Lancet* 336:8728 (December 1990), 1427-1432.

16 Ann Louise Gittleman, M.S. *Guess What Came To Dinner: Parasites and Your Health* (Garden City Park, NY: Avery Publishing Group, 1993), 94-95. Gary Null, Ph.D. *The Woman's Encyclopedia of Natural Healing* (New York: Seven Stories, 1996), 285. Pavel I. Yutsis, M.D. "Intestinal Parasites at Large." *Explore!* 7:1 (1996), 27-31.

17 Ann Louise Gittleman, M.S. *Guess What Came To Dinner: Parasites and Your Health* (Garden City Park, NY: Avery Publishing Group, 1993), 97.

18 Ann Louise Gittleman, M.S. *Guess What Came To Dinner: Parasites and Your Health* (Garden City Park, NY: Avery Publishing Group, 1993), 96.

19 Pavel I. Yutsis, M.D. "Intestinal Parasites at Large." *Explore!* 7:1 (1996), 27-31.

20 Ann Louise Gittleman, M.S. *Guess What Came To Dinner: Parasites and Your Health* (Garden City Park, NY: Avery Publishing Group, 1993), 80-86. Hermann Bueno, M.D. *Uninvited Guests* (New Canaan, CT: Keats: 1996), 33.

21 Pavel I. Yutsis, M.D. "Intestinal Parasites at Large." *Explore!* 7:1 (1996), 27-31.

22 Ann Louise Gittleman, M.S. *Guess What Came To Dinner: Parasites and Your Health* (Garden City Park, NY: Avery Publishing Group, 1993), 108-114.

23 J. Bland. "Aloe Vera to Treat Gastrointestinal Problems." *Journal of Alternative Medicine* (1985).

24 V.P. Choudhry, M. Sabir, and V.N. Bhide. "Berberine in Giardiasis." *Indian Pediatrics* 9:3 (March 1972), 143-146.

Chapter 15: Cleanse the Liver

1 Jack Tips, N.D., Ph.D. *Your Liver...Your Lifeline* (Ogden, UT: Apple-A-Day Press, 1995), 90.

2 Ibid., 2.

3 Paul Yanick, Jr., PhD. "The Amazing Chemical Plant of Our Bodies: The Liver." *Let's Live* (August 1987), 59.

4 Ralph Golan, M.D. *Optimal Wellness* (New York: Ballantine, 1995), 173.

5 F. Nomura et al. "Liver Function in Moderate Obesity—Study in 534 Moderately Obese Subjects Among 4,613 Male Company Employees." *International Journal of Obesity* 10 (1986), 349-354.

6 Jorge H. Mestman, M.D. "Perinatal Thyroid Dysfunction: Prenatal Diagnosis and Treatment." *Medscape Women's Health* 2:7 (1997).

7 Stephen Langer, M.D., with James F. Scheer. *Solved: The Riddle of Illness* (New Canaan, CT: Keats, 1995), 86-87.

8 Anthony Cichoke, D.C. *Enzymes & Enzyme Therapy* (New Canaan, CT: Keats, 1994), 51.

9 Ralph Golan, M.D. *Optimal Wellness* (New York: Ballantine, 1995), 177.

10 Ralph Golan, M.D. *Optimal Wellness* (New York: Ballantine, 1995), 172-175. Jack Tips, N.D., Ph.D. *Your Liver...Your Lifeline* (Ogden, UT: Apple-A-Day Press, 1995), 105, 115.

11 Daniel Reid. *The Complete Book of Chinese Health and Healing* (Boston: Shambhala, 1994), 78. Harriet Beinfeld, L.Ac., and Efrem Korngold, L.Ac., O.M.D. *Between Heaven and Earth: A Guide to Chinese Medicine* (New York: Ballantine, 1991), 107.

12 Jack Tips, N.D., Ph.D. *Your Liver...Your Lifeline* (Ogden, UT: Apple-A-Day Press, 1995), 13-15.

13 Ralph Golan, M.D. *Optimal Wellness* (New York: Ballantine, 1995), 177.

14 Paul Yanick, Jr., Ph.D. "The Amazing Chemical Plant of Our Bodies: The Liver." *Let's Live* (August 1987), 57.

15 Ralph Golan, M.D. *Optimal Wellness* (New York: Ballantine, 1995), 174. Donna Gates with Linda Schatz. *The Body Ecology Diet* (Atlanta, GA: B.E.D. Publications, 1996), 136-137.

16 Christopher Hobbs, L.Ac. Foundations of Health. *Healing With Herbs & Foods* (Loveland, CO: Botanica, 1994).

17 W. John Diamond, M.D., and W. Lee Cowden, M.D., with Burton Goldberg. *Alternative Medicine Definitive Guide to Cancer* (Tiburon, CA: Future Medicine Publishing, 1997), 101-102.

18 Stephen Langer, M.D., and James F. Scheer. *Solved: The Riddle of Weight Loss* (Rochester, VT: Healing Arts Press, 1989), 91.

19 Michael T. Murray, N.D. *Natural Alternatives for Weight Loss* (New York: William Morrow, 1996), 125.

20 Jay Lombard, M.D., and Carl Germano. *The Brain Wellness Plan* (New York: Kensington Books, 1997), 188.

21 Sandra Cabot, M.B.B.S., D.R.C.O.G. *Liver Cleansing Diet* (Paddington, New South Wales, Australia: Women's Health Advisory Service, 1996), 66-67.

22 Bernard Jensen, D.C., Ph.D. *Chlorella, Jewel of the Far East* (Escondido, CA: Bernard Jensen International, 1992), 40-46.

23 Sandra Cabot, M.B.B.S., D.R.C.O.G. *Liver Cleansing Diet* (Paddington, New South Wales, Australia: Women's Health Advisory Service, 1996), 66.

24 Michael T. Murray, N.D., and Joseph E. Pizzorno, Jr., N.D., eds. *Encyclopedia of Natural Medicine* (Rocklin, CA: Prima, 1991), 445-446.

25 Lesley Tierra, L.Ac. *The Herbs of Life* (Freedom, CA: Crossing Press, 1992), 73.

26 Sandra Cabot, M.B.B.S., D.R.C.O.G. *Liver Cleansing Diet* (Paddington, New South Wales, Australia: Women's Health Advisory Service, 1996), 70.

27 Ralph Golan, M.D. *Optimal Wellness* (New York: Ballantine, 1995), 178. Donna Gates

with Linda Schatz. *The Body Ecology Diet* (Atlanta, GA: B.E.D. Publications, 1996), 140.

28 Suzanne Skinner, Ph.D. "Is Distilled Water Healthy?" *Perceptions* (May/June 1995), 30.

Chapter 16: Get the Lymph Flowing

1 Morton Walker, D.P.M. *Jumping for Health* (Garden City Park, NY: Avery, 1989).

2 Kathy A. Conti. "Cellulite Solution." *Delicious!* (January/February 1993), 56-58.

3 Sky David, R.P.T., M.P.T., and Courtland Reeves, M.S. "Lymph Dysfunction and Its Role in Breast Cancer." *Explore!* 6:2 (1995), 19-22.

4 Lita Lee, Ph.D. "The 24-Hour Urinalysis According to Loomis." *Earthletter* 4:2 (Summer 1994), 2.

5 Robert Gray. *The Colon Health Handbook* (Reno, NV: Emerald Publishing, 1990), 24.

6 Kathy A. Conti. "Cellulite Solution." *Delicious!* (January/February 1993), 56-58.

7 W. John Diamond, M.D., W. Lee Cowden, M.D., with Burton Goldberg. *Alternative Medicine Definitive Guide to Cancer* (Tiburon, CA: Future Medicine Publishing, 1997), 969-971.

8 Arthur C. Guyton. *Basic Human Physiology* (Philadelphia, PA: W.B. Saunders, 1971).

9 John Anderson. "Rebounders: Bounce Your Way to Better Health." *Alternative Medicine Digest* 20 (October/November 1997), 42-46.

10 Robert Gray. *The Colon Health Handbook* (Reno, NV: Emerald Publishing, 1990), 23, 47-51.

11 Kathy A. Conti. "Cellulite Solution." *Delicious!* (January/February 1993), 56-58.

12 J.W. Shields, M.D. "Lymph, Lymph Glands, and Homeostasis." *Lymphology* 25:4 (December 1992), 147-153.

13 Inge Dougans. *The Complete Illustrated Guide to Reflexology* (Rockport, ME: Element, 1996), 87.

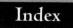

Index

BOOKS *your* *health* depends on

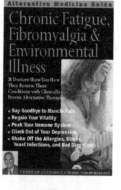
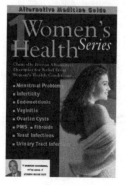
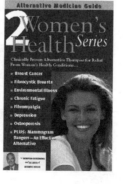
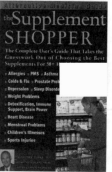
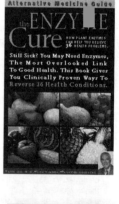

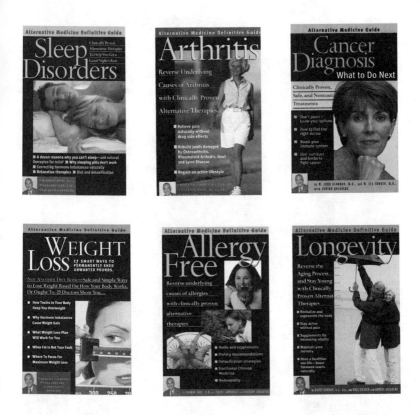

These titles are part of our *Alternative Medicine Guide* paperback series—healing-edge advice that may mean the difference between sickness and robust health. We distill the advice of hundreds of leading alternative physicians from all disciplines and put it into a consumer-helpful format—medical knowledge without the jargon. Essential reading before—or instead of—your next doctor's visit. Because you need to know your medical alternatives.

To order, call 800-841-BOOK or visit www.alternativemedicine.com.
You can also find our books at your local health food store or bookstore.

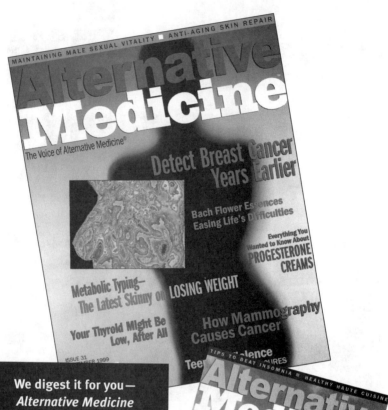

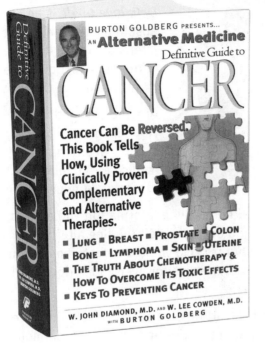

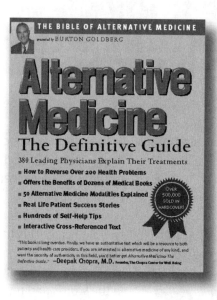